The Daily Telegraph

The
COMPLETE
Guide to
ALLERGIES

D0993867

The Daily Telegraph

The
COMPLETE
Guide to
ALLERGIES

Pamela Brooks

ROBINSON
London

Constable Publishers
3 The Lanchesters
162 Fulham Palace Road
London W6 9ER
www.constablerobinson.com

A copy of the British Cataloguing in Publication Data for this title is
available from the British Library.

ISBN 1-84119-161-2

Important note:
This book is not intended to be a substitute for medical advice or
treatment. Any person with a condition requiring medical attention
should consult a qualified medical practitioner or suitable therapist.

Edited and designed by Grapevine Publishing Services
Printed and bound in the EC

Contents

Acknowledgements

Many people have been generous with time and information during the production of this book.

First of all, I'd like to thank Fiona Robertson of the BMA library and the staff of Norfolk County Council Library at Costessey for help in obtaining reference material.

For pointing me in the right direction, I owe thanks to Maureen Jenkins and the immunology department at the Norfolk and Norwich Hospital

Thanks also to the following companies who kindly sent me information about allergens and testing: ALK-Abello, Aller-ayde, Cogent Diagnostics, Pharmacia & Upjohn, Quest Biomedical.

And, last but definitely not least, special thanks to Gerard and Christopher for giving me the time and space to work, keeping me supplied with glasses of water, and not minding about all the piles of paper...

Pamela Brooks
June 2000

Foreword

Allergic reactions have become increasingly common as a result of ill-understood interactions between our immune system and our 21st-century diet, lifestyle and environment.

The Complete Guide to Allergies by Pamela Brooks is the most comprehensive and impressive book I have seen on this subject. It contains a wealth of information useful to everyone who suffers from a potentially allergic symptom or condition, ranging from asthma, eczema and contact dermatitis to conjunctivitis, migraine, psoriasis, rhinitis and a variety of digestive disorders.

As well as explaining what happens in allergic reactions, it provides in-depth information on symptoms, diagnostic tests and treatments for each condition, explores the orthodox drug treatments your doctor or pharmacist may recommend, and the complementary self-help approaches that are becoming increasingly popular.

One of the most useful sections is the complete A to Z of potential allergens found in cosmetics, household products and our diet. Each entry lists related items to which there may be a cross reaction. If you know you are allergic to avocado, for example, it is useful to know you may also be sensitive to apple, bay leaves, cinnamon and latex so you can take steps to avoid these additional substances where possible.

If a severe allergic reaction develops, the book explains what to do in an emergency, giving first aid tips and advice on how to avoid recurrences. If someone in your family has severe allergic reactions, read this section regularly so you are always prepared and know what to do.

The appendices contain vital information, such as details of self-help groups, alternative therapy organisations and lists of food additives (E numbers), including where they are found and the allergic symptoms they can cause. The lists of allergens linked with occupational asthma or occupational contact dermatitis – conditions causing growing concern to industry – are applicable to workers everywhere.

If you suffer from an allergy, or suspect one may be possible, this is a must-have reference book for your shelves. While you are unlikely to read it from cover to cover, it will soon become well-thumbed. I found myself checking labels on products as diverse as skin cream, bubble bath and tinned soup to look up their contents and assess their allergic potential.

Dr Sarah Brewer

How to use this book

If you think you may have an allergy but you don't know what's causing it:
- Look up your symptoms in Chapter 2. It will suggest potential allergens and give suggestions for treatments, including medication, alternative therapies and self-help tips.

If you think you might be allergic to a particular substance:
- Keep a symptom diary
- Try elimination tests (see page 73)
- Consult your GP and ask him or her to refer you for allergy tests. Chapter 4 gives more detail about the tests available.

If you know you are allergic to something:
- Look up the substance in Chapter 8. It will tell you what kind of allergies the substance provokes and how they can be treated, as well as warning you about other related substances you might also react to.
- For specific treatments, you can then refer to chapter 5 and decided which one suits you best.

If you suffer from allergic illness:
- Read chapter 7 for ways of coping with recurrent illnesses.
- For specific treatments, you can then refer to chapter 5 and decided which one suits you best.

For babies, children, pregnant women, the elderly and those with weakened immune systems:
- Chapter 6 gives advice about precautions you need to take.

For everyone:
- Chapter 3 gives advice on dealing with severe allergic reactions.
- Throughout the book, cross references in *italics* refer you to other sections containing relevant information.
- The comprehensive index will also help guide you to the information you need.

Introduction

An allergy is the overreaction of the body's defence mechanism to something that's usually harmless; the most common reactions include sneezing, watery eyes, itchy rashes and swelling of the lips and tongue.

The allergen, or substance that causes the reaction, usually contains a protein – that is, the part of a living organism that includes hydrogen, oxygen and nitrogen. There are non-protein allergens (including penicillin and other prescription drugs) which cause an allergic response once they bind with protein in your body.

A common reaction

Allergies are very common; the British Allergy Foundation says that one in four people in the UK suffers from an allergy at some time in their life. This figure is increasing by roughly 5 per cent a year, and almost half of all allergy sufferers are children. And a study conducted in Leicester for the National Asthma Campaign found that asthma and wheezing in children under five years have almost doubled since 1990.

Increase in allergies

One of the reasons why allergy is increasing is because allergies run in families. The allergy gene that controls the production of the allergy antibody immunoglobulin E (IgE) can be passed on, so your genetic make-up will influence whether you get allergy problems.

The other key factor is when and how you're exposed to the substance that causes the allergic reaction. Younger children in large families have fewer allergies than the first-born children in the family, and it's believed that this is related to viral infections passed between children. Because the first-born children are exposed to fewer viral infections, their immune systems take longer to develop; and so the general trend for smaller families is leading to a higher proportion of children developing allergies.

Other factors that influence the development of allergies include:

- *Where you live* – studies in Japan and Germany show that allergies are more common in children and adults who live near busy roads rather than in less polluted parts of cities.
- *Air exchange* – before double glazing and insulation became widespread, houses were draughty and the air in rooms

changed up to seven times an hour; in insulated houses with double glazing and central heating, it's likely to be less than once an hour, so the air is more humid.

• *Furnishings* – houses with lots of soft furnishings and fitted carpets are the ideal environment for the house dust mite (a major allergen) and will also trap more allergens such as pet fur, cigarette smoke and vapour from household chemicals.

Becoming allergic in later life

Although most allergies (with the exception of asthma) tend to develop before the age of forty, you may suddenly become sensitive to something after years of low-level exposure. It's worth keeping a symptom diary to help pinpoint what's caused your allergy; remember that although you may be exposed to an allergen at work, your symptoms might not start until a couple of hours after you finish work.

Extreme cases

There have been reported cases of people who are allergic to almost everything – the so-called "allergic to twentieth-century life" syndrome. However, these are very rare and there is a possibility that some of the symptoms have a psychological basis.

1

What happens in allergic reactions?

How your body comes in contact with an allergen

There are four main ways that your body will come into contact with an allergen (i.e. the substance that causes your immune system to overreact to it – usually a protein). These are:

- *Contact* – you're likely to experience a rash, skin irritation, swelling and reddening; your eyes and mouth may be affected as well as your skin.
- *Inhaling* (either fumes or very small particles) – the proteins enter your body through the cells lining the eyes, nose, sinuses and bronchial tubes, so you're likely to experience reactions in your nose, eyes, throat and lungs; you may also come out in a rash, suffer from headaches, migraine, palpitations or muscular pain, or feel faint. The allergens are also absorbed into the bloodstream, so you may have a whole body reaction.
- *Consuming* (usually food or drink) – this means that the proteins enter your body through the cells lining the mouth, oesophagus, stomach and intestines, so you may experience problems first with itching of the palate and mouth, then swelling of the lips and tongue, then gastrointestinal problems such as nausea, vomiting, diarrhoea and wind; you may also have reactions in your nasal system, such as sneezing or rhinitis, respiratory problems such as coughing, wheezing or breathing problems, and you may also come out in a rash.
- *Injectant* – where substances are introduced directly into the circulation, such as injected drugs or insect stings.

The difference between allergies, intolerances and sensitivities

The term "allergy" is often used to describe the body's unpleasant reaction to a food, insect sting, chemical or other substance that enters the body or touches the skin. This term can be misleading because if your body doesn't produce the IgE antibody, the unpleasant symptoms you experience may be due either to sensitivity or intolerance rather than to true allergy.

Sensitivity

This is when your body's reaction to a substance is similar to a normal side-effect produced by that substance, but is exaggerated – for example, someone who uses too high a dose of a reliever inhaler for asthma and is sensitive to the prescribed medicine may start to "shake".

Intolerance

This usually refers to foods – often dairy products. If you're intolerant to a particular food and eat it without realizing, your digestive system doesn't produce enough of the right enzyme or chemical to break the food down, and this causes your body to react badly.

Because the treatments for allergy, sensitivity and intolerance differ, the cause of your symptoms needs to be diagnosed correctly, so you can be given the right treatment. See the section on *Identifying allergens*.

What happens in an allergic reaction?

First contact – sensitization

When your body comes into contact with an allergen (a normally harmless substance which contains a protein) for the first time, your immune system – the part of the body that protects you against harmful bacteria, viruses and other foreign invaders – believes that the allergen is damaging, so it produces large quantities of the antibody Immunoglobulin E (IgE) in order to attack it.

The IgE antibodies latch on to the substance, mark it, and immobilize it; the phagocytes (the scavenging cells) in your system are then able to deal with the invader. At the same time, your body produces memory B-cells (or white blood cells) which can produce more of the specific IgE antibody when stimulated.

At this stage, you will not experience any symptoms of an allergic reaction because the IgE attaches only to the allergen, not to mast cells (see *below*); the symptoms begin to appear when you are re-exposed to the allergen.

Second contact

The next time you come into contact with the allergen, the memory B-cells (white blood cells) "remember" the allergen and produce more IgE antibodies – 2,000 per second are produced by each B-cell – and the IgE antibodies then attach themselves to the mast cells and basophils (the part of the cells which release histamine during an allergic reaction).

IgE attaches to the mast cells

Mast cells are found in your skin, the lining of your nose, your mouth, your tongue, the airways in your lungs (particularly in asthma sufferers) and your intestines. They are filled with granules which contain histamine, leukotriene and chemo-attractants. On the surface, the mast cells have receptor sites, which allow IgE antibodies to attach to them easily.

The allergen attaches to the IgE antibodies and causes the mast cell to burst

When the allergen attaches to the IgE antibodies, it causes the mast cell to burst and release three types of chemical: histamine, leukotriene and chemoattractants. The release of these chemicals is also known as degranulation.

Histamine and leukotrienes cause itching, sneezing and swelling (or inflammation) in the skin, the airways and the lining of the nose; this results in itchy red blotches on your skin, wheezing and a blocked nose. Histamine is a vasoactive amine created from the reaction of the amino acid histidine and makes the cells produce more mucus, causing watering eyes and a stuffy nose. Leukotrienes can cause more inflammation than histamine, and are created when arachidonic acid, a fatty acid found in animal fats, is exposed to oxygen in the body.

Prostaglandin is also activated when the mast cells burst. Prostaglandins are hormone-like substances metabolized from dietary fats; some relieve inflammation, but others (such as Prostaglandin E2, or PGE2, converted from arachidonic acid) cause inflammation.

Eosinophils or white blood cells are also attracted to the broken mast cells. Eosinophils cause inflammation and make your airways and the lining of your nose more sensitive.

Lymphocyte cells (white blood cells manufactured in bone marrow) are also attracted by the broken mast cells, and they cause further inflammation, particularly in skin conditions such as eczema and contact dermatitis.

More serious symptoms can occur, leading to anaphylactic shock – see the section on *what to do in an emergency*.

The four types of hypersensitivity

The four main types of allergy are:

Type I (IgE-mediated) Allergic Hypersensitivity

This type of allergy is also known as "immediate onset" and develops in response to repeated exposure to specific allergens such as animal dander, pollen, dust mites, drugs and food. Once you become sensitized to the allergen, as soon as you are exposed to it again, your immune system will react within minutes, and the severity can range from mild sneezing through to anaphylactic shock.

Types II and III (Antibody-mediated, non-IgE) Hypersensitivity

Type II, or antibody-mediated cytotoxic hypersensitivity, occurs when antigens lodge in the body's cells – for example, antibiotics may be absorbed into the red blood cells. The antibodies then bind to the cells and destroy them.

Type III, or immune-complex-mediated hypersensitivity, is when antibodies and antigens are too large to be destroyed by the leukocytes; they end up in tissues (such as the lungs, arteries and skin) and cause inflammation – for example, causing extrinsic allergic alveolitis or rheumatoid arthritis.

Type IV (Delayed) Hypersensitivity (DTH)

The symptoms of Type IV hypersensitivity appear between 24 and 72 hours after exposure to the allergen. It's more likely to be a contact allergen (such as nickel or plants) affecting the skin, or an inhaled allergen affecting the lungs (such as latex or formaldehyde).

2

Symptoms that can be manifested

For more detailed information about triggers and treatments, please see the sections on *Treatments* and *A–Z allergens*. Entries referred to in these sections are marked in small capitals.

Abdominal pain and swelling

What is it?

Abdominal pain and swelling is discomfort in the stomach and a feeling of distension. Pain may be "colicky" (that is, a pain every few minutes as muscular spasm occurs) if part of the intestine is inflamed.

Other symptoms that may occur with it

Angioedema, colitis, constipation, cystitis, diarrhoea, gastric upset/irritation, heartburn, indigestion, nausea, rumbling noises in the stomach, vomiting, weight gain, weight loss, wind (belching and flatulence)

Possible triggers

AMINES

DRINK: beer, tea

FOOD: avocado, banana, beetroot, blackberries, carrot, celery, cheese, chick pea, chocolate, corn, egg, fish, gooseberries), kiwi fruit, mango, milk, oats, orange, pea, peach, peanuts, peppers, pineapple, pork, redcurrant, rhubarb, rye, shellfish, soya, spinach, strawberry, wheat

FOOD ADDITIVES: preservatives, emulsifiers/stabilizers/ thickeners, flavour enhancers

HERBS/SPICES: cayenne pepper, coriander, pepper

MEDICATION: dichlorophen

Treatments

Aromatherapy
- Use one of the following oils as a compress with a hot water bottle placed on top (use 6 drops of essential oil in 500ml hot water, dip a cloth into it and wring it out, then lay the cloth on the affected area until it has cooled to body temperature), or massage your stomach (using 1 drop of essential oil to 5 ml of a carrier oil such as sweet almond): lavender, Roman camomile

Herbal remedies
- Teas (use 1–2 tsp of dried herb to 1 cup of boiling water, steeped for 10–15 minutes): camomile, ginger, peppermint

Homeopathic remedies
- Magnesium phosphoricum – for cramping abdominal pain

Over-the-counter remedies
- Antacids

Prescription medication
- Antacids
- Anti-spasmodic drugs

Self-help tips
- A hot water bottle placed across the abdomen may help
- A milky drink or live yoghurt may soothe the stomach

Angioedema

What is it?
Angioedema, also known as angioneurotic oedema, is a swelling in the deeper layers of the skin. It tends to occur in soft tissue, such as the eyelids, face, mouth, hands, feet or genitals, and is a result of the action of histamine. It can also affect the voicebox (larynx); if it affects the gastrointestinal tract, you may also have abdominal pain and feel sick. Women tend to suffer more than men, and it's more common in adults than in children. It may last for anything from a couple of hours to three days.

Other symptoms that may occur with it
Abdominal pain, itching/burning mouth, nausea, urticaria, vomiting

Possible triggers

ANIMAL DANDER

CHEMICALS: persulphate, volatile organic compounds

COSMETICS: AHAs, deodorants, depilatories, douche preparations, eye liner, eye shadow, face powder, foundation, hair care products, hand cream, lip balm, lipstick, mascara, moisturizer, mouthwash, nail varnish, perfume, shampoo, shaving products, skin care products, soap, suncream, toothpaste

DRINK: cider, tea

DUST MITES

FOOD: apple, apricot, asparagus, banana, barley, blackberries, blackcurrant, blueberries, carrot, celery, cheese, cherries, chick pea, cider vinegar, citrus fruit, corn, cranberry, cucumbers, currants, dates, egg, fish, gooseberries, grapes, kiwi fruit, lentil, lettuce, liquorice, mango, melon, milk, mushrooms, mustard, nectarine, oats, orange, parsnip, passion fruit, pea, peach, peanuts, pear, peppers, pineapple, plum, potato, prune, raisin, raspberry, rice, rye, sauerkraut, sausages, shellfish, soya, spinach, strawberry, sunflower seeds, tomato, wheat, wine vinegar, Worcestershire sauce

FOOD ADDITIVES: colours, preservatives

HERBS/SPICES: anise, aniseed, clove, coriander, cumin, curry powder, dill, fennel, fenugreek, horseradish, oregano, paprika, parsley, rosemary, tarragon, thyme, turmeric

HISTAMINE

INFECTION

INSECT STINGS

LATEX

LINSEED OIL

MEDICATION: ACE-inhibitors, aspirin, codeine, frusemide, ibuprofen, insulin, iodine, paracetamol, penicillin

MENTHOL

MOULDS

POLLEN

SALICYLATES

SANITARY PRODUCTS

SEMEN

STRESS

TEMPERATURE (heat or cold)

Treatments

Over-the-counter remedies
• Antihistamines

Prescription medication
- Swelling in larynx or throat – adrenaline, intubation (a breathing tube put through the mouth into the windpipe) or tracheostomy (breathing hole cut into the windpipe)
- Swelling in the skin – corticosteroid drugs, antihistamines

Anxiety

What is it?
Anxiety is an emotional response to worry or stress; it may present as a sense of dread, fear and mental upset.

Other symptoms that may occur with it
Breathing difficulties, headaches, palpitations, sleeping problems, sweating, tremors

Possible triggers
TURPENTINE
See also the section on *Psychological problems* in this chapter

Treatments
Aromatherapy
- Use one of the following oils for massage (use 1 drop of essential oil to 5 ml of a bland carrier oil such as sweet almond oil), in a vaporizer (use 6 drops oil in 2 tsp water for a 3 metres-square room) or in a bath (four drops to a full bath – add when the water has run and disperse vigorously!): bergamot, camomile, frankincense, juniper, lavender, melissa, neroli, ylang ylang

Bach flower remedies
- Rescue remedy
- Rock rose – for extreme anxiety and panic
- White chestnut – for persistent nervous thoughts

Herbal remedies
- Teas (use 1–2 tsp of dried herb to 1 cup of boiling water, steeped for 10–15 minutes): camomile, linden, orange blossom, passiflora, valerian, vervain

Homeopathic remedies
- Calc Phos
- Kalium phosphoricum

• Magnesium phosphoricum

Prescription medication
• Benzodiazepines – these are thought to increase the chemical gamma-aminobutyric acid in the brain, preventing excessive brain activity that causes anxiety. They also have a sedative effect
• Beta blockers – these block the action of the chemical transmitter noradrenaline (which stimulates the heart and digestive system)

Self-help tips
Relaxation techniques (such as breathing exercises) may help.

Asthma
See section on *Asthma* in chapter on *Allergic illnesses*

Blisters
What is it?
A blister is fluid that collects beneath the outer layer of the skin to form a raised area. The fluid is serum leaked from blood vessels. It may be a complication of eczema and dermatitis herpetiformis.

Other symptoms that may occur with it
Rash

Possible triggers
COSMETICS: deodorants, depilatories, douche preparations, eye liner, eye shadow, face powder, foundation, hair care products, hand cream, lip balm, lipstick, mascara, moisturizer, mouthwash, nail varnish, perfume, shampoo, shaving products, skin care products, soap, suncream, toothpaste
MEDICATION: sulphonamides
SANITARY PRODUCTS
SEMEN

Treatments
Aromatherapy
• Add 2 drops of Roman camomile to half a cup of water and use it as a skin wash

Over-the-counter remedies:
• Antihistamines

Prescription medication
• Antihistamines

Self-help tips
• Let the blister heal on its own
• If it's likely to burst through friction, sterilize a needle (with alcohol or in a flame) and puncture the blister; drain the fluid, leaving the skin intact, and cover with a sterile dressing during the day. Remove the dressing at night so the blister can dry out.

Bloating

What is it?
Bloating is when your abdomen feels swollen; it is usually caused by wind or fluid retention. It's often part of irritable bowel syndrome.

Other symptoms that may occur with it
Constipation, heartburn, wind

Possible triggers
CHEESE (lactose intolerance)

Treatments
Herbal remedies
• Teas (use 1–2 tsp of dried herb to 1 cup of boiling water, steeped for 10–15 minutes): camomile, fennel

Over-the-counter remedies
• See *Constipation, Wind*

Prescription medication
• See *Constipation, Wind*

Self-help tips
• *Drink*: cinnamon milk (soak a cinnamon stick in a glass of hot milk or add half a teaspoon of ground cinnamon);
• *Food*: live yoghurt can help to settle your stomach

Breathing difficulty

What is it?

Breathing difficulty is when your rate and depth of breathing changes. It can vary in severity, from a brief period of breathlessness after exercise, through to severe difficulties that make it hard to speak or walk; it may be a symptom of asthma. If you have angioedema in the mouth or throat, it can also cause breathing difficulties.

Other symptoms that may occur with it

Anxiety, cough, wheezing

Possible triggers

Anything that triggers asthma may cause breathing difficulties, i.e.:

AIRBORNE PARTICLES

ALLERGENS: pollen; animal fur or feathers, saliva and urine; house dust mite; moulds

ARTIFICIAL FIBRES

CHEMICALS: butyl alcohol, formaldehyde, isocyanates, volatile organic compounds

COLDS, FLU, SINUSITIS OR VIRAL INFECTIONS

DUST MITES

EMOTIONAL UPSET AND EXCITEMENT (PARTICULARLY IN SMALL CHILDREN)

EXERCISE

FOOD: barley, beef, celery, corn, egg, milk, oats, orange, pork, soya, wheat

FOOD ADDITIVES: colours, preservatives

INSECT BITES AND STINGS

MEDICATION: ACE inhibitors, amoxycillin, antibiotics, anti-emetics, aspirin, beta-blockers, cephalosporins, frusemide, ibuprofen, insulin

MOULDS

OCCUPATIONAL EXPOSURE TO ALLERGENS, VAPOURS, DUST, GASES OR FUMES

OZONE

SOLVENTS: amyl alcohol, isopropanol, methyl alcohol, aromatic hydrocarbons, chlorinated hydrocarbons, esters, glycols, glycol ethers, halogenated solvents, ketone solvents

STRONG SMELLS

SULPHUR DIOXIDE

TEMPERATURE CHANGES
WOOL

Treatments
Prescription medication
• Bronchodilators – sympathomimetics, xanthines, anticholinergics and corticosteroids

Colitis

What is it?
Colitis is inflammation of the large intestine. Ulcerative colitis is the most common form of inflammatory bowel disease, and symptoms tend to come and go.

Other symptoms that may occur with it
Abdominal pain, diarrhoea (often blood-stained), fever

Possible triggers
FOOD: milk, papaya, soya, strawberry
FOOD ADDITIVES: emulsifiers/stabilizers/thickeners

Treatments
Herbal remedies
• Teas (use 1–2 tsp of dried herb to 1 cup boiling water, steeped for 10–15 minutes): meadowsweet infusion
• Slippery elm (use 1 heaped tsp in a cup of warm water)

Prescription medication
• Aminosalicylates
• Corticosteroids (these reduce the ability of white blood cells to pass into the bowel wall)
• Immunosuppressants
• Sulphasalazine (this prevents prostaglandins forming round damaged tissue, which in turn reduces inflammation)

Conjunctivitis, allergic

What is it?
Allergic conjunctivitis is irritation of the transparent membrane that covers the white of your eye and the inside of your eyelids. Your eyes will look red and feel sore and itchy, with a clear

discharge; your eyelids will be swollen; and you may become sensitive to bright light. Hot and dry weather can make it worse.

Other symptoms that may occur with it
Rhinitis (runny nose), sneezing

Possible triggers
AIRBORNE PARTICLES: particularly animal dander, chalk dust, coal dust, coffee, cork dust, cotton dust (affects smokers more), feathers, flour, grains, house dust mite, mould spores, pollen, powdered drugs, silk dust, soya bean dust, talcum powder, tea dust, tobacco dust, vegetable dust, wood dust

CHEMICALS: acetate, ammonia, benzyl acetate, chlorine, formaldehyde, isocyanates, volatile organic compounds

CONTACT LENS CLEANING SOLUTION

CONTACT IRRITANTS: matches, newsprint, carbon paper, household sprays, insecticides

COSMETICS: deodorants, depilatories, eye liner, eye shadow, face powder, foundation, hair care products, hand cream, lip balm, lipstick, mascara, moisturizer, mouthwash, nail varnish, perfume, shampoo, shaving products, skin care products, soap, suncream, toothpaste

FOOD: asparagus, avocado, buckwheat, celery, chick pea, egg, fish, kiwi fruit, lentil, mango, milk, onion, peanuts, potato, rice, soya, wheat

HERBS/SPICES: fennel, parsley

LATEX

MEDICATION: aspirin, sedatives

MOULDS

PETS

POLLEN

RAPE SEED

SOLVENTS: amyl alcohol, isopropanol, methyl alcohol, alcohol solvents, aliphatic hydrocarbons, esters

TURPENTINE

OCCUPATIONAL ALLERGENS (see *Appendix* page 609)

Treatments
Herbal remedies:
- Eye wash: camomile tea, fennel tea
- Compress – use a cold used teabag: camomile tea, fennel tea
- Compress – soak a pad of cotton wool in a tincture and use as a compress: calendula, eyebright, golden seal

Homeopathic remedies
- Euphrasia – for conjunctivitis with watering eyes
- Apis – for swollen, red, puffy eyelids

Over-the-counter remedies
- Antihistamines

Prescription medication
- Antihistamine eye drops (first-line)
- Corticosteroid eye drops, provided there is no other infection (as the drugs will make it worse)
- Cromoglycate
- Nedocromil sodium
- Steroids
- Sympathomimetics

Self-help tips
- Wear dark glasses
- Avoid eye make-up and contact lenses until the conjunctivitis has cleared up
- Rinse the eyes frequently with warm water, using separate compresses and eye baths for each eye.
- Cold compresses: using other ingredients as eyewashes or compresses can also help sore eyes:
- Diluted witch hazel (good for sore, red, closed eyes – witch hazel is mildly astringent and contains tannins, which constrict the blood vessels below the skin's surface: this reduces swelling and itching)
- Salt water eyewash: 1 teaspoon bicarbonate of soda in a pint of cooled boiled water
- Placing either of the following over the eyes can help to relieve itching:
  - raw grated carrot (spread it on a piece of gauze and place it gauze-side down on the eyelids) – it has antiseptic and disinfectant properties
  - chilled cucumber slices – cucumber juice has anti-inflammatory properties

Constipation
What is it?

Constipation is when the bowel movements are less frequent, harder or dryer than usual, making them difficult to pass. It's often a symptom of irritable bowel syndrome and can be caused by a poor diet, not enough fluid intake and lack of exercise.

Other symptoms that may occur with it

Abdominal pain, bloating, depression, weight gain, weight loss

Possible triggers

FOOD: milk

Treatments

Aromatherapy

- Try abdominal massage (in clockwise direction) with one of the following oils (diluted with 1 drop of essential oil to 5 ml of a bland carrier oil such as sweet almond oil): black pepper, fennel, ginger, lemongrass, mandarin, marjoram, orange, rosemary

Herbal remedies

- Teas (use 1–2 tsp of dried herb to 1 cup of boiling water, steeped for 10–15 minutes): fennel, ginger, liquorice, psyllium seeds, senna leaves (infusion)

Homeopathic remedies

- Calcarea carbonica – contains senna and aloes
- Graphites
- Ignatia
- Natrum muriaticum
- Nux vomica
- Silica

Over-the-counter remedies

- Laxatives (check with your doctor, first, to make sure there isn't an underlying problem such as an underactive thyroid – especially if you're vomiting as well – and don't use for more than 2–3 days); there are four types:
- bulk-forming laxatives, e.g. isphaghula husk, methylcellulose, sterculia – these increase the bulk of the stools and make them softer; the increased bulk also causes more pressure in the bowel, which makes the muscles contract more strongly. They

should always be taken with lots of fluid, and you may suffer from wind and flatulence. The action is not as rapid as with a stimulant laxative, but they are safer for longer-term use

– *stimulant laxatives* e.g. senna, biascodyl – these irritate the lining of the bowel, making the bowel muscle contract and increasing the speed of the faeces moving through the intestine; they may cause stomach cramps and should not be used regularly as your body can become dependent on them

– *osmotic laxatives* e.g. lactulose, magnesium hydroxide, magnesium sulphate, sodium sulphate – these draw water into the bowel, which softens the stools and makes them easier to pass; as with bulk-forming laxatives, action is not as rapid as with a stimulant laxative, but they are safer for longer-term use

– *lubricating agents* e.g. glycerin suppositories (rectal use) or liquid paraffin (oral use) – these line the bowel with lubricant, easing the passage of faeces. They work more quickly than other methods but, as with stimulant laxatives, they should not be used regularly as your body can become dependent on them.

Prescription medication
• As OTC remedies

Self-help tips
• Eat more foods rich in fibre (particularly bran), which will help to speed up the elimination of food waste; it also absorbs more water, making the stools softer and easier to pass.
• Foods which have a laxative effect include liquorice, unsweetened dried fruits (apricots, raisins, sultanas, figs and prunes) and molasses; if you have asthma, check that the dried fruit has not been preserved with sulphites
• Hot drinks may stimulate bowel movements
• Drink more fluids (particularly orange or prune juice), i.e. six to eight large glasses of water a day; fennel tea, camomile tea, ginger tea, lemon balm tea and peppermint tea can also help (the fluid gives the natural laxatives greater effect)
• Castor oil is a remedy for constipation used since the time of the ancient Egyptians. The oil is soothing until it reaches the intestine and is split by the enzyme lipase; then it releases ricinoteic acid, an irritant, which stimulates the intestines and softens the stools

Coughing

What is it?

A cough is the body's reflex action to clear the airways of an irritant or blockage. It is characteristic of lung conditions such as bronchitis or chest infection as well as asthma, so the cause can be difficult to diagnose; in young children, bronchiolitis (caused by the respiratory syncytial virus) mimics the symptoms of asthma. You should check with your doctor as the treatment for bronchitis/bronchiolitis is antibiotics, whereas an asthmatic cough responds to anti-asthma treatment.

Other symptoms that may occur with it

Breathing difficulties, rhinitis, postnasal drip, sinusitis

Possible triggers

CHEMICALS: formaldehyde, isocyanates
DUST MITES
ENVIRONMENTAL POLLUTANTS: nitrogen dioxide, sulphur dioxide
FOOD: asparagus, barley, cheese, chick pea, corn, grapes, lentil, milk, oats, soya, wheat
MEDICATION: ACE inhibitors, aspirin
MOULDS
RAPE SEED

Treatments

Aromatherapy

- Steam inhalation can help to make breathing easier and relieve coughing (unless you suffer from asthma, in which case avoid steam inhalation: use a few drops of decongestant essential oil on a tissue, instead). Simply add one of the mixtures below to a small bowl of freshly boiled water, then lean over the bowl, cover your head with a towel, and breathe in the steam as deeply as you can for several minutes.
- one drop each of essential oil of camomile, eucalyptus, lavender and peppermint
- cinnamon
- eucalyptus (leaves will also work)
- grapefruit
- lavender
- lemon
- tea tree
- Direct inhalation: place a couple of drops of essential oil of frankincense on a tissue and inhale

Homeopathic remedies
- Aconite – for dry, barking coughs
- Bryonia – for dry, irritating coughs
- Calcarea fluorica – for coughs with yellow mucus
- Carbo vegetalis – for violent coughs
- Drosera – for tickly coughs
- Euphrasia – for daytime coughs with mucus
- Hepar sulphuris – for coughing that is worse with cold air
- Ignatia – for irritating coughs
- Nux vomica – for violent coughs
- Phosphorus – for coughs with breathing difficulties

Over-the-counter remedies
- Check with the pharmacist, who will need to know whether it's:
- *a dry cough* – you will be given either a demulcent (containing ingredients such as glycerine) to soothe it or an antitussive (such as codeine, pholcodine or dextromethorpan) to suppress it by reducing the activity of the cough centre in the brain
- *a cough producing mucus* – you will be given an expectorant which will break up the mucus and make it easier to remove from your airways when you cough. Common expectorant ingredients include ammonium chloride, guaiphenesin, diphenhydramine and ipecacuanha.

Prescription medication
- Antihistamines
- Bronchodilator drugs
- Corticosteroid drugs

Self-help tips
- Increase the humidity in the air – use a humidifier or hang wet towels over radiators
- Drink extra fluids

Cystitis
What is it?
Cystitis is inflammation of the inner lining of the bladder. Symptoms include needing to pass urine frequently, and only being able to pass a small amount of urine each time; this is often accompanied by a burning or stinging sensation, and you may also have blood in the urine. You may feel abdominal pain or discomfort, and have a fever.

Other symptoms that may occur with it
Abdominal pain, fever

Possible triggers
SCENTED BATH AND PERSONAL CARE PRODUCTS: soaps, powders, bath oils, vaginal deodorants, douche preparations
WASHING POWDER
FOOD AND DRINK: coffee, carrot, fruit juice, spicy foods, tea
SANITARY PRODUCTS

Treatments
Aromatherapy
• Use four drops of essential oil of Roman camomile, lavender, myrrh, juniper or sandalwood or tea tree in a full bath – add when the water has run and disperse vigorously

Herbal remedies
• Teas (use 1–2 tsp of dried herb to 1 cup of boiling water, steeped for 10–15 minutes): yarrow

Homeopathic remedies
• Apis mellifica – for stinging pain when urinating
• Belladonna – for cystitis with high temperature and/or headache
• Cantharis – for pain when urinating
• Nux vomica – for bladder irritation
• Sepia – for pain when urinating

Over-the-counter remedies
• Potassium citrate (this makes the urine less acid)

Prescription medication
A doctor may prescribe antibiotics to cure any infection.

Self-help tips
• Drink lots of water to flush out the bladder; keep the urine alkaline by drinking a teaspoon of bicarbonate of soda in water every six hours
• Bed rest may help
• Place a hot water bottle over your abdomen; it can help to relieve pain in the lower back or pelvic region
• Drink a glass of cranberry juice daily to prevent cystitis

- Apply a compress of witch hazel to help relieve the burning sensation of cystitis. Witch hazel is mildly astringent and contains tannins, which constrict the blood vessels below the skin's surface: this reduces swelling and itching
- Live yoghurt applied directly to the affected area has a soothing effect and the bacteria can help to fight germs

Diarrhoea

What is it?

Diarrhoea is when the bowel movements are more fluid or frequent than usual, or have a greater volume. It's often a symptom of Crohn's disease, colitis and irritable bowel syndrome.

Other symptoms that may occur with it

Abdominal pain and swelling, colitis, gastric upset/irritation, headaches, nausea, vomiting, weight loss, wind

Possible triggers

AMINES
DRINK: beer, tea
FOOD: apple, banana, beef, beetroot, blackberries, blackcurrant, carrot, cheese, chocolate, cranberry, egg, fish, gooseberries, kiwi fruit, melon, milk, orange, passion fruit, pea, peach, peanuts, peppers, pineapple, pork, redcurrant, rhubarb, rye, shellfish, soya, spinach, strawberry, sunflower seed, wheat
FOOD ADDITIVES: colours, preservatives, emulsifiers/stabilizers/ thickeners
HISTAMINE
HERBS/SPICES: garlic
MEDICATION: antibiotics, cephalosporins, tetracycline
SALICYLATES

Treatments

Aromatherapy

- Use a warm compress (use 6 drops of oil in 500 ml of hot water, dip a cloth into it and wring it out, then lay the cloth on the affected area until it has cooled to body temperature): camomile, ginger, marjoram, neroli, peppermint, sandalwood, sweet thyme

Herbal remedies
- Teas (use 1 tsp of dried herb to 1 cup of boiling water, steeped for 10–15 minutes): camomile, ginger, marshmallow, meadowsweet
- Slippery elm (use 1 heaped tsp in a cup of warm water)
- Black tea (high tannin levels have an astringent effect)

Homeopathic remedies
- Argentium nitricum
- Arsenicum album – for sudden diarrhoea with vomiting
- Colocynthis – for diarrhoea with abdominal cramps
- Mercurius solubilis
- Natrum sulphuricum – for yellow diarrhoea
- Sulphur

Over-the-counter remedies
- Kaolin (aluminium silicate) and morphine – this absorbs anything in the bowel that causes the diarrhoea, while the morphine relaxes the bowel muscles, slowing down the passage of food and allowing more water to be absorbed; you should take this with plenty of fluids and ensure the bottle is shaken well before each dose
- Calcium carbonate
- Pectin

Prescription medication
- Antidiarrhoeal drugs – codeine phospate, diphenoxylate, loperamide. Loperamide relaxes the bowel muscles, slowing down the passage of food and allowing more water to be absorbed; you should take it with plenty of fluids

Self-help tips
- Don't eat solid foods for 24 hours
- To prevent dehydration, drink plenty of clear fluids, preferably with a rehydration formula (either bought commercially, or dissolve one teaspoon of salt with eight teaspoons of sugar in a litre of water).

Foods that can help settle your stomach include:
- live yoghurt
- bananas
- grated apple can help diarrhoea: apples contain malic and tartaric acid, which regulate stomach acidity and help with the

digestion of protein and fat. An old remedy recommends letting the grated apple turn brown, first

• blackberries – they come from the same family as apples, and both fruits contain the water-soluble fibre pectin, which can help bind bile acid. Pectin is used an ingredient in several over-the-counter remedies.

Ears – blocked or painful, hearing difficulties

What is it?
When your ears feel blocked or painful, you may also find that your hearing is dulled as well.

It usually goes with a runny nose; when the mucous membranes in the nose and sinuses swell, the mucous membranes in the Eustachian tubes (which equalize pressure in the ears and allow the liquid from the middle ear to drain into the throat) also swell, causing pain and dulled hearing.

Other symptoms that may occur with it
Nose running, faintness, fatigue

Possible triggers
DUST MITES
FOOD: milk, chocolate, tomatoes, citrus fruits, wheat, eggs

Treatments
Aromatherapy
• Put one drop of lavender on some cotton wool and place it in the ear; or use Roman camomile in a warm compress on the side of the face

Herbal remedies
• Essential oil of St John's wort – use 2 drops in each ear

Homeopathic remedies
• Argentum nitricum – for earache and buzzing in the ears
• Belladonna – for throbbing earache
• Chamomilla – for children's earache
• Hepar sulphuris
• Mercurius solubilis

Over-the-counter remedies
• Painkillers

Prescription medication
• Sympathomimetics

Self-help tips
• Hold a warm flannel or hot water bottle over your ear (use a cold compress instead if your ear is red and swollen)

Eczema See section on *Eczema* in *Allergic illnesses*

Eyes, sore or itchy See *Conjunctivitis, allergic*

Eyes, watering
What is it?
Tears wash away particles and foreign bodies from the eyes. If you are allergic to something, your tear production may be overstimulated, causing watery eyes

Other symptoms that may occur with it
Conjunctivitis, allergic

Possible triggers
AIRBORNE ALLERGENS: animal dander, chalk dust, coal dust, coffee, cork dust, cotton dust (this affects smokers more), feathers, flour, grains, house dust mite, mould spores, pollen, powdered drugs, silk dust, soya bean dust, talcum powder, tea dust, tobacco dust, vegetable dust, wood dust

Treatments
See *Conjunctivitis, allergic*

Faintness
What is it?
Faintness is caused by a drop in blood pressure and a reduction in your heart rate, meaning that not enough blood or oxygen is reaching your brain. As a symptom of allergy, it can be a warning

signal of anaphylactic shock – see the section on *What to do in an emergency*.

Other symptoms that may occur with it
Dimmed vision, dizziness, fatigue, nausea, ringing in the ears, sweating

Possible triggers
The most common causes of anaphylactic shock are:
FOOD: dairy products, eggs, fish and shellfish, fruit, peanuts and other nuts, sesame seeds
LATEX (rubber)
PRESCRIBED DRUGS such as penicillin
WASP OR BEE STINGS

Treatments
Aromatherapy
- Essential oil of peppermint contains menthols, which is a stimulant with restorative properties; sniffing one drop on a handkerchief may stop you feeling faint. Basil, lavender and rosemary may also help.

Bach flower remedies
- Rescue remedy

Prescription medication
- Adrenaline

Self-help tips
- If you feel faint, sit down with your head between your knees until the symptoms subside. Drink some cool water and open the windows for more oxygen.
- If you can, lie flat on your back with your legs raised – this will help blood flow to the brain.

Fatigue
What is it?
Fatigue or tiredness is when you feel that you don't have the energy to do anything. If you can't put it down to lack of sleep, overwork, depression, anaemia or the early stages of pregnancy, it could be a symptom of allergy. As a symptom of allergy, a sudden

feeling of fatigue (particularly if combined with other symptoms such as dizziness or nausea) can be a warning signal of anaphylactic shock – *see* the section on *What to do in an emergency*.

Other symptoms that may occur with it
Dimmed vision, dizziness, faintness, nausea, ringing in the ears, sweating

Possible triggers
CHEMICALS: isocyanates
AMINES (including tyramine)

Treatments
Aromatherapy
- Essential oil of peppermint – inhale 2 drops on a tissue or add to a bath with 4 drops rosemary; add when the water has run and disperse vigorously (it has stimulating and refreshing properties as the oil is roughly a third menthol)
- Essential oils of lavender and camomile are also soothing in the bath (four drops to a full bath) and can help you relax.
- Essential oils of rosemary and basil are a good stimulant, though avoid rosemary if you have high blood pressure or suffer from epilepsy

Bach flower remedies
- Olive

Homeopathic remedies
- Gelsemium
- Sepia

Fever/high temperature
What is it?
Fever is when your body temperature is above 37°C.

Other symptoms that may occur with it
Colitis, cystitis, flushed face, headache, hot skin, rapid breathing, shivering, sweating

Possible triggers
BACTERIA
CHEMICALS: anhydrides, epoxy resin, isocyanates

FOOD: mushrooms, oats
MEDICATION: ACE inhibitors, amoxycillin, antibiotics, cephalosporins, macrolides, penicillin, sulphonamides

Treatments
Herbal remedies
• Teas (use 1 tsp of dried herb to 1 cup of boiling water, steeped
for 10–15 minutes): camomile, catmint

Homeopathic remedies
• Ferrum phos – for fever with throbbing headache

Over-the-counter remedies
• Aspirin
• Ibuprofen
• Paracetamol

Prescription medication
• As OTC remedies

Self-help tips
• Drink plenty of cold fluids
• Sponge the body with tepid water
• Take a warm (not hot) bath

Flushing
What is it?
Flushing is reddening of the skin, caused by blood vessels dilating
near the surface of the skin. It tends to show mainly in the face
and neck.

Other symptoms that may occur with it
Fever, migraine

Possible triggers
FOOD: alcohol, aubergine, avocado, banana, beans, beef, beer,
broad beans, caffeine, cheese, chocolate, citrus fruit, eggs,
fermented foods, figs, fish, pickled fish, game, parsley, peperoni,
plums, prunes, sauerkraut, sausages, shellfish, soy sauce,
spinach, strawberries, tomatoes, yeast
FOOD ADDITIVES: flavour enhancers

Treatments

Flushing will disappear of its own accord within a couple of hours; vitamin E tablets may help

Gastric upset/irritation

What is it?

Inflammation of the stomach and intestine.

Other symptoms that may occur with it

Abdominal pain and bloating, diarrhoea, nausea, vomiting

Possible triggers

CHEMICALS: isocyanates, volatile organic compounds

FOOD: barley, beef, blackcurrant, buckwheat, celery, chick pea, corn, cranberry, fish, kiwi fruit, mustard, oats, onion, orange, passion fruit, peach, potato, rice, rye, shellfish, soya, sunflower seed

FOOD ADDITIVES: preservatives, antioxidants, emulsifiers/ stabilizers/ thickeners, anti-caking agents

HERBS/SPICES: cinnamon, coriander, horseradish

MEDICATION: tetracycline

SALICYLATES

SULPHUR DIOXIDE

TURPENTINE

Treatments

Aromatherapy

- Use 1 drop of the following essential oils to 5 ml of a bland carrier oil such as sweet almond oil and massage over your abdomen: camomile, marjoram, orange

Herbal remedies

- Teas (use 1–2 tsp of dried herb to 1 cup of boiling water, steeped for 15 minutes): meadowsweet
- Slippery elm (1 teaspoon powdered herb into a cup of warm water)

Over-the-counter remedies

- Use paracetamol rather than aspirin

Prescription medication

- As OTC remedies

Self-help tips
- Avoid alcohol
- Drink lots of fluid during the attack to avoid dehydration
- Live yoghurt and banana can help to settle the stomach

Hay fever
See section on *Hay fever* in chapter on *Allergic illnesses*

Headaches
What is it?
A headache is a feeling of pain in the head or back of the neck. It's caused by tension in or stretching of the membranes around the brain (the meninges) or the blood vessels or muscles of the scalp. See also *Migraine*, below

Other symptoms that may occur with it
Anxiety, diarrhoea, fever, heartburn, nausea, vomiting

Possible triggers
AMINES including phenylethylamine, tyramine
ARTIFICIAL FIBRES
BACTERIA
CHEMICALS: formaldehyde, isocyanates, some volatile organic compounds
DUST MITES
FOOD: aubergines, avocado, bananas, beef, beer, broad beans, canned meats, cheese, chicken liver, chocolate, citrus fruit, eggs, figs, game, pickled fish, pineapple, prunes, plums, salami, sesame, soy sauce, soya, sunflower seed, tomato, yeast, yeast extract (e.g. Marmite)
FOOD ADDITIVES: preservatives, emulsifiers/stabilizers/ thickeners, flavour enhancers
HISTAMINE
SCENT/FLAVOURING: amyl acetate
TURPENTINE
WOOL

Treatments
Acupuncture

Aromatherapy
- Use one of the following oils for inhalation (1 drop on a handkerchief) or as a cold compress (use 6 drops of oil in 500ml cold water, dip a cloth into it and wring it out, then lay the cloth on the affected area until it has reached body temperature): camomile, clary sage, eucalyptus, lavender, peppermint, rosemary

Herbal remedies
- Teas (use 2 tsp of dried root or herb to 1 cup of boiling water, steeped for 15 minutes): meadowsweet, skullcap, valerian, wood betony
- Feverfew – chop leaves and add to food
- Elderflower has anti-inflammatory properties; try placing fresh elder leaves on the temples to relieve a headache.

Homeopathic remedies
- Actaea racemosa – for headache with severe pain starting at the back of the head and spreading upwards
- Belladonna – for severe, throbbing headache
- Coffea – for one-sided headache
- Gelsemium – for general headache
- Ignatia – for piercing headache
- Kalium phosphoricum – for headache with humming in the ears
- Lachesis – for throbbing headache
- Natrium muriaticum – for severe headache
- Nux vomica – for headache with nausea or vomiting
- Thuja – for severe headache

Over-the-counter remedies
- Pain relievers (ibuprofen, paracetamol)
- Non-steroidal anti-inflammatories (NSAIDs – aspirin)

Prescription medication
As OTC remedies

Self-help tips
- A hot bath may help
- Lying down in a dark room can help
- Brushing your hair gently can also help, because it stimulates blood flow to the area.

Heartburn

What is it?

Heartburn is a burning pain in the centre of the chest; it may travel from the tip of the breastbone to the throat. Acid may also rise into the throat. The pain is often worse at night, or if you lie flat or bend over.

Other symptoms that may occur with it

Abdominal pain, bloating, headaches, indigestion, wind (belching)

Possible triggers

FOOD: caffeine, chocolate, citrus fruits, fish, milk, onion, orange, peppermint, shellfish, sugar

MEDICATION: antibiotics, aspirin

Treatments

Aromatherapy

• Use one of the following oils as massage (use 1 drop of essential oil to 5 ml of a bland carrier oil such as sweet almond oil): black pepper, fennel, ginger, peppermint, Roman camomile

Herbal remedies

• Teas (use 1–2 tsp of dried herb to 1 cup of boiling water, steeped for 10–15 minutes): camomile, ginger (use 1½ teaspoons of freshly grated root), meadowsweet infusion (1–2 teaspoons of dried herb in a cup of boiling water, infused for 15 minutes)
• Marshmallow – take as capsules
• Slippery elm – take as capsules

Homeopathic remedies

• Argentum nitricum
• Natrum phosphoricum
• Obina – particularly for heartburn with wind and headaches

Over-the-counter remedies

• Antacid medications, such as magnesium hydroxide, magnesium trisilicate and sodium bicarbonate, neutralize the acid in the stomach
• Alginates – these form a layer on top of the stomach contents and form a barrier between the acid in the stomach and the oesophagus

Prescription medication
- As OTC remedies
- Acid-blocking drugs – such as ranitidine

Self-help tips
- Eat small meals and avoid eating just before bedtime
- Raise the head of your bed or sleep propped up on pillows
- Maintain your recommended weight (being overweight makes it worse)
- Eat live plain yoghurt
- Drinks: try lemon juice in hot water (the acids are metabolized to produce potassium carbonate, which helps to neutralize excess acidity and protect the lining of the digestive tract), or a teaspoon of cider vinegar in hot water

Hives   See *Urticaria*

Hyperactivity in children
What is it?
This is also known as attention deficit disorder (ADD), when children over the age of four find it difficult to concentrate and always seem on the go, sleep less than other children, fidget, have no sense of danger, and are often impulsive or reckless.

Possible triggers
DRINK: cider, tea
FOOD: apple, apricot, asparagus, banana, blackberries, blackcurrant, blueberries, cherries, cider vinegar, citrus fruit, cranberry, cucumbers, currants, dates, gooseberries, grapes, liquorice, melon, nectarine, orange, passion fruit, pea, peach, peppers, pineapple, plum, prune, raisin, raspberry, strawberry, sugar, tomato, wine vinegar, Worcestershire sauce
FOOD ADDITIVES: colours
HERBS/SPICES: aniseed, clove, cumin, curry powder, dill, mace, oregano, paprika, rosemary, tarragon, thyme, turmeric
SALICYLATES

Treatments
Herbal remedies
- Evening primrose oil

Prescription medication
• Stimulant drugs

Self-help tips
The Hyperactive Children's Support Group recommends that the following are avoided:

• *Colours*:
  E102 Tartrazine
  E104 Quinoline yellow
  107 Yellow 2G
  E110 Sunset yellow FCF
  E120 Cochineal
  E122 Carmoisine
  E124 Ponceau
  E127 Erythrosine
  E128 Red 2G
  E132 Indigo carmine
  E133 Brilliant blue FCF
  E150 Caramel
  E154 Brown FK
  E155 Brown HT
  E160(b) Annatto

• *Preservatives*:
  E210 Benzoic acid
  E111 Sodium benzoate
  E220 Sulphur dioxide
  E250 Sodium nitrite
  E251 Sodium nitrate
  E320 Butylated hydroxyanisole
  E321 Butylated hydroxytoluene

Indigestion
What is it?
Indigestion is a group of conditions (including bloating, wind and heartburn) that affect the upper abdomen; it is often associated with excess stomach acid following a heavy or spicy meal. There may be a burning or gnawing sensation in the stomach.

Other symptoms that may occur with it
Abdominal pain, heartburn, nausea and wind

Possible triggers
See *Heartburn*

Treatments
Aromatherapy
- Abdominal massage (in clockwise direction) with one of the following oils (diluted as 1 drop essential oil to 5 ml carrier oil): black pepper, camomile, clary sage, coriander, fennel, ginger, marjoram, peppermint

Herbal remedies
- Teas (use 1–2 tsp of dried herb to 1 cup of boiling water, steeped for 15 minutes): aniseed, camomile, dill, fennel, ginger, lemon balm, meadowsweet, peppermint tea
- Seeds, chewed after a meal: aniseed, cardamom, fennel

Homeopathic remedies
- Carbo vegetalis – for indigestion with flatulence
- Kalium muriaticum – for indigestion caused by fatty foods

Over-the-counter remedies
- Antacid medications e.g. magnesium hydroxide, magnesium trisilicate, sodium bicarbonate – these neutralize the acid in the stomach by reacting with it to form weaker acids which are not as damaging to the stomach
- Alginates – these are derived from seaweed; when they react to the stomach acid, they form a layer of small bubbles on top of the stomach contents which acts as a barrier between the acid in the stomach and the oesophagus
- Prokinetics – these make the stomach muscles contract, which in turn makes the contents of the stomach move down. They're fairly new to the market (at the time of writing), so check with your pharmacist or GP before using them

Prescription medication
- As OTC remedies
- H2 agonists – these slow the production of stomach acid rather than neutralizing it (e.g. ranitidine, cimetidine)
- Proton pump inhibitors (omeprazole, lansoprazole)

Self-help tips
- Drinks: milk; 1 tsp bicarbonate of soda in a glass of water; a tea-spoon of cider vinegar in a glass of water can sometimes help; soda water
- Food: chewing cardamom seeds can help – the spice contains oils that relieve nausea, soothe intestinal spasms and promote the expulsion of gas; eat 2 tsp honey (a remedy used by the ancient Egyptians)
- Eat slowly and chew food thoroughly; eat small meals regularly

Inflammation

What is it?
Inflammation is when body tissues are red, hot, swollen and painful. It occurs when histamine is released; blood flow to the area is increased and the blood vessels leak, causing the heat and redness.

Other symptoms that may occur with it
Itching, rash

Possible triggers
- *On the skin* – anything that causes contact dermatitis
- *Other parts of the body* – likely to be food allergy

Treatments
Over-the-counter remedies
- Emollients
- Antihistamines

Prescription medication
- As OTC remedies
- Corticosteroids

Insomnia   See *Sleep problems*

Irritation of mucous membranes
What is it?
Irritation of the mucous membranes is when the membranes that line the throat and eyelids become swollen, inflamed and painful.

Possible triggers

CHEMICALS: benzyl alcohol, chlorine, formaldehyde, phthalic acid, phthalic anhydride, volatile organic compounds

FOOD: apple, grapes, kiwi fruit, mango

FOOD ADDITIVES: emulsifiers/stabilizers/thickeners, anti-caking agents

HERBS/SPICES: garlic

LATEX

Treatments

Herbal remedies
- Eyebright – take an infusion or capsules

Over-the-counter remedies
- Painkillers

See also *Conjunctivitis*

Prescription medication
- As OTC remedies

Itching/burning mouth/palate

What is it?

Itching/burning mouth or palate is also known as "oral allergy syndrome"; it is a sensation of itching or burning in the mouth and palate.

Other symptoms that may occur with it

Angioedema

Possible triggers

ARTIFICIAL FIBRES

FOOD: apple, banana, buckwheat, carrot, celery, cherries, grapes, guava, kiwi fruit, lettuce, mango, melon, mustard, orange, parsnip, pea, peach, pear, plum, pork, potato, spinach, strawberry, swede

HERBS/SPICES: clove, fennel, parsley

HISTAMINE

MEDICATION: antibiotics

SCENT/FLAVOURING: menthol

Treatments

The problem will resolve on its own.

Over-the-counter remedies
• Painkillers

Prescription medication
As OTC remedies

Itching
What is it?
Itching is an irritating or tickling sensation in the skin. It may be felt in one particular area or all over the body. It tends to be worse at night, when the skin is warm and there are fewer distractions. It tends to occur with eczema, dermatitis, psoriasis and urticaria. Scratching gives temporary relief but may make the condition worse in the long term – for example, if you have eczema, scratching may damage the skin further, leading to infection.

Other symptoms that may occur with it
Dry skin, inflammation, rash, skin irritation (e.g. after insect bites), urticaria

Possible triggers
AMINES

ARTIFICIAL FIBRES

CHEMICALS: chromate, formaldehyde, mercaptobenzothiazole, volatile organic compounds

COSMETICS: AHAs, deodorants, depilatories, douche preparations, eye liner, eye shadow, face powder, foundation, hair care products, hand cream, lip balm, lipstick, mascara, moisturizer, mouthwash, nail varnish, perfume, shampoo, shaving products, skin care products, soap

FLEAS

FOOD: apple, barley, blackcurrant, buckwheat, celery, cranberry, fish, kiwi fruit, malt, mango, melon, oats, orange, passion fruit, peanuts, pear, pineapple, rice, rye, shellfish, soya, sunflower seed, wheat

FOOD ADDITIVES: colours

INSECT STINGS

MEDICATION: amoxycillin, antibiotics, antifungals, aspirin, cephalosporins, frusemide, gentamycin, insulin, tetracycline

METALS: nickel

PLANTS
PLASTERS/BAND AIDS (THE ADHESIVE)
SALICYLATES
SANITARY PRODUCTS
SEMEN
SOLVENTS: alcohol solvents
THURIAMS
WOOL

Treatments

Aromatherapy
• Use essential oil of lavender or lemon balm in the bath (four drops to a full bath – add when the water has run and disperse vigorously!)

Herbal remedies
• Chickweed – pour 3 cups of boiling water on 10 tsp of dried herb, infuse for 15 mins and add to the bath

Over-the-counter remedies
• Antihistamines
• Calamine lotion
• Emollients

Prescription medication
• As OTC remedies

Self-help tips
• Avoid soap
• Wear cool, light clothing – choose cotton rather than wool, as it's less irritating
• Press rather than scratch the itch so you don't damage your skin
• Apply cold compresses to your skin
• Ground oatmeal – add 2 cups to warm bath
• A tepid (not hot) bath can help to ease itchiness. Additives to the bath that can help moisturize the skin and ease itchiness include:
– apricot kernel oil
– a few drops of cider vinegar – it acts as an astringent and helps to reduce inflammation and swelling
– sesame oil

Joint pain and swelling

What is it?

Joint pain and swelling is a form of arthritis. Rheumatoid arthritis is when the body's immune system acts against the joints and their surrounding soft tissues.

Other symptoms that may occur with it

Muscle pain

Possible triggers

DUST MITES
MEDICATION: antifungals, cephalosporins, penicillin
SEROTONIN
WOOL

Treatments

Aromatherapy

• Use the following essential oils in a bath (four drops to a full bath – add when the water has run and disperse vigorously!): lavender, camomile, eucalyptus, ginger, juniper

Herbal remedies

• Cabbage leaves – bruise them, warm them in a microwave and wrap around the affected joint; cover with a towel and leave for 15 minutes

Homeopathic remedies

• Apis mellifica – for arthritis with red and swollen joints
• Bryonia – for arthritis
• Calcarea fluorica – for arthritis responding to warmth
• Ferrum phosphoricum – for rheumatism
• Kalium muriaticum – for rheumatic swelling
• Kalium sulphuricum – for rheumatism that moves from joint to joint
• Ledum – for rheumatism in the lower limbs
• Natrum phosphoricum – to remove excess lactic acid, helping rheumatism
• Phytolacca – for rheumatism and shooting pains in the body
• Pulsatilla – for arthritis
• Rhus toxicodendron – for joint stiffness
• Ruta graveolens – for rheumatism

Over-the-counter remedies
- Aspirin
- Paracetamol

Prescription medication
- Anti-inflammatory drugs

Self-help tips
- Weight control – try to maintain your recommended weight

Migraine
What is it?
Migraine is a severe headache which lasts from between two hours and two days; vision is usually disturbed (e.g. the sufferer may see flashing lights).

Other symptoms that may occur with it
Depression, fatigue, flushing, nausea, sensitivity to light, vomiting

Possible triggers
ALCOHOL
AMINES including phenylethylamine, tyramine
DRINK: beer, wine
FOOD: aubergine, avocado, banana, beans, beef, broad beans, caffeine, cheese, chocolate, chicken liver, citrus fruit, egg, fermented food, figs, fish, fish (pickled), game, plum, prune, sauerkraut, sausages, shellfish, soy sauce, spinach, strawberry, tomato, yeast, yeast extract
FOOD ADDITIVES: colours, preservatives
HERBS/SPICES: parsley
HISTAMINE
SEROTONIN
TOBACCO

Treatments
Acupuncture

Alexander technique

Aromatherapy
- Use one of the following essential oils as a hot or cold compress

(use 6 drops of oil in 500ml cold water or hot, dip a cloth into it and wring it out, then lay the cloth on the affected area until it has reached body temperature): camomile, coriander, clary sage, lavender, marjoram, melissa, peppermint

Chiropractic

Herbal remedies
- Feverfew to reduce frequency and severity – add chopped leaves to a sandwich

Homeopathic remedies
- Kalium bichromicum – for migraine with blurred vision before an attack
- Pulsatilla – for migraine made worse by fatty foods
- Sanguinaria – for migraine on right side
- Silicea – for migraine that settles above one eye
- Thuja – for migraine on left side

Hypnosis

Osteopathy

Over-the-counter remedies:
- Aspirin
- Ibuprofen
- Paracetamol

Prescription medication
- Beta blockers
- Sumatryptan
- Ergotamine
- 5HT agonists
- Sodium valproate
- Anti-sickness drugs

Reflexology

Self-help tips
Lie down in a dark room

Mouth ulcers

What is it?

Mouth ulcers are small lesions on the tongue, inside of the cheeks or roof of the mouth

Possible triggers

FOOD ADDITIVES: preservatives
SCENT/FLAVOURING: menthol

Treatments

Aromatherapy

- 1 drop essential oil of cypress, myrrh or tea tree in two teaspoons of cider vinegar – use as mouthwash
- A little essential oil of tea tree, dabbed neat on to the sore, can also help, as tea tree oil has antiseptic properties

Herbal remedies

- Garlic – cut it in half, squeeze until the oil beads on the surface, then dab on the ulcer 2–3 times a day (it will sting!)
- Marigold (use as a mouthwash)
- Myrrh (use as a mouthwash, diluted)
- Purple sage (use as a mouthwash)
- Thyme (use as a mouthwash)
- Vitamin E oil may help healing

Homeopathic remedies

- Hypericum and calendula tincture – use as a mouthwash

Over-the-counter remedies

- Antiseptic mouthwash
- Folic acid (may shorten attack or prevent another one)
- Hydrocortisone pellets

Prescription medication

As OTC remedies

Self-help tips

Compresses

- Holding a warm used tea bag against the sore may help, as the tannic acid in the tea is an astringent, reducing inflammation, and will help to make the sore heal more quickly

- Putting a pinch of bicarbonate of soda directly on to the sore will sting, but will help to heal it because it reduces the amount of bacteria in the mouth. Or try making a paste of the bicarbonate of soda and a little water, for ease of application.

Mouthwashes
- Mix a pinch of turmeric with a little glycerine and dab on to mouth ulcers to soothe them
- Rinsing the mouth with cabbage juice can also help to soothe them. Cabbage juice has anti-inflammatory properties, which are soothing and encourage healing; its sulphur compounds give it antiseptic properties, and it also stimulates the immune system and antibody production.
- A spoonful of lemon juice in water, used as a mouthwash, will help the sore remain clean – the antiseptic nature of the acid will kill any bacteria in the sore and lemon acts as an astringent, reducing bleeding, inflammation and swelling.
- A salt mouthwash or a gargle of one teaspoon of salt in a glass of warm water will help heal mouth ulcers. It will sting but the salt water will help to draw fluid through the tissues, which will help to speed the healing process.

Muscle pain

What is it?
Muscles are fibres in the body which contract and relax to create movement; pain – also known as myalgia – occurs when the muscle tissues are inflamed.

Other symptoms that may occur with it
Joint pain

Possible triggers
CHEMICALS: anhydrides, isocyanates
DUST MITES

Treatments
Homeopathic remedies
- Actaea racemosa – for stiff neck and muscle ache
- Arnica – for aching muscles
- Magnesia phosphoricum – for muscular spasms

Over-the-counter remedies
• Aspirin
• Ibuprofen

Prescription medication
As OTC remedies

Self-help tips
• Ice pack to reduce pain and swelling
• Avoid hot baths (will make it worse)
• Raise the affected part to reduce swelling

Nausea

What is it?
Nausea is a feeling that you are going to be sick.

Other symptoms that may occur with it
Abdominal pain and swelling, angioedema, diarrhoea, faintness, fatigue, gastric upset/irritation, headaches, indigestion, migraine, vomiting, weight loss, wind

Possible triggers
ALCOHOL
AMINES including tyramine
CHEMICALS: formaldehyde, methylene blue, volatile organic compounds
FOOD: beef, carrot, corn, egg, fish, milk, oats, orange, pea, peach, peanuts, pork, rye, shellfish, strawberry, sunflower seed, wheat
FOOD ADDITIVES: colours, preservatives, antioxidants, emulsifiers/stabilizers/thickeners, anti-caking agents, flavour enhancers
HERBS/SPICES: anise, garlic
MEDICATION: antibiotics, dichlorophen, frusemide
SOLVENTS: amyl alcohol, alcohol solvents, aliphatic hydrocarbons

Treatments
Aromatherapy
• Inhale two drops of one of the following oils on a handkerchief: cardamom, coriander, fennel, ginger, lavender, nutmeg, peppermint

Herbal remedies
- Teas (add 1–2 tsp of dried herb to 1 cup of boiling water and infuse for 10–15 minutes): camomile, ginger (use 1 tsp fresh grated root), lemon balm, peppermint, vervain
- Cloves – take 1–2 drops clove oil on a sugar lump
- Ginger, crystallized

Homeopathic remedies
- Ipecacuanha
- Sepia

Over-the-counter remedies
- *Antihistamines*

Prescription medication
- As OTC remedies

Self-help tips
- Food – try nibbling dry biscuits or toast to help relieve nausea. Ginger is known to help nausea; try eating ginger biscuits or crystallized ginger
- Drinks – drink plenty of fluids, particularly water; drinking slowly can help the fluid to stay down. Ginger beer can also help, if sipped slowly; some people recommend that you should allow the drink to go flat, first. Lemon juice in hot water can also help. During digestion, the acids are metabolized to product potassium carbonate, which helps to neutralize excess acidity and protect the lining of the digestive tract. A tablespoon of cider vinegar in hot water can also help.

Neurological problems

What is it?
Nerve fibres carry information from a receptor or sense organ to the nervous system, or from the nervous system to a muscle. Types of neurological problem include migraine, pain in the ears and pain in the back of the tongue. See *Ear problems, Migraine, Itching/burning mouth*

Possible triggers
FOOD ADDITIVES: preservatives
SULPHUR DIOXIDE

Nose, running or blocked
What is it?
If your nose is blocked or congested, the mucus membrane lining your nose may be swollen, causing it to feel "stuffy"; blowing it doesn't have much effect. Your nose may also produce a runny discharge. If the discharge is clear, the problem is likely to be allergic rhinitis or hay fever; if it's thicker or discoloured, it's more likely to be a cold or viral infection.

Other symptoms that may occur with it
Allergic conjunctivitis, breathing problems, coughing (caused by the mucus), ear pain (caused by blocked Eustachian tubes), post-nasal drip (caused by the mucus), sinusitis, sneezing

Possible triggers
AIRBORNE ALLERGENS: pollen; animal fur or feathers, saliva and urine; house dust mite; cockroaches; moulds

ARTIFICIAL FIBRES

BACTERIA

BIRD DROPPINGS

COCKROACHES

COSMETICS: Balsam of Peru, bitter almond oil, cassia oil, citronella oil

DUST MITES

DYES

FOOD: apple, asparagus, avocado, bamboo shoots, banana, barley, blackcurrant, buckwheat, carrot, celery, chick pea, corn, cranberry, egg, fish, flour, grapes, guava, lentil, lettuce, mandarin, milk, mustard, oats, onion, orange, parsnip, passion fruit, pea, peach, peanuts, pork, potato, rice, rye, shellfish, soya, strawberry, swede, wheat, yeast

FOOD ADDITIVES: colours, emulsifiers/stabilizers/thickeners

HERBS/SPICES: cayenne pepper, coriander, fennel, garlic, pepper

MEDICATION: aspirin, sedatives

MOULDS

PETS

POLLEN

RAPE SEED

SALICYLATES

SCENT/FLAVOURING: balsam of Peru, cassia oil

SOLVENTS: esters

TURPENTINE

WOOL

Treatments
Aromatherapy
• Steam inhalation can also help to relieve the symptoms, particularly if decongestant oils such as eucalyptus or peppermint are added to the warm water

Over-the-counter remedies:
• Antihistamines (to stop the allergic reaction)
• Decongestants (to shrink the mucus membrane)

Prescription medication
• As OTC remedies
• Sodium cromoglycate

Self-help tips
• Drink plenty of clear fluids – this will help to keep the mucus thin and avoid complications such as ear pain and sinusitis
• Use petroleum jelly around your nose, to stop it becoming sore.
• Drink cider vinegar and honey in hot water to relieve nasal congestion – they both have decongestant properties

Palpitations
What are they?
Palpitations make you feel as if your heart is beating fast or irregularly.

Other symptoms that may occur with them
Anxiety

Possible triggers
FOOD: caffeine
FOOD ADDITIVES: flavour enhancers
MEDICATION: insulin

Treatments
Aromatherapy
• One of the following oils in a vaporizer (use approximately 6 drops of oil and 2 dessertspoons of water in a room 3 metres square): lavender, melissa, neroli, ylang ylang

Herbal remedies
• Teas (add 1–2tsp of the dried herb to 1 cup boiling water and

infuse for 10–15 minutes): choose camomile, lime flower, passiflora, valerian

Homeopathic remedies
• Nux vomica – after food, alcohol or coffee

Prescription medication
• Beta blockers
• Calcium channel blockers
• Digitalis drugs

Psychological problems
What are they?
Mood swings, irritability, food cravings, panic attacks, depression, tension

Other symptoms that may occur with them
Constipation, migraine, sleep problems

Possible triggers
FOOD ALLERGY

Treatments
Aromatherapy
• For depression, use one of the following oils for massage (1 drop oil to 5 ml carrier oil), in a vaporizer (6 drops oil in 2 tsp water for a 3 metre-square room) or in a bath (four drops to a full bath – add when the water has run and disperse vigorously!): basil, citrus, clary sage, lavender, neroli, sandalwood

Bach flower remedies
• Rock rose

Herbal remedies
• Teas (add 1–2tsp dried herb to 1 cup boiling water and infuse for 10–15 minutes): linden, valerian, vervain
• St John's Wort

Prescription medication
• For depression: antidepressants increase the level of neurotransmitters in the brain. The most common types of drugs

prescribed are tricylics, serotonin re-uptake inhibitors (SRIs) and monoamine oxidase inhibitors (MOAIs)

Skin irritation/sensitivity

What is it?
Skin irritation or sensitivity can present itself as stinging, burning or peeling.

Other symptoms that may occur with it
Itching, rash

Possible triggers
CHEMICALS: chloroform, chromate, cobalt, mercaptobenzothiazole (rubber boots, gloves and catheters)

COSMETICS AND PERFUME including the following ingredients: benzoyl peroxide, benzyl acetate, benzyl alcohol, colophony (cosmetics and soaps), epoxy resin (adhesives, vinyl, plastic); AHAs, deodorants, depilatories, douche preparations, eye liner, eye shadow, face powder, foundation, hair care products, hand cream, lip balm, lipstick, mascara, moisturizer, nail varnish, perfume, shampoo, shaving products, skin care products, soap, suncream, toothpaste

ETHYLENE DIAMINE (creams, paints), formaldehyde (cosmetics), phthalic acid (cosmetics and nail polish), phthalic anhydride (cosmetic dyes)

DRINK: tea

FLEAS

FOOD: mango

FOOD ADDITIVES: preservatives, antioxidants, emulsifiers, stabilizers and thickeners

HERBS/SPICES: aniseed, cumin, mace, oregano, rosemary, tarragon

MEDICATION: insulin

METALS: cobalt

PLANTS

SANITARY PRODUCTS

SCENT/FLAVOURING: Amyl acetate, balsam of Peru, clove oil

SEMEN

SOLVENTS: alcohol solvents, aromatic hydrocarbons, chlorinated hydrocarbons, esters, glycols, glycol ethers, halogenated solvents, ketone solvents

THURIAMS

Treatments
Over-the-counter remedies
• Emollients

Prescription medication
As OTC remedies

Self-help tips
See *Skin rash*, below

Skin rash

What is it?
A rash is a group of spots; it may also show as an area of red or inflamed skin. It may affect only a small area of skin or it may affect the entire body.

Rashes are associated with the allergic conditions of eczema, dermatitis, psoriasis and urticaria. Scratching gives temporary relief but may make the condition worse in the long term – for example, if you have eczema, scratching may damage the skin further, leading to infection.

Types of rash
• Blisters
• Bullae (large blisters)
• Macules
• Papules
• Vesicles
• Dry or weeping
• Itchy or non-itchy

Other symptoms that may occur with it
Inflammation, irritation, itching, stinging

Possible triggers
Contact dermatitis:
ADHESIVES
AIRBORNE PARTICLES
ALCOHOL
BATTERIES
BLEACH
CEMENT

CHEMICALS: acid, alkalis, ammonia, antimony, alkalis, benzoyl peroxide, butyl alcohol, chlorocresol (glues), chromate (cement, dyeing, tanning, printing), chromium, cobalt (including chloride and sulphate, in adhesives), glutaraldehyde (sterilizing fluid), gum acacia (printing), epoxy resin (adhesives, vinyl, plastic), ethylene diamine (paints), formaldehyde (cosmetics, textiles, home construction), isocyanates, mercapto-benzothiazole (rubber boots, gloves and catheters), paraphenylenediamine or PPDA (textiles, inks, rubber), phenylenediamines, thiurams (rubber, paint), turpentine (polishes, varnishes, paint thinners, pine-scented cleaners)

METALS: beryllium, chromium, chromate, cobalt, copper sulphate (insecticides, dyes, coins), gold, iron, lead, mercury bichloride (thermometers, batteries, silk, disinfectants), nickel (jewellery, dyes, stainless steel wire), palladium, platinum salts, potassium dichromate (photographic supplies, leather goods, bleaches, tanning agents, yellow paint), selenium, silver, tellurium, zinc

COSMETICS: aluminium chloride (deodorants), ammonia, ammonium carbonate, ammonium dichromate, amyl acetate, balsam of Peru, benzocaine, benzophenones, benzoyl peroxide, bitter almond oil (eye cream, perfume, soaps), butyl alcohol (shampoos), camphor oil (skin cream), caraway oil (soaps), cinnamon bark (cosmetics), cinnamon oil (cosmetics), citronella oil (insect repellent), cobalt (hair dyes), coconut oil (soaps and toiletries), coriander oil (cosmetics), colophony (cosmetics and soaps), ethylene diamine (creams), formaldehyde (cosmetics), glutaraldehyde (hand cleaners), menthol, nickel sulphate (hair dyes), parabens – including butylparaben, methylparaben and propylparaben (preservative in cosmetics), patchouli oil (cosmetics and soaps), perfumes, pheneythl alcohol (cosmetic preservative and scent), phenol, phenylenediamines (hair dye), paraphenylenediamine or PPDA (hair dye), silver nitrate (hair dyes), thiurams (soap)

DUST

DYES

ENZYMES: benzophenones

FOODS: bamboo shoots, beef, buckwheat, carrot, cashew nuts, chicken, chicory, citrus fruit, duck, egg, endive, fish, flour, goose, kiwi fruit, lemon, lettuce, lime, mustard, onion, orange, parsnip, pea, peanuts, pear, peppers, potato, radish, rice, rye, soya, strawberry, swede, wheat

FOOD ADDITIVES: colours, preservatives, antioxidants

HERBS/SPICES: allspice, caraway, cardamom, cayenne pepper, cinnamon, clove, cumin, curry powder, horseradish, garlic, ginger, nutmeg, oregano, paprika, parsley, pepper, rosemary, turmeric

INSECTICIDES

INSECT BITES AND STINGS: fleas

LATEX

LEATHER GOODS

MEDICATION: antifungals, antihistamines, antimitotic compounds, antiseptic, arnica, benzocaine, frusemide, iodine, penicillin

NYLON

PAINT AND PAINT THINNER

PARABENS

PLANTS: carrots, celery, chives, chrysanthemums, daisies, daffodils, garlic, hops, hyacinth, ivy, narcissi, nettles, oleander, onion, philodendron, pine trees, poison ivy, poison oak, primrose, primula, pyrethrum, ragweed, tulips, yarrow

PLASTIC

SANITARY PRODUCTS

SCENT/FLAVOURING: balsam of Peru, menthol

SEMEN

SESAME

SOLVENTS: alcohol solvents, aromatic hydrocarbons, chlorinated hydrocarbons, esters, glycols, glycol ethers, halogenated solvents, ketone solvents

TALC

THURIAMS

TURPENTINE

WOOD

WOOL

Irritant dermatitis:

ACIDS

ALKALIS

AIRBORNE ALLERGENS: coal dust, stone dust, talc, dust mites

CLAY

CLEANING MATERIALS: detergent, disinfectant

FOODS: flour

GLUE

PAINT

PAINT THINNERS

SOLVENTS

Photoallergenic contact dermatitis:

COSMETICS AND PERFUME, including the following ingredients: acridine (lipsticks, dyes); benzyl salicylate (perfumes, sunscreens), bithionol (antiseptic soap, cosmetics), cedarwood oil (perfumes and soaps), cinnamon bark (cosmetics), dichlorophen (antiseptic soaps and cosmetics), digalloyl trioleate (antiseptic soaps and cosmetics), eoisin (lipsticks), fluorescin (lipsticks, chemical dyes), formaldehyde (cosmetics), hexachlorophene (antiseptic soaps, cosmetics), lavender oil, methylene blue (chemical dyes, lipsticks), para-aminobenzoic acid or PABA (sunburn products), parsley oil, perfume, petitgrain oil, quinine, rose Bengal (lipsticks, chemical dyes), salicylanides (antiseptic soaps, cosmetics), sulphonamides (antibiotic creams and ointments)

CHEMICALS: acridine, benzyl salicylate, chlorsalicylamide (fungicides), eosin, fluorescein, formaldehyde (textiles, home construction), methylene blue, rose Bengal

FOODS: carrot, celery, lemon, lime, parsnip, spinach

HERBS/SPICES: angelica, coriander, dill, parsley (oil)

MEDICATION: bithionol, dichlorophen, digaylloyl trioleate, hexachlorophene, quinine, salicylanides, sulphonamides

SCENT/FLAVOURING: petitgrain oil

General rash:

AROMATHERAPY OILS

CHEMICALS: benzyl salicylate, phenol

COSMETICS: bitter almond oil, cedarwood oil, cinnamon bark, coconut oil, patchouli oil, phenethyl alcohol

FOOD ADDITIVES: colours, preservatives, antioxidants

GUM ACACIA

HERBS/SPICES: angelica

HISTAMINE

MEDICATION: ACE inhibitors, amoxycillin, antibiotics, antiemetics, aspirin, cephalosporins, ibuprofen, insulin, iodine, macrolides, penicillin, phenoxymethilpenicillin, sedatives, sulphonamides, tetracycline

MOULDS (penicillium)

SCENT/FLAVOURING: peppermint oil, petitgrain oil

WOOL

Treatments
Aromatherapy
• Essential oil of tea tree – it has antiseptic properties

• Essential oil of lavender
Note that some oils may act as allergens for some people

Over-the-counter remedies
• Topical steroids
• Coal tar
• Emollients

Prescription medication
• Steroids
• Antihistamines

Self-help tips
• Topical applications of the following can help:
– Aloe vera cream or gel – it contains salicylates, the painkilling
  and anti-inflammatory compound found in aspirin
– Calendula cream or oil – it is anti-inflammatory
– Cucumber juice – it has anti-inflammatory properties, soothing
  the skin and encouraging healing
– Evening primrose oil
– Olive oil
• Cool water soaks – will relieve itching
• Protect skin from sunburn
• Use barrier to allergen such as gloves, preferably cotton-lined;
  discard them if they get a hole; wear gloves when
  peeling/preparing fruit and vegetables
• When washing:
– Use glycerine-based soap
– Pat skin dry rather than rubbing
– Bathe in lukewarm rather than hot water
– Remove rings before washing up
– Switch to loose-fitting cotton clothing rather than wool or
  synthetics

Sleep problems
What is it?
Problems with sleeping – usually insomnia – tend to be a result of
the allergy rather than a symptom on its own.

Other symptoms that may occur with it
Anxiety, depression

Possible triggers
CAFFEINE

Treatments
Aromatherapy
- Use one of the following oils for massage (1 drop to 5 ml carrier oil), in a vaporizer (6 drops oil in 2 tsp water for a 3 metres-square room), in a bath (4 drops to a full bath – add when the water has run and disperse vigorously!) or add 1 drop to a handkerchief placed under or near your pillow: camomile, lavender, mandarin, marjoram, melissa, neroli, sandalwood, ylang ylang

Bach flower remedies
- Olive, vervain or white chestnut

Herbal remedies
- Teas (add 1–2 tsp of dried herb to 1 cup of boiling water and infuse for 10–15 minutes): camomile, lemon balm, limeflower, hops, passionflower, valerian, vervain

Homeopathic remedies
- Calcarea carbonica
- Sulphur
- Nux

Over-the-counter remedies
- Most OTC remedies for sleep problems contain antihistamines. Avoid alcohol if you use them.

Prescription medication
- Benzodiazepines – these reduce communication between nerve cells in the brain, leading to a lower level of brain activity which lets you fall asleep

Self-help tips
- Avoid eating and drinking alcohol/coffee/tea before bed
- Hot bath
- Milky drink
- Establish a calming routine to follow in the evening before going to bed
- Don't nap during day

- If you can't settle, get up and read for 30 minutes, then go back to bed; if you're still awake 30 minutes later, get up and read
- Relaxation or meditation exercises

Sneezing

What is it?
Sneezing is the expulsion of air through the nose and mouth when the upper respiratory tract has been irritated, either as a result of allergic rhinitis or inhalation of a substance such as pepper or dust.

Other symptoms that may occur with it
Conjunctivitis, nose running

Possible triggers
AIRBORNE PARTICLES
AIR POLLUTANTS
ALCOHOL
ALLERGENS: pollen; animal fur or feathers, saliva and urine; house dust mite; moulds
BACTERIA
DYES
FOOD: banana, barley, corn, grapes, milk, mustard, pork, potato, rice, rye, wheat
HERBS/SPICES: garlic
OCCUPATIONAL EXPOSURE to allergens, vapours, dust, gases or fumes
RAPE SEED

Treatments
Acupuncture

Over-the-counter remedies
- Decongestants

Prescription medication
- As OTC remedies
- Antihistamines
- Sodium cromoglycate

Self-help tips
- Use petroleum jelly around your nose, to stop it becoming sore.

- Drink cider vinegar and honey in hot water to relieve nasal congestion – they both have decongestant properties
- Steam inhalation can help

Stinging (skin)

What is it?

Skin stinging is a form of skin irritation – see *Skin rash*

Possible triggers

COSMETICS are the most likely cause of stinging and it usually starts as soon as you use the cosmetics; certain ingredients are known as "stingers" (such as AHAs, propylene glycol and perfume) but they are still widely used because they have desirable qualities.

Treatments

The only treatment is avoidance.

Swelling, face
See *Angioedema*

Swelling, lips
See *Angioedema*

Swelling, tongue
See *Angioedema*

Urticaria

What is it?

Urticaria – also known as hives or nettle rash – is a red, itchy, swollen skin reaction. The weals vary in size and can appear anywhere on the body. It is caused by histamine in the upper layers of the skin. It is often due to a viral infection or a reaction to a drug, food or latex, and the reaction starts within less than an hour of taking the drug or eating food.

Other symptoms that may occur with it

Angioedema, itching, hay fever

Possible triggers

AMINES

CHEMICALS: acetic acid, butyl alcohol, chloramphenicol, dimethyl sulphoxide, ethyl alcohol, formaldehyde (found in cosmetics, textiles, home construction), persulphate, phenol

COSMETICS: benzophenones, cetyl alcohol, cinnamic acid, cinnamic aldehyde, phenol

COLDS (in children)

DRINK: beer, cider, tea, wine

ENZYMES: benzophenones

FOOD: apple, apricot, asparagus, aubergine, avocado, banana, barley, beans, beef, blackberry, blackcurrant, blueberry, broad beans, buckwheat, caffeine, carrot, celery, cheese, cherry, chick pea, chocolate, cider vinegar, citrus fruit, corn, cranberry, cucumber, currants, dates, eggs, fermented foods, figs, fish, pickled fish, game, gooseberries, grape, kiwi fruit, lentil, lettuce, liquorice, malt, mango, melon, milk, mushrooms, mustard, nectarines, nuts, oats, orange, papaya, passion fruit, peach, peanuts, peas, peperoni, peppers (capsicum), pineapple, plums, pork, potato, prunes, raisin, raspberry, sauerkraut, sausages, shellfish, soy sauce, soya, spinach, strawberries, sunflower seed, tomatoes, wheat, wine vinegar, Worcestershire sauce, yeast

FOOD ADDITIVES: colours, preservatives, emulsifiers/stabilizers/thickeners

HERBS/SPICES: aniseed, clove, cumin, curry powder, dill, fennel, horseradish, mace, oregano, paprika, parsley, rosemary, tarragon, thyme, turmeric

INSECT BITES AND STINGS

LATEX

LINSEED OIL

MEDICATION: antibiotics (particularly penicillin, aspirin, other non-steroidal anti-inflammatory drugs such as ibuprofen), high blood pressure medicines (known as ACE-inhibitors), painkillers containing codeine, insulin, benzocaine, frusemide, gentamycin, neomycin, streptomycin

POLLEN

ANIMAL DANDER

PHYSICAL CAUSES: rubbing or chafing of the skin, physical exertion or exercise, pressure

TEMPERATURE: cold, heat (cholinergic urticaria), sunlight (solar urticaria)

SCENT/FLAVOURING: balsam of Peru, butyric acid, menthol

SALICYLATES

Treatments
Aromatherapy
- Use one of the following essential oils in a bath (four drops to a full bath – add when the water has run and disperse vigorously!): Roman camomile, lavender or melissa

Herbal remedies
- Aloe vera
- Cabbage – apply a fresh leaf to the affected part
- Heartsease – use as a skin wash
- Sliced onion

Homeopathic remedies
- Urtica urens – for itchy rash (especially caused by shellfish)
- Apis – for swelling and puffiness, with stinging, burning pain
- Natrum mur – for urticaria made worse by exercise
- Pulsatilla – for urticaria made worse by fatty foods

Over-the-counter remedies
- Calamine lotion
- Witch hazel

Prescription medication
- Antihistamines
- Emollients
- Steroids

Self-help tips
- Use aqueous or emollient cream on the affected area instead of soap, until the rash has cleared up.
- Other gels and pastes that can soothe the rash and remove itching include:
  - aloe vera gel (it contains salicylates, the painkilling and anti-inflammatory compound found in aspirin, so it is soothing and cooling; clinical studies have shown that aloe vera can boost tissue regeneration and speed up the healing process)
  - calendula cream
  - a paste of bicarbonate of soda
  - honey – it has antiseptic properties and can aid healing
- Try cold compress/ice pack to relieve itching
- Baths – a tepid to warm bath can help to ease the itching, particularly if one of the following ingredients is added:

– bicarbonate of soda
– oatmeal
– cider vinegar – this restores the skin's pH. You could also dab cider vinegar on to the affected area with cotton wool.

Vomiting
What is it?
Vomiting is when the stomach contents are expelled through the mouth.

Other symptoms that may occur with it
Abdominal pain and swelling, angioedema, diarrhoea, gastric upset/irritation, headaches, migraine, nausea, weight loss, wind

Possible triggers
ALCOHOL
AMINES including tyramine
CHEMICALS: methylene blue, volatile organic compounds
DRINK: beer, tea
FOOD: apple, banana, beef, beetroot, blackberries, carrot, cherries, chocolate, corn, egg, gooseberries, kiwi fruit, lentil, melon, milk, mustard, oats, orange, pea, peach, peanuts, peppers, pineapple, pork, redcurrant, rhubarb, rye, shellfish, soya, spinach, strawberry, sunflower seed, wheat
FOOD ADDITIVES: colours, preservatives, antioxidants, emulsifiers/ stabilizers/thickeners, anti-caking agents, flavour enhancers
HERBS/SPICES: horseradish
MEDICATION: antibiotics, frusemide
SOLVENTS: amyl alcohol, alcohol solvents, aliphatic hydrocarbons

Treatments
Herbal remedies
• Teas (use 1½ tsp grated root to 1 cup of boiling water, steeped for 10–15 minutes): camomile, ginger, peppermint

Over-the-counter remedies
• Oral rehydration solution

Prescription medication
• Anti-emetic drugs – often antihistamines, phenothiazines and metoclopramide

Self-help tips
- Drink lots of water to avoid dehydration – small frequent sips are more likely to stay down
- Eat live yoghurt

Weight gain

What is it?
Weight gain is when your body mass increases. Unexplained weight gain should always be checked with your GP; establishing the cause will help to stop the symptoms.

Other symptoms that may occur with it
- Abdominal pain, constipation

Possible triggers
FOOD: pork

Weight loss

What is it?
Weight loss is when your body mass decreases. Unexplained weight loss should always be checked with your GP; establishing the cause will help to stop the symptoms.

Other symptoms that may occur with it
Abdominal pain, diarrhoea, constipation, nausea or vomiting; it may be a symptom of Crohn's disease or IBS.

Possible triggers
CHEMICALS: isocyanates
FOODS: soya, wheat
HERBS/SPICES: cinnamon

Wheezing

What is it?
A whistling sound that occurs when air is forced through swollen airways in the lungs – may be a symptom of asthma. It tends to be more obvious when breathing out.

Other symptoms that may occur with it
Breathing difficulties

Possible triggers

CHEMICALS: benzyl acetate, chlorine, chloroform, formaldehyde, isocyanates, volatile organic compounds

DRINK: cider, tea

DUST MITES

FOOD: apple, apricot, asparagus, banana, barley, beef, blackberries, blackcurrant, blueberries, buckwheat, celery, cherries, chick pea, cider vinegar, citrus fruit, corn, cranberry, cucumbers, currants, dates, egg, fish, gooseberries, grapes, liquorice, mango, melon, milk, nectarine, oats, orange, passion fruit, pea, peach, peanuts, peppers, pineapple, plum, pork, prune, pumpkin, raisin, raspberry, rye, shellfish, soya, spinach, strawberry, sunflower seed, tomato, wheat, wine vinegar, Worcestershire sauce

HERBS/SPICES: aniseed, clove, coriander, cumin, curry powder, dill, fenugreek, garlic, mace, oregano, paprika, parsley, rosemary, tarragon, thyme, turmeric

INSECT STING

MEDICATION: antibiotics, aspirin, beta-blockers, ibuprofen, insulin, phenoxymethilpenicillin

MENTHOL

MOULDS

OZONE

RAPE SEED

SALICYLATES

SULPHUR DIOXIDE

WOOD DUST

Treatments

Prescription medication
• Bronchodilator
See also *Asthma*

Wind

What is it?

Wind is the noisy return of air from the stomach – either as belching or flatulence.

Other symptoms that may occur with it

Abdominal pain and swelling, bloating, diarrhoea, heartburn, indigestion, nausea, rumbling noises, vomiting

Possible triggers
FOOD: cheese, fish, milk, shellfish, wheat
FOOD ADDITIVES: emulsifiers/stabilizers/thickeners

Treatments
Aromatherapy
- Use one of the following essential oils and massage over abdomen massage (use 1 drop of essential oil to 5 ml of a bland carrier oil such as sweet almond oil): aniseed, coriander, fennel, ginger, marjoram, peppermint

Herbal remedies
- Teas (add 1–2 tsp of dried herb to 1 cup of boiling water and infuse for 10–15 minutes): aniseed, caraway, fennel, ginger (1 tsp of grated fresh root rather than dried), lemon balm, peppermint, sweet flag

Homeopathic remedies
- Carbo Vegetalis – for belching, bloating and flatulence
- China – for bloating and flatulence
- Magnesium phosphoricum – for flatulence, belching and abdominal pain

Over-the-counter remedies
- Antacids – aluminium hydroxide, calcium carbonate, hyfrotalcite, magnesium hydroxide, sodium bicarbonate

Prescription medication
- As OTC remedies

Self-help tips
- Drinks – sip hot water very slowly; ½ tsp bicarbonate of soda in a glass of water
- Try to eat without talking – you may be swallowing large amounts of air without realizing

3

What to do in an emergency

Anaphylaxis or anaphylactic shock

What is it?

Anaphylaxis is a severe allergic reaction which affects the whole body, usually within a few minutes (although occasionally after some hours) of exposure to the allergen.

As with any allergic reaction, the body's immune system releases histamine and other chemicals which make the blood vessels leak (causing swelling), cause low blood pressure, and make the bronchial tissues swell (causing asthma). However, in cases of anaphylactic shock, this allergic reaction spirals out of control and causes inflammation throughout the body – also known as systemic inflammation. The blood vessels widen and become leaky, so there is less blood available for your heart to pump; if the heart can't pump enough blood to meet your body's needs, you may suffer from medical shock, where vital organs such as the lungs, liver, kidneys and brain are starved of oxygen and nutrients. This could ultimately be fatal.

If you have suffered a bad allergic reaction in the past, any future reaction may also be severe. You should see your doctor and insist on a referral to a specialist allergy clinic, especially if you have asthma as well as allergies – people with asthma have a higher risk of developing anaphylaxis.

What are the symptoms?

Not everyone experiences all the symptoms, and some people find that their symptoms are very mild, such as tingling or itching in the mouth. However, future attacks could be much more severe, so if you experience any of the following symptoms, you should ask your doctor for referral to an allergy specialist:

- swollen throat and mouth (this can restrict swallowing and breathing)

- difficulty in swallowing or speaking
- difficulty in breathing – due either to severe asthma or throat swelling
- urticaria anywhere on the body (particularly large hives)
- flushed skin
- abdominal cramps, nausea and vomiting
- a sudden feeling of weakness or sense of doom (caused by a drop in blood pressure)
- faster or slower heart rate
- collapse and unconsciousness

If you find it very difficult to breathe or swallow, or suffer from a sudden weakness or floppiness, it's a serious reaction and you need immediate treatment.

What is the treatment?

Call an ambulance and give an adrenaline (or epinephrine) injection under the skin or into a muscle as soon as you suspect a serious reaction. The adrenaline will counteract your body's response to the overload of histamine by:

- Constricting your blood vessels – which stops them leaking more fluid
- Relaxing the smooth muscles in your lungs (which helps to improve breathing)
- Stimulating your heartbeat
- Helping to stop swelling around the face and lips (angioedema)

Even after you've had adrenaline and the symptoms seem to be abating, it's best to go to hospital in case you have a secondary response, which could be fatal. You may also need oxygen and bronchodilator drugs to help your breathing.

What to do if there isn't any adrenaline available

The major problem is swelling of the tongue and throat – this can cause suffocation. In an emergency, slide the smooth handle of a spoon over the top of the affected person's tongue and into his throat, then press down gently but firmly to keep the airway open.

What are the most common causes of anaphylactic shock?

The most common causes include:

DUST: cotton seed

EXERCISE

EXPOSURE TO COLD

FOODS: camomile tea, chicken, dairy products (milk – usually in the under-fives; cheese), eggs, enzymes (chymopapain), fish (cod, crab, halibut) and shellfish (molluscs and crustaceans); fruit (apple, banana, cherry, grapes (particularly red), kiwi, mango, melon, orange, papaya, peach, pear, pineapple, plum, tangerine); grains (barley, buckwheat, corn, oats, rice, rye, wheat); herbs/spices (anise, coriander, cumin, curry powder, fennel, garlic, mustard, oregano, parsley); legumes (beans, chick peas, lentil, peas, soya); peanuts and other nuts (almonds, Brazils, cashews, hazelnuts, pecans, pistachios and walnuts); seeds (millet, pine nut, sesame, sunflower); vegetables (avocado, carrot, celery, courgette, lettuce, mushroom, parsnip, potato, tomato); wine; yeast; enzymes (papain)

INSECTS: cockroaches; wasp or bee stings

MALT

MEDICATION: antibiotics, aspirin, insulin, penicillin, phenoxy-methilpenicillin, sedatives, tetracycline, vaccines, x-ray dyes

NATURAL LATEX (rubber)

SULPHUR DIOXIDE

Exercise-induced anaphylaxis

Exercise-induced anaphylaxis is due to the direct stimulation of the mast cells, rather than a true IgE-related reaction. The symptoms are similar to that of anaphylactic shock induced by an allergen (see above).

Attacks can last from between thirty minutes and four hours, and you may have a severe headache for up to 72 hours afterwards. The reaction may be serious enough to need an injection of adrenaline.

Exercise-induced anaphylaxis is also associated with food and medication; the reaction only sets in if you exercise strenuously after eating a specific food (such as celery or shellfish) or taking a particular medication.

It's more likely to happen if you exercise in humid conditions, in very cold air, during the pollen season or (for women) during a menstrual period.

Diagnosis is by "challenge" – that is, exercising on a treadmill under medical conditions, after eating the suspected foods, to see if symptoms appear. Blood tests may show raised levels of histamine.

If you're prone to exercise-induced anaphylaxis, always carry adrenaline and always exercise with someone who is aware of the problem and knows how to cope with an emergency.

Avoiding anaphylactic shock
Minimize the risk
Food
Check food labels for anything you know you are allergic to. Check with staff in restaurants; some chains may have ingredient lists. Foods to watch out for include:

Peanuts
- Peanut butter
- Groundnuts
- Earth nuts
- Monkey nuts
- Mixed nuts
- Cakes
- Biscuits
- Pastries
- Ice cream
- Desserts
- Cereal bars
- Confectionery (including praline and marzipan)
- Vegetarian products (such as veggie burgers)
- Salads and salad dressings
- Satay sauce
- Curries
- Chinese, Thai or Indonesian dishes

Sesame
- Tahini
- Gomashio
- Hummus
- Chinese stir fry oils

Egg
- Albumen
- Lecithin (an emulsifier)

Milk
- Whey
- Whey powder
- Whey solids
- Lactose
- Casein
- Caseinates
- Non-milk fat

The Leatherhead Food Intolerance Databank provides product information relating to milk, egg, wheat, soya, BHA and BHT, sulphur dioxide, benzoate and azo colours; your GP can refer you to a registered dietician, to take advantage of this service.

Avoiding insect bites
- Insect repellents: use a commercial brand or eat raw garlic – insects don't like it
- Clothing: avoid wearing black, flowery, shiny or brightly coloured clothing, which attracts insects; wear shoes so you don't accidentally tread on a wasp or bee barefoot; wear long-sleeved tops and trousers to make your skin less vulnerable
- Gardening: wear gloves while gardening
- Avoid strong perfumes (including those in sunscreen products, hairspray, make-up and deodorant), which attract bees
- Avoid drinking/eating sweet things outside, which attract insects
- Don't panic or swat insects – move away quietly; if the insect lands on you, sit still as it will usually fly away again within a few seconds
- If you think there might be a nest near your house, ask your local council to remove it and make sure you're well out of the way while it's removed
- Remove the sting carefully

Cosmetics
If you are allergic to peanuts or tree nuts (such as almonds), check cosmetics and toiletries (such as soaps, aromatherapy base oils and pharmaceutical products) for arachis oil or nut oil; if any is absorbed through cracked skin, you may react badly to the allergen.

Watch for symptoms

If you think you're starting to show the signs of a severe reaction, don't wait – use adrenaline and call an ambulance.

Know how to use your adrenaline kit

Make sure that your kit is one you find easy to use and, if not, ask for a different type. Make sure your family and friends know how and when it should be administered.

Make sure people know about it

Tell family and friends, so they know about the risks – particularly in cases of children, where teachers and playgroup staff need to know about the allergy in case of problems with school meals.

Plan for a crisis

Write a list of how to handle the emergency and keep it with you. If your child is the one at risk, make sure that his or her teachers and the parents of friends know what to do and where the adrenaline is kept.

Wear a MedicAlert bracelet

This will help medical staff.

First aid tips

Artificial respiration

If someone stops breathing, call the emergency medical services immediately and start resuscitation. Put the affected person on his or her back on a hard surface; if there are no signs of neck injury, tilt the head backwards to open the airway, by pressing on the forehead and lifting the chin.

This may start the affected person breathing again; check to see if the chest rises and falls, and listen/feel for exhaled air.

If there are no signs, you need to start artificial respiration – make sure the patient's chin is lifted and his or her head is tilted throughout, so that air enters the lungs.

Pinch the nose shut with the thumb and index finger. Take a deep breath and seal your mouth around the patient's. Give a full breath, wait for the patient's chest to deflate, and give a second full breath.

Remove your mouth and check the pulse in the neck. If there is a pulse but the patient still isn't breathing, continue giving one breath every five seconds until medical help arrives.

Cardiopulmonary resuscitation (cardiac massage)

Check the patient's airways are clear, check for breathing, and check the pulse. If the patient is breathing, place him or her in the recovery position. Turn the patient's head towards you and tilt it back to open the airway. Put the arm nearest you by the patient's side and slide it under his or her bottom. Put the other arm across the chest and cross the leg furthest from you over the other ankle. Grasp the patient's clothing at the hip furthest from you, support the head, and pull the patient towards you to rest against your knees. Bend the upper arm and leg to support the body and stop the patient rolling on to his or her face. Check that the head is tilted well back and the airways are clear.

If the patient is not breathing, call for help and begin artificial resuscitation as above.

If breathing doesn't start and you can't feel a pulse or heartbeat, start cardiac compression. Press on the lower part of the breastbone with the heel of one hand placed on top of the other, making sure you keep the pressure clear of the patient's ribs. Give 80 compressions per minute, giving two breaths after every 15 compressions.

If there are two people able to resuscitate the patient, one should give artificial respiration (one breath to five compressions) and the other should perform cardiac compressions, at a rate of sixty per minute with a one-second pause after every five compressions.

4

How can you tell if you have an allergy?

Your history

If you think that you have an allergy, you should see your GP. He or she will want to know more about your symptoms before he or she can start to identify the allergen. The kind of information he or she will want to know includes:

- What your symptoms are
- When your symptoms occur – any particular time of day or year?
- How often your symptoms occur
- Which part of your body is affected
- How severe your symptoms are
- Your family history (i.e. does anyone else in your family suffer similar symptoms?)
- If any self-help remedies relieve the symptoms (and, if so what)
- "Triggers" – anything that makes your symptoms worse
- Whether your symptoms are worse in particular places (e.g. work, home, outdoors) and if they improve when you're away from those places

Testing methods – general rules

Before you take any kind of allergy test, your doctor may ask you to stop using any medication that could affect the test. This includes antihistamines, some antidepressants and some cortico-steroids. You also need to tell your doctor if you are pregnant, because testing may cause uterine contractions.

Any allergen extracts used should be of known composition and potency, and should be kept in optimum conditions – allergen extracts deteriorate with age, dilution and exposure to high temperatures.

Skin tests will not be performed on places where you have dermatitis.

Positive (histamine) and negative (diluent) controls need to be in place, so the tester can interpret the results properly.

Emergency equipment and medication should be on hand, in case you have a severe reaction (*see* the section on *What to do in an emergency*).

WHAT YOU CAN DO AT HOME

Elimination tests

When you suspect only one or two foods of triggering your symptoms, you can try an elimination test. However, as reintroducing the food can lead to an asthma attack or anaphylactic shock, this is best done under medical supervision. *Don't try eliminating foods if you have had a severe reaction in the past.*

How the test is done

You simply stop eating the types of food that you think cause your symptoms, and then reintroduce them one by one to see whether your symptoms reappear.

How the test works

If your symptoms disappear once the food is eliminated and recur when it's reintroduced, your allergy is confirmed.

Symptoms diary

When you suspect certain substances of triggering your allergy symptoms or making them worse, you can try keeping a diary.

How the test is done

You keep a note of when your symptoms are worse – including peak flow meter readings, if possible, for asthma symptoms – and what they might have been triggered by. Then discuss it with your doctor.

How the test works

If there is a distinct pattern which shows that you always come into contact with a substance just before your symptoms worsen, it's likely that an allergy is involved and your GP may recommend further tests such as skin prick tests, blood tests or inhalational challenges.

WHAT YOUR DOCTOR WILL TRY

Skin prick test

Because there are mast cells in your skin as well as the lining of your nose, your mouth, your tongue, the airways of your lungs and your intestines, skin tests can stimulate what's happening in the rest of your body.

The skin prick test is usually the first test recommended when your doctor suspects an allergy. It's simple, quick and inexpensive, provides results within about twenty minutes, and can be carried out within your local hospital or GP's surgery by specially trained nurses or doctors. Because the amount of allergens used in the test is so small, it can be used for all age groups, including babies, although it's not quite as reliable in the elderly and small children.

If there is a risk that you might have an anaphylactic shock reaction, your doctor will suggest doing a blood test instead. The test is also not suitable if you are taking antihistamine drugs to control your allergy, as this will block the skin test reaction – you will be asked to avoid taking antihistamines, cough medicine and some antidepressants for five or six days before the test (though some non-sedating antihistamines, such as astemizole, may have a suppressant action for several months). It is also unsuitable if you have very bad eczema as it would make test conditions too difficult.

The skin prick test is very good for inhalant allergies, but may be positive for foods which your body can tolerate, particularly if it's an allergy you've grown out of.

Not all allergies can be identified through skin prick testing.

How the test is done

The test is usually done on your inner forearm (palm uppermost) or, if you have bad eczema in that area, on your back. Your doctor will code your arm with a marker pen for each allergy to be tested, then put a tiny drop of allergen on to your skin, next to the appropriate code, and then prick your skin through the drop, using a prick needle or lancet. The procedure is uncomfortable but shouldn't hurt, and the point of the lancet doesn't go deep enough to draw blood.

Up to twenty-five allergens can be tested at the same time, and these will be placed at least 4 cm apart to make sure that the reaction to one allergen doesn't influence the reaction to another.

There also will be a "positive and negative control" at the top and bottom of the test row, to make sure that the test is working properly. The "negative control" is a plain saline or salt-water solution (which is also used to dilute the allergen); most people will not react to salt water, but if you do, it tells the doctor that your skin is extremely sensitive and the results of the allergen tests need to be interpreted very carefully. The "positive control" solution contains histamine, to which everyone should react. If you don't, it could mean that any medication you're taking is blocking the response to the histamine and allergens.

How the test works
If the allergen stimulates histamine, your skin will become itchy within a few minutes, and then it will become red and swollen with a blister-like weal in the middle – very much like a nettle sting reaction. This is known as the "weal and flare" response. The size of the weal (which reaches its maximum after about 20 minutes and should clear within an hour) will show the level of your reaction to that particular allergen.

Allergens that can be tested
ANIMAL HAIR/DANDER: cat, camel, cow, dog, goat, guinea pig, hamster, horse, mouse, pig's bristles, rabbit, rat, sheep
COCOA
FABRIC: cotton, wool
FEATHERS: budgerigar, chicken, duck, goose, pigeon, poultry
FISH AND SHELLFISH: carp, cod, crab, eel, halibut, herring, lobster, mackerel, mussels, plaice, salmon, shrimp, sole, spiny lobster, trout, tuna
FRUIT: apple, banana, cherry, grape, grapefruit, lemon, orange, peach, pear, pineapple, strawberry, tangerine/clementine
GRAIN: barley, barley bran, barley flour, corn bran, corn flour, gluten (wheat), maize, oat, oat flour, rape seed oil, rice, rye bran, rye flour, wheat, wheat bran, wheat flour
HERBS/SPICES: aniseed, camomile, caraway, celery root, coriander, cumin, curry powder, paprika, parsley, pepper (white)
HOPS
LATEX (*Hevea brasiliensis*)
LEGUMES: soya bean
MEAT AND EGGS: beef, chicken, duck, goose, egg (whole, white or yolk), horse, lamb, mutton, pork, turkey, veal

MILK AND RELATED PRODUCTS: casein, raw cow's milk, pasteurized cow's milk, cheese

MITES: dust mite (*Dermatophagoides pteronyssinus*), grain mite (*Dermatophagoides farinae*)

MOULDS AND FUNGI: *Alternaria alternata, Alternaria tenuis, Aspergillus fumigatus, Aspergillus niger, Aureobasidium pullulans, Botrytis cinerea, Candida albicans, Chaetomium globosum, Cladosporium cladosporioides, Cladosporium herbarum, Curvularia lunata, Fusarium culmorum, Fusarium moniliforme, Fusarium roseum, Helminthosporium halodes, Merulius lacrymans, Mucor mucedo, Mucor racemosus, Neurospora sitophila, Penicillium brevicompactum, Penicillium commune, Penicillium notatum, Phoma betae, Pullularia pullulans, Rhizopus nigricans, Saccharomyces carlsbergensis, Saccharomyces cerevisiae, Saccharomyces mellis, Serpula lachrymans, Stemphylium botryosum, Trichopyton rubrum, Trichophyton mentagrophytes, Ustilago tritici*

NUTS: almond, brazil nut, hazelnut, peanut, walnut

PLANTS/TREES: ash, beech, dandelion, dock, English plantain, mugwort, nettle, pine, plane tree, poplar, willow

POLLEN: alder (*Alnus glutinosa*), ash (*Fraxinus excelsior*), barley (*Hordeum vulgare*), beech (*Fagus sylvatica*), bent grass (*Agrostis stolonifera*), bermuda (*Cynodon dactylon*), black locust (*Robinia pseudoacacia*), daisy (*Chrysanthemum leucanthemum*), dandelion (*Taraxacum officinale*), elderberry (*Sambucus nigra*), elm (*Ulmus campestris*), English plantain (*Plantago lanceolata*), goat willow (*Salix caprea*), goosefoot (*Chenopodium album*), hazel (*Corylus avellana*), horse chestnut (*Aesculus hippocastanum*), linden (*Tilia cordata*), maize (*Zea mays*), maple (*Acer sp*), meadow fescue (*Festuca rubra*), meadow foxtail (*Alopecurus pratensis*), meadow grass (*Poa pratensis*), mugwort (*Artemisia vulgaris*), nettle (*Urtica dioica*), oak (*Quercus robur*), oat (*Arrhenatherum elatius* and *Avena sativa*), olive (*Olea europea*), orchard (*Dactylis glomerata*), pellitory (*Parietaria*), poplar (*Populus sp*), ragweed (*Ambrosia elatior*), red sorrel (*Rumex acetosella*), rye (*Secale cerale*), rye grass (*Lolium perenne*), silver birch (*Betula verrucosa*), sweet vernal (*Anthoxanthum odoratum*), sycamore (*Platanus acerifolia*), timothy grass (*Phleum pratense*), velvet (*Holcus lanatus*), wheat (*Triticum satium*)

VEGETABLES: asparagus, carrot, cauliflower, celery, cress, green bean, white bean, green pea, horseradish, onion, potato (with peel), radish, spinach, tomato

VENOM: bee, wasp

Intradermal test

If a skin prick test is negative, but your symptoms and medical history strongly suggest a specific allergy, your doctor may suggest an intradermal test, which is more sensitive than the skin prick test. As with the skin prick test, you will be asked to avoid taking antihistamines, cough medicine and some antidepressants for five or six days before the test to make sure that the medication doesn't affect the test results.

The test is particularly good for drug and sting allergies, though isn't reliable for food allergy. It may also show that you're allergic to a substance when it doesn't cause any symptoms, and the risk of anaphylactic shock is slightly higher than for the skin prick test, so it's rarely used in the UK.

How the test is done

The doctor will inject between 0.01 and 0.05ml of a diluted extract of an allergen just below your skin. Ten or more allergens can be tested at the same time.

How the test works

If the test is positive, swelling, itching and a red welt will develop within 20 minutes.

Allergens that can be tested

ANIMAL HAIR: camel, cat, cow, dog, goat, guinea pig, hamster, horse, mouse, rabbit, rat, sheep

FEATHERS: budgerigar, chicken, duck, goose

FISH AND SHELLFISH: cod, carp, eel, halibut, lobster, mussels, salmon, shrimp, sole, spiny lobster, trout, tuna

FRUIT: apple, banana, grape, grapefruit, lemon, orange, peach, pear, pineapple, strawberry, tangerine/clementine

GRAIN: barley bran, barley flour, corn bran, corn flour, oat flour, rye bran, rye flour, wheat bran, wheat flour

HERBS/SPICES: paprika, parsley

MEAT AND EGGS: beef, chicken, duck, egg (whole), egg white, egg yolk, goose, horse, mutton, pork, turkey

MITES: dust mite (*Dermatophagoides pteronyssinus*), grain mite (*Dermatophagoides farinae*)

MOULDS AND FUNGI: *Alternaria tenuis, Aspergillus fumigatus, Botrytis cinerea, Candida albicans, Chaetomium globosum, Cludosporium herbarum, Curvularia lunata, Fusarium moniliforme, Helminthosporium halodes, Microsporium canis, Mucor mucedo, Neurospora sitophila, Penicillium notatum, Phoma betae,*

Pullularia pullulans, Rhizopus nigricans, Saccharomyces cere-visiae, Serpula lacrymans, Sporothrix schenckii, Trichophyton mentagrophytes, Ustilago tritici

NUTS: brazil nut, hazelnut, peanut, walnut

POLLENS: acacia, alder (*Alnus glutinosa*), ash (*Fraxinus excelsior*), barley (*Hordeum vulgare*), beech (*Fagus sylvatica*), birch (*Betula verrucosa*), dandelion (*Taraxacum officinale*), elderberry (*Sambucus nigra*), elm (*Ulmus campestris*), grass, English plantain (*Plantago lanceolata*), hazel (*Corylus avellana*), linden (*Tilia cordata*), mugwort (*Artemisia vulgaris*), nettle (*Urtica dioica*), oak (*Quercus robur*), oat (*Avena sativa*), plane, poplar (*Populus sp*), red sorrel (*Rumex acetosella*), rye (*Secale cerale*), sallow, silver birch (*Betula verrucosa*), wheat (*Triticum satium*)

VEGETABLES: asparagus, cauliflower, pea, potato, spinach, tomato

Skin patch test

This tests for allergens that cause contact dermatitis – such as nickel, preservatives and detergents. It is not used to test for food intolerance but it may be used to test for contact dermatitis caused by foods (usually occupational, for example fish and shellfish). Your doctor will treat your symptoms and bring them under control before you can be tested, otherwise the results may be unreliable. You'll also need to stop using any steroid creams for three to four weeks before the test, to avoid the steroids affecting the test result. Try to minimize sun exposure on the test site before the test, and don't apply any lotions, creams or ointments to the test area before the test.

It is not usually carried out on babies, because they are unlikely to suffer from allergic contact dermatitis. The test is best avoided during pregnancy.

The skin patch test can be useful before a food challenge, to check for a possible anaphylactic reaction; if applying the food to your skin causes urticaria, a food challenge is not advisable.

How the test is done

It usually takes place at the dermatology (skin) department in your local hospital, as interpretation can be difficult. The allergen solution is put into white soft paraffin (such as Vaseline) and spread on to 1cm discs – which are made of a special metal that won't provoke a reaction. The doctor will then put the discs on your back, coding your skin for each allergen tested, and tape the discs to your skin using hypoallergenic tape. You'll need to keep your skin dry for the next 48 hours, so avoid any exercise that's likely to cause you to sweat, and wear loose clothing.

If the patch test becomes loose, or the test area feels itchy or burns severely, call your doctor.

How the test works

After 48 hours, the doctor will remove the discs, examine your skin and note if there is any redness or swelling – signs of eczema. You'll be examined again 48 hours after that, to check for any remaining redness or swelling. It's difficult to tell the difference between an irritant reaction and an allergic reaction, though some experts say that an irritant reaction is more likely to have a sharp outline which corresponds to the outline of the patch test, whereas an allergic reaction is more likely to have vesicles or papules, and a more blurred outline which goes beyond the outline of the patch test.

As with the skin prick test, this test is not suitable if you are taking antihistamine drugs to control your symptoms or you have very bad eczema.

Blood test (CAP-RAST)

Blood tests are also known as "in vitro" tests.

RAST stands for Radio AllergoSorbent Test; it tests for the presence of IgE antibodies in your blood. It is more accurate than skin tests because it can measure the exact amount of the allergen antibody in your blood. It is not, however, used for food intolerance reactions (which do not involve IgE antibodies).

It's generally used if a skin prick test can't be done – for example, if you have bad eczema, your symptoms are so severe that you can't stop taking antihistamine medication, or you're at risk of anaphylactic shock – or where your doctor suspects that you're reacting to unusual or rare allergens.

How the test is done

Your doctor will take a small sample of blood, usually from a vein in your forearm. The sample is then sent to a hospital laboratory. An extract of allergen is applied to an inert carrier substance called sepharose, and the liquid part of the blood (serum) is poured over the sepharose. If there are any IgE antibodies in the blood, they will bind to the antigens. The sample is rinsed (to remove everything apart from the IgE molecules) and then another liquid (anti-IgE antibody, which has been marked with a radioactive label) is poured over it. The anti-IgE binds to the IgE molecules, so the amount of IgE in the blood can be measured.

The results come back to your doctor within two weeks. There is also a testing kit available in pharmacies, but the blood sample will still need to be sent to a laboratory for testing.

How the test works

The results are usually shown on a scale of 0 to 6, and up to 30 allergens can be tested in one sample. Scale 0–1 means that there is little or no antibody in your blood and you are probably not allergic to the allergen. Moderate to high levels (scale 2–3) mean that you have an allergy, and extremely high levels (scale 4–6) are when you're very sensitive to an allergen.

Allergens that can be tested

ANIMAL HAIR/EPIDERMALS: budgerigar droppings, cat dander, chicken droppings, chinchilla epithelium, cow dander, deer epithelium, dog dander, dog epithelium, ferret epithelium, fox epithelium, gerbil epithelium, goat epithelium, guinea pig epithelium, hamster epithelium, horse dander, mink epithelium, mouse epithelium, pigeon droppings, rabbit epithelium, rat epithelium, reindeer epithelium, sheep epithelium, swine epithelium

ANIMAL PROTEINS: budgerigar serum, cat serum albumin, chicken serum, dog serum albumin, horse serum, mouse serum, mouse urine, rabbit serum, rabbit urine, rat serum, rat urine, swine serum albumin, swine urine

ANTIBIOTICS: penicilloyl, ampicilloyl

CHEMICALS: alpha-amylase, chloramin T, ethylene oxide, formaldehyde, phthalic anhydride, trimetellic anhydride (TMA)

COFFEE

DAIRY PRODUCTS: casein, cheese (cheddar), cheese (mould), cow's milk (raw and boiled), cow's whey, goat milk, sheep milk, sheep whey, a-lactalbumin, ß-lactoglobulin

DUST: castor bean, cotton seed, green coffee bean, sunflower seed

FABRIC: cotton, silk, silk waste

FEATHERS: budgerigar, canary chicken, duck, goose, finch, parrot, pigeon, turkey

FISH AND SHELLFISH: anchovy, blue mussel, chub mackerel, clam, cod, crab, crayfish, eel, hake, herring, jack mackerel, langoustines (spiny lobster), mackerel, megrim, octopus, oyster, pilchard, plaice, salmon, sardine, scallop, shrimp, snail, sole, squid, swordfish, trout, tuna

FOOD ADDITIVES: cochineal, guar gum, gum Arabic, tragacanth

FRUIT: apple, apricot, avocado, banana, blackberry, blueberry, carambola, cherry, cranberry, date, fig, grape, grapefruit, guava, jack fruit, jujube, kiwi, lemon, lime, mandarin, mango, melon, orange, papaya, passion fruit, peach, pear, persimmon, pineapple, plum, redcurrant, strawberry, watermelon

GELATIN

GRAIN: barley, buckwheat, corn, gluten, maize, oat, rye, wheat

HERBS/SPICES: allspice, anise, basil, bay leaf, caraway, cardamom, chilli pepper, cinnamon, clove, coriander, curry, dill, fennel (seed and fresh), fenugreek, ginger, lovage, mace, marjoram, mint, mustard, nutmeg, oregano, paprika, parsley, pepper (black), saffron, tarragon, thyme, vanilla

HONEY

HOPS

INSECTS AND PARASITES: anisakis, ascaris, bee (*Bombus terrestris*), Berlin beetle (*Trogoderma angustum*), blood worm (*Chironomus thummi*), cockroach (*Blatella germanica*), echinococcus, fire ant (*Solenopsis invicta*), grain weevil (*Sitophilus granarius*), green nimitti (*Cladotanytarsus Lewisi*), horse bot fly (*Gasterophilus intestinalis*), horse fly (*Tabanus sp*), mediterranean flour moth (*Ephestia kuchniella*), mosquito (*Aedes communis*), moth (*Bombyx mori*)

INSULIN (bovine, human, porcine)

ISPHAGULA

ISOCYANATES (HDI, MDI, TDI)

LATEX

MALT

MEAT AND EGGS: beef, chicken, cows' whey, egg white, egg yolk, elk meat, horse meat, mutton, ovalbumin, ovomucoid, pork, rabbit, turkey

MITES: dust mite (*Dermatophagoides farinae, Dermatophagoides microceras, Dermatophagoides pteronyssinus, Euroglyphus maynei*), storage mite (*Acarus siro, Glycyphagus domesticus, Lepidoglyphus destructor, Tyrophagus putrescentiae*)

MOULDS AND FUNGI: *Alternaria alternata, Alternaria tenuis, Aspergillus fumigatus, Aspergillus niger, Aureobasidium pullulans, Botrytis cinerea, Candida albicans, Cephalosporium acremonium, Chaetomium globosum, Cladosporium herbarum, Curvularia lunata, Epicoccum purpurascens, Fusarium moniliforme,*

Helminthosporium halodes, Micropolyspora faeni, Mucor racemosus, Penicillium notatum, Phoma betae, Pityrosporum orbiculare, Rhizopus nigricans, Stemphylium botryosum, Trichoderma viride, Trichophyton rubrum

NUTS, PULSES AND SEEDS: almond, brazil nut, carob, cashew, chestnut, chick pea, cocoa, coconut, hazelnut, linseed, lentil, millet (common, foxtail, Japanese), peanut, pecan, pine nut, pistachio, poppy seed, pumpkin seed, rape seed, red kidney bean, rose hip, sesame, walnut

POLLEN: acacia (*Acacia longifolia*), American beech (*Fagus grandifolia*), Australian pine (*Casuarina equisetifolia*), bahia grass (*Paspalum notatum*), barley (*Hordeum vulgare*), bent grass or redtop (*Agrostis stolonifera*), bermuda grass (*Cynodon dactylon*), box elder (*Acer negundo*), Brome grass (*Bromus inermis*), camomile (*Matricaria chamomilla*), canary grass (*Phalaris arundinacea*), cedar (*Libocedrus decurrens*), chestnut (*Castanea sativa*), cocklebur (*Xanthium commune*), cocksfoot grass (*Dactylis glomerata*), common pigweed (*Amaranthus retroflexus*), common ragweed (*Ambrosia elatior*), common reed (*Phragmites communis*), cottonwood (*Populus deltoides*), cypress (*Cupressus sempervirens*), dandelion (*Taraxacum officinale*), date (*Phoenix canariensis*), Douglas fir (*Pseudotsuga taxifolia*), elder (*Sambucus nigra*), elm (*Ulmus americana*), English plantain or ribwort (*Plantago lanceolata*), eucalyptus (*Eucalyptus sp*), false oat grass (*Arrhenatherum elatiu*), false ragweed (*Franseria acanticarpa*), firebush or kochia (*Kochia scoparia*), giant ragweed (*Ambrosia trifida*), golden rod (*Solidago virgaurea*), goosefoot or lamb's quarters (*Chenopodium album*), grey alder (*Alnus incana*), hazel (*Corylus avellana*), hornbeam (*Carpinus betulus*), horse chestnut (*Aesculus hippocastanum*), Japanese cedar (*Cryptomeria japonica*), Johnson grass (*Sorghum halepense*), linden (*Tilia cordata*), London plane or maple-leaf sycamore (*Platanus acerifolia*), lupin (*Lupinus sp*), maize (*Zea mays*), meadow fescue (*Festuca elatior*), meadow foxtail (*Alopecurus pratensis*), meadow grass or Kentucky blue (*Poa pratensis*), melaleuca or cajeput tree (*Melaleuca leucadendron*), mesquite (*Prosopis juliflora*), mountain juniper (*Juniperus sabinoides*), mugwort (*Artemisia vulgaris*), mulberry (*Morus alba*), nettle (*Urtica diocia*), oak (*Quercus alba*), oat (*Avena sativa*), olive (*Olea europaea*), oxeye daisy (*Chrysanthemum leucanthemum*), paloverde (*Cercidium floridum*), pecan (*Carya pecan*), pepper tree (*Schinus molle*), pine (*Pinus radiata*), prickly saltwort or Russian thistle (*Salsola kali* and *Salsola pestifer*), privet (*Ligustrum vulgare*), queen palm (*Arecastrum romanzoffianum*), rape (*Brassica napus*), rough marshelder (*Iva ciliata*), rye (*Secale cerale*), rye grass (*Lolium perenne*), salt grass (*Distichlis spicata*), scale or lenscale (*Atriplex lentiformis*), sheep sorrel (*Rumex acetosella*), silver birch (*Betula verrucosa*), spruce (*Picea excelsa*), sugar beet (*Beta vulgaris*), sunflower (*Helianthus annuus*), sweet gum (*Liquidambar styracuflua*), timothy grass (*Phleum pratense*), velvet grass (*Holcus lanatus*), vernal grass (*Anthoxanthum odoratum*), Virginia live oak (*Quercus virginiana*), wall pellitory (*Parietaria officinalis* and *Parietaria judaica*), walnut (*Juglans californica*), western ragweed (*Ambrosia psilostachya*), wheat (*Triticum sativum*), white ash (*Fraxinus americana*), white pine (*Pinus strobus*), wild rye grass (*Elymus triticoides*), willow (*Salox carpea*), wormwood (*Artemisia absinthium*)

SEMINAL FLUID

SOYA

TEA

VEGETABLES: asparagus, aubergine, bamboo shoot, beetroot, broccoli, Brussels sprouts, cabbage, carrot, cauliflower, celery, cucumber, garlic, green bean, green pepper, lettuce, mushroom, onion, pea, potato, pumpkin, sweet potato, spinach, tomato

VENOM: bee, hornet (white-faced, yellow, European) wasp (common, paper)

YEAST

Blood test – ELISA

ELISA stands for Enzyme-Linked ImmunoSorbent Assay; it tests for the presence of antibodies. It can identify allergens for all kinds of pollens, mites, dander and fungal spores.

How the test is done

Your doctor will take a sample of blood and add it to a sample of the suspected allergen on a plate. If antibodies are present, they will link to the antigens in the allergen. He will then add a substance called a ligand which attaches to the antibodies and is linked to an enzyme called peroxidase. The plate is washed, and a solution of chromogen is added.

How the test works

If the solution changes colour, it proves that the enzyme is there (the colour change only occurs in the presence of the enzyme) and the result is positive.

Allergens that can be tested

AIRBORNE PARTICLES: green coffee bean, castor bean, cotton seed, isphagula, orris root, sunflower seed

ALKALASE

ALPHA-AMYLASE

ANIMAL HAIR/EPIDERMALS: angora epithelium, camel epithelium, cat hair, cat scurf, chinchilla, cow dander, deer hair/dander, dog dander, dog epithelium, ferret epithelium, fox epithelium, gerbil epithelium, goat epithelium, guinea pig epithelium, golden hamster epithelium, hare epithelium, horse dander, human hair, llama epithelium, mink hair, mouse epithelium, pig epithelium, rabbit epithelium, rat epithelium, sheep epithelium

ANIMAL PROTEINS: bovine serum, bovine serum albumin, budgerigar serum, canary serum, chicken serum, horse serum, mouse droppings, mouse epithelium protein, mouse serum, mouse urine, parrot serum, pigeon serum, rat droppings, rat epithelium protein, rat serum, rat urine

ARTIFICIAL FIBRES: acrylon, kapok, nylon, rayon, terylene

BIRD DROPPINGS: budgerigar droppings, canary droppings, duck droppings, finch droppings, goose droppings, lovebird droppings, parrot droppings, pigeon droppings

BROMELAIN

CASTOR BEAN OIL

DAIRY PRODUCTS: butter, casein, cheese (parmesan, ewe's, goat's, cheddar, mould, Edam, Roquefort, Camembert, Swiss, Gouda, Leerdam), cow's milk (raw and boiled), goat milk, a-lactalbumin, ß-lactoglobulin, sheep milk, whey, yoghurt

CHLORAMINE T

CHOCOLATE

COFFEE

COLLAGEN

DRUGS: acetyl salicylic acid, amoxycillin, ampicillin, cephalo-sporin, chymopapain, doxyclycline, erythromycin, furosemide, gentacycin, insulin (pork, bovine, human), penicillin, phena-cetin, polylysine, pyrazolon, succinyl choline, sulfamethoxazol, tetracycline, trimethroprim

ETHYLENE OXIDE

FEATHERS: budgerigar, chicken, canary, duck, duck down, finch, goose, goose down, lovebird, parrot, pigeon, turkey

FOOD: licorice

FORMALDEHYDE

FISH AND SHELLFISH: anchovy, carp, caviar, clam, cod, crab, crayfish, eel, haddock, halibut, herring, langoustines (spiny lobster), lobster, mackerel, mussel, oyster, perch, pike, plaice, salmon, sardine, shrimp, snail, squid, sole, trout, tuna

FRUIT: apricot, avocado, apple, banana, blackberry, blackcurrant, blueberry, canteloupe, cherry, cranberry, date, fig, gooseberry, grape, grapefruit, guava, kiwi, lemon, mandarin, mango, melon, nectarine, orange, papaya, peach, pear, pineapple, plum, raisin, raspberry, redcurrant, rhubarb, strawberry, tangerine, watermelon

GELATIN

GRAIN: barley, bran, buckwheat, corn (flour), gluten, malt, oat, rice, rye, sago, spelt (*Triticum spelta*), wheat, wheat bran

HAY DUST, STRAW DUST

HERBS/SPICES: allspice, aniseed, basil, bay leaf, camomile, cardamom, cayenne pepper, chervil, chilli pepper, chives, cinnamon, clove, comfrey, coriander, cumin, curry, dill, fennel (fresh), garlic, ginger, juniper berry, lovage, marjoram, mustard, nutmeg, oregano, paprika, parsley, pepper (black and white), peppermint, rosemary, saffron, sage, tarragon, thyme, turmeric, vanilla

HONEY

HOPS

HUMAN SERUM ALBUMIN

INSECTS AND PARASITES: fire ant (*Solenopsis invicta*), ascaris, Berlin beetle (*Trogoderma angustum*), bumblebee, cockroach (*Blatella germanica*), echinococcus, fly, honeybee (*Apis mellifera*), hornet (*Vespa crabro*), white-faced hornet (*Dolichovespula maculata*), yellow hornet (*Dolichovespula arenaria*), horse fly (*Gasterophilus intestinalis*), midge (*Aedes sp*), red midge larva, schistosoma, common wasp (*Vespula vulgaris*), paper wasp (*Polistes sp*), water flea (*Daphnia cladocera*)

ISOCYANATES (TDI, MDI, HDI)

LATEX

LYSOZYME

MEAT AND EGGS: beef, chicken, deer, duck, egg (white, yolk, whole), goose, horse meat, lamb, ovalbumin, ovomucoid

MITES: dust mite (*Dermatophagoides farinae, Dermatophagoides microceras, Dermatophagoides pteronyssinus, Euroglyphus maynei*), storage mite (*Acarus siro, Lepidoglyphus destructor*), *Glycyphagus domesticus, Tyrophagus putrescentiae*

MOULDS AND FUNGI: *Aspergillus amstelodami, Aspergillus clavatus, Aspergillus flavus, Aspergillus fumigatus, Aspergillus nidulans, Aspergillus niger, Aspergillus oryzae, Aspergillus terreus, Aspergillus versicolor, Aspergillus repens, Alternaria tenuis, Aureobasidium pullulans, Botrytis cinerea, Candida albicans, Cephalosporium acremonium, Chaetomium globosum, Cladosporium cladospor, Cladosporium fulvum, Cladosporium herbarum, Curvularia lunata, Curvularia spicifera, Epicoccum purpurascens, Fusarium culmorum, Fusarium moniliforme, Fusarium oxysporum, Helminthosporium halodes, Helminthosporium sp, Micropolyspora faeni, Microspora canis, Mucor mucedo, Mucor racemosus, Mucor spinosus, Neurospora sitophila, Paecilomyces sp, Penicillium brevicompactum, Penicillium citrinum, Penicillium commune, Penicillium expansum, Penicillium notatum, Penicillium roqueforti, Penicillium viridicatum, Phoma betae, Pullularia pullans, Rhizopus nigricans, Saccharomyces carlsbergensis, Saccharomycescerevisiae, Serpula lacrymans, Sporobolomyces roseus, Stemphylium botryosum, Thermopolyspora, Trichoderma viridae, Trichophyton mentagrophytae, Trichophyton rubrum, Trichophyton verrucosum, Ustilago tritici*

NUTS, PULSES AND SEEDS: almond, brazil nut, carob flour, cashew, chestnut, chick pea, chilli bean, cocoa, coconut (inc. desiccated), flax, hazelnut, lentil, millet, peanut, pecan, pine nut, pistachio, red kidney bean, rose hip, sesame, sunflower seed, walnut

OLIVE

OTHER FIBRES: flax, jute, linen, wool (treated and untreated), silk

PAPAIN

PECTIN

PHTHALIC ACID ANHYDRIDE

PLANTS: cyclamen, cut grass, pine

POLLEN

GRASS: bahia grass (*Paspalum notatum*), barley (*Hordeum vulgare*), bent grass or redtop (*Agrostis alba*), Bermuda grass (*Cynodon dactylon*), Brome grass (*Bromus inermis*), common reed (*Phragmites communis*), dog's tail grass (*Cynosurus cristatus*), Johnson grass (*Sorghum halapense*), maize (*Zea mays*), meadow fescue (*Festuca elatior*), meadow foxtail (*Alopecurus pratensis*), meadow grass or Kentucky blue (*Poa pratensis*), oat (*Avena sativa*), oat grass tail (*Arrhenatherum elatis*), orchard grass (*Dactylis glomerata*), red top (*Agrostis stolonifera*), rye (*Secale cerale*), rye grass (*lolium perenne*), salt grass (*Distichlis spicata*), timothy grass (*Phleum pratense*), velvet grass (*Holcus lanatus*), vernal grass (*Anthoxanthum odoratum*), wheat (*Triticum aestivum* and *Triticum sativum*), wheat grass (*Agropyron smithii*), wheat grass (*Agropyron repens*)

TREES: acacia (*Acacia longifolia*), agave, American beech (*Fagus grandifolia*), Arizona ash (*Fraxinus velutina*), Australian pine (*casuarina equisetifolia*), bayberry (*Myrica* gale), black walnut (*Juglans nigra*), black willow (*Salix nigra*), box elder (*acer negundo*), Brazilian pepper tree, broom (*Genista anglica*), common yew (*Taxus baccata*), cottonwood (*Populus deltoides*), Chinese/Siberian elm (*Ulmus pumila*), daphne (*Daphne mezereum*), elder (*Sambucus nigra*), elm (*Ulmus americana*), eucalyptus (*Eucalyptus sp*), European beech (*Fagus silvatica*), golden chain (*Laburnum sp*), hackberry (*Celtis occidentalis*), hawthorn (*crataegus sp*), hazel (*Corylus avellana, Corylus americana*), hibiscus (marshmallow), horse chestnut (*Aesculus hippocastanum*), Italian cypress (*Cupressus sempervirens*), Japanese cedar (*Cryptomeria japonica*), jasmine (*Jasminum sp*), juniper (*Juniperis monosperma*), lilac (*Syringa vulgaris*), linden (*Tilia cordata*), Loblolly pine (*Pinus taeda*), locust tree (*Robinia pseydoacadia*), London plane or maple-leaf sycamore (*Platanus acerifolia*), magnolia (*Magnolia grandiflora)*, melaleuca (*Melaleuca leucadendron*), mesquite (*Prosopis juliflora*), mistletoe (*Viscum album*), mountain cedar (*Juniperus sabinoides/ sabina*), mulberry (*Morus alba*), oak (*quercus alba*), oleander, olive (*Olea europaea*), orange tree (*Citrus sp*), pecan (*Carya pecan*), pepper tree (*Schinus molle*), privet (*Ligustrum vulgare*), queen palm (*Arecastrum roman, Cocus plumosa*), red alder (*Alnus rubra*), red cedar (*Juniperus virginiana*), red oak (*Quercus rubra*), salt cedar (*Tamarix gallica*), Scotch pine (*Pinus silvestris*), scrub elm (*Ulmus carrisfolia*), smooth alder (*Alnus rugosa*), speckled alder (*Alnus glutinosa*), spruce (*Picea abies*), sweet chestnut (*Castanea sativa*), sweet gum (*Liquidambar styaciflua*), sycamore (*Plantanus occidentalis*), tree of heaven (*Alianthus altissima*), tree of life (*Thuja occidentalis*), Virginia live oak (*Quercus virginiana*), walnut (*Juglans regia*), white ash (*Fraxinus sp*), white bald cypress (*Taxodium distichum*), white birch (*Betula verrucosa/alba, Betula populifolia*), white hickory (*Carya alba*), white pine (*Pinus strobus*), willow (*Salix carpea*)

WEEDS: alfalfa (*Medicago sativa*), burrobrush (*Hymenoclea salsola*), careless weed (*Amaranthus palmcri*), cocklcbur (*Xanthium commune and Xanthium strumarium*), coltsfoot (*Tussilago farfara*), common ragweed (*Ambrosia elatior*), common sagebrush (*Artemisia tridentata*), dandelion (*Taraxacum officinalis*),

English plantain or ribwort (*Plantago lanceolata*), false ragweed (*Franseria acanticarpa*), firebush or kochia (*Kochia scoparia*), giant ragweed (*Ambrosia trifida*), golden rod (*Solidago virgaurea*), goosefoot or lamb's quarters (*Chenopodium album*), ironwood (*Ostrya virginiana*), knotgrass (*Polygonum sp*), lenscale (*Atriplex lentiformis*), Mexican tea (*Chenopodium ambrosiodes*), mugwort (*Artemisia vulgaris*), nettle (*Urtica diocia*), oxeye daisy (*Chrysanthemum leucanthemum*), poverty weed (*Iva azillaris*), rabbit bush (*Franseria deltoides*), rough marshelder (*Iva ciliata*), rough pigweed (*Amaranthus retroflexus*), Russian thistle (*Salsola kali*), salt bush (*Atriplex sp*), sheep sorrel (*Rumex acetosella*), spiny pigweed (*Amaranthus spinosus*), sweet clover (*Trifolium pratense*), wall pellitory (*Parietaria officinale* and *Parietaria judaica*), western ragweed (*Ambrosia psilostachya* and *Ambrosia coronopifolia*), western water hemp (*Acnida tamariscina*), wing scale (*Atriplex* canescens), wormwood (*Artemisia absinthium*), yellow dockweed (*Rumex crispus*)

HERBS/FLOWERS: aster (*Callistephus chinensi*), azalea, balm (*Melissa officinalis*), cactus, camellia, camomile (*Camomilla*), carnation (*Dianthus sp*), chrysanthemum (*Chrysanthemum sp*), cornflower (*Centaurea cyanus*), dahlia (*Dahlia variabilis*), heather (*Calluna vulgaris*), forsythia (*Forsythia suspensa*), French marigold, gerbera (*Gerbera sp*), geranium (*Geranium* sp), gillyflower (*Matthiola incana*), golden rod (*Solidago sp*), hyacinth (*Hyacinthoides sp*), ivy (*Hedera helix*), lily of the valley (*Convallaria majalis*), lily (*Lilium sp*), lupin (*Lupinus sp*), marigold (*Calendual officinalis*), narcissus (*Narcissus sp*), pansy (*Viola tricolar*), primrose (*Primula variabilis*), rape (*Brassica* napus), rose (Rosa sp), St John's wort (*Hypericum sp*), sugar beet (*Beta vulgaris*), sunflower (*Helianthus annuus*), tulip (*Tulipa gesneriana* and *Tulipa sp*), willow herb (*Epilobium angustifolium*), yarrow (*Achillea sp*)

SOYA

SUGAR

TEA

TRIMETALLIC ACID ANHYDRYDE

VEGETABLES: artichoke, asparagus, aubergine, bamboo shoot, bean (white, pinto), beetroot, broccoli, Brussels sprouts, cabbage (red, Chinese, pickled, savoy), carrot, cauliflower (boiled and raw), celery, courgette, cress, cucumber, green bean, green pepper, kohlrabi, leek, lettuce, mushroom (oyster), mushroom,

onion, pea, potato, radish (giant), red pepper, spinach, squash (summer), sweetcorn, sweet potato, tomato
WINE (white and red)
WINE VINEGAR
WOOD: abechi wood (dust), ash, beech, birch, red cedar, cherry wood, kambala wood, limba, mahogany, makore, maple, meranti, white pine, oak, ramin, silver fir, spruce, teak, walnut
WOOL FAT (lanolin)
YEAST (baker's, brewer's, wine)

Food challenge tests

If your symptoms aren't typical of an allergy but may be due to a food intolerance, or there's a positive skin prick test and the doctor wants to determine which particular food is the allergen, he or she may suggest a food challenge test. This is either a "single-blind" test (when the doctor knows what is in the capsule and you don't) or a "double-blind" test (when the test records are kept by someone else, and neither the doctor nor you knows what is in the capsule). The "double-blind" test is considered the best possible test for food allergies.

The test should always be done under medical conditions, as you may suffer a severe asthma attack or anaphylactic shock. If you have had anaphylactic shock in the past, you should never take a food challenge test.

How the test is done

All foods that are associated with your symptoms are temporarily eliminated from your diet (for up to two weeks); this is because if you are regularly taking a food which may be an allergen (such as milk), it could mask the reaction to a single dose. You should also stop taking any antihistamines twelve hours before a challenge test.

If your symptoms disappear, the foods will be reintroduced one at a time, every few days, in the form of a capsule. You will be given a very low dose of the food to start with, and then the dose will be doubled every 15–20 minutes. You will also be given placebo capsules (i.e. that do not contain an allergen) as a check. Any reaction should start to show by eight hours after the trial.

How the test works

If you develop symptoms in response to the capsule containing the food allergen but not to the placebo capsules, you have an allergy. If you don't develop any symptoms, your doctor may suggest trying the food for the next 24–48 hours.

Peak Flow Meter

If you suspect that you have asthma, your doctor may measure your PEFR or "peak expiratory flow rate" (i.e. how you breathe) using a peak flow meter. Your maximum PEFR depends on your age, your height and whether you're male or female. For non-asthmatics, it's usually 400–600 litres per minute; asthmatics have a peak flow of 200–400 litres per minute, and it can fall to only 100 litres per minute in severe attacks. It can be used by anyone over the age of about seven.

How the test is done

A peak flow meter is a small tube with a marker at the side that that slides up and down as you blow into it. You need to stand (or sit upright with your head lifted), hold the tube horizontally (without touching the marker) and make sure it's set at zero before you start, then put the mouthpiece between your lips, make sure the seal is good, and blow out as hard and fast as you can.

How the test works

The marker stops at the point when you blow hardest. It's usually repeated twice and the highest reading of the three is noted on a chart. Your doctor may ask you to keep a diary of readings (usually morning and evening) so he or she can see how your breathing is affected by asthma. It is also used to record how any treatment is working.

Spirometer

This measures your breathing against time; normally, as you breathe out, the air comes out quickly at first and then slows down. Your doctor measures two things:

• your "forced expiratory volume in one second" (FEV1) – that is, the amount of air you breathe out in one second
• your "forced vital capacity" (FVC) – that is, how much air you breathe out until you can't breathe out any more.

How the test is done

You inhale as deeply as you can and then breathe into the spirometer as hard or as completely as you can. Your breath is then "traced" as a curve by the monitor.

How the test works

If you have asthma, the amount of air you breathe out and the rate at which you breathe it out will be reduced. In general, non-asthmatics take about four seconds to breathe out, and about three-quarters of the breath is expelled in the first second; that gives an FEV1 of around 70 per cent. Asthmatics may have an FEV1 of 20–50 per cent.

Exercise challenge test

If you suspect certain foods of causing exercise-induced anaphylaxis, your doctor will ask you to perform an exercise challenge – that is, exercising on a treadmill either before or after eating the suspected allergen (depending on your previous experience). This needs to be done under medical conditions so that you can be treated for anaphylactic shock immediately.

Inhalation challenge tests

These tests are also known as broncho-provocation, and involvesyou being exposed to an allergen and then seeing whether it causes an attack of asthma. It's always done under medical conditions, in case of anaphylactic shock.

How the test is done

You sit in a sealed chamber and an allergen is introduced into it, which you then breathe in. A very dilute allergen will be tested at first (such as 1:10,000), and the concentration will increase in a series of steps – often 1:1,000, 1:100, 1:10 and then undiluted.

There are three main ways of testing your airways:
- *histamine or methacholine challenge* – although non-asthmatics do not react to these chemicals, asthma sufferers do; the drugs act on the muscles surrounding the airways and make them tighten
- *non-allergic triggers* – usually exercise and a fine spray of salt solution

• *specific triggers* – this is particularly useful for occupational asthma and sensitivity to aspirin

How the test works

The doctor will give you a lung function test – either a peak flow meter or a spirometer – and if the challenge causes your "normal" readings to drop by around 20 per cent, you're allergic to the particular trigger.

You will be kept under observation for the next twenty-four hours, in case of a delayed reaction.

Allergens that can be tested

GRAIN: barley bran, barley flour, corn bran, corn flour, oat bran, oat flour, rye bran, rye flour, wheat bran, wheat flour

Nasal challenge test

This test involves you being exposed to an allergen and then seeing whether it causes a reaction. It's always done under medical conditions, in case of anaphylactic shock. A maximum of two allergens will be tested on any one day. A control test (using saline, which should not cause a reaction) will be done first.

How the test is done

There are two main ways of testing:
• single-dose pump sprays – you will be asked to blow your nose, put your head back, breathe in and hold your breath. The solution (either saline or the allergen) will be applied to a nostril (don't breathe it in), and you will be asked to breathe out through your nose.
• syringe and speculum – using a syringe and speculum, roughly 2 drops of the test solution are trickled into your nasal concha.

Whichever test is used, you will then be asked to breathe through a special mask for "rhinomanometric evaluation" – the quantity of air you breathe and the pressure difference are measured.

Allergens that can be tested

ANIMAL HAIR: cat, dog, guinea pig, horse
GRAIN: barley bran, barley flour, corn bran, corn flour, oat bran, oat flour, rye bran, rye flour, wheat bran, wheat flour
MITES: dust mite (*Dermatophagoides pteronyssinus*), grain mite (*Dermatophagoides farinae*)

MOULDS AND FUNGI: *Alternaria alternata*, *Aspergillus fumigatus*, *Cladosporium cladosporioides*, *Penicillium notatum*

POLLEN: alder (*Alnus glutinosa*), English plantain (*Plantago lanceolata*), goosefoot (*Chenopodium album*), hazel (*Corylus avellana*), mugwort (*Artemisia vulgaris*), red sorrel (*Rumex acetosella*), silver birch (*Betula verrucosa*), timothy grass (*Phleum pratense*)

Conjunctival challenge test

This test involves your eyes being exposed to an allergen and then seeing whether it causes an allergic reaction. It's always done under medical conditions, in case of anaphylactic shock.

How the test is done

You will be asked to sit down and put your head back slightly. A drop of saline will be put in your eye. If there is no reaction after ten minutes, one drop of the diluted allergen will be put in the other eye. If there is no reaction after ten to twenty minutes, one drop of a higher concentration of the allergen will be put in the other eye, and higher concentrations will be tested on alternate eyes every twenty minutes until there is a reaction. If there is no reaction to the undiluted allergen, the test is negative.

How the test works

A positive test often occurs after two to three minutes. Your reaction will be evaluated as:

- mild, if your eye looks red, itches and you feel as if there's a piece of grit in your eye
- moderate, as above plus the conjuctiva bulbi (the membrane covering the white of your eye) will be swollen
- strong, if there's a strong itching sensation plus the conjuctiva bulbi is extremely swollen
- severe, if it also causes tears and photosensitivity

Other tests

There are other tests available, but they are not recognized by conventional medical practitioners because they are not standardized or have not had any valid clinical trials. These include:

Applied kinesiology

A sample of food is placed under your tongue or held in a glass container in your hand. You are then asked to push your free arm against that of the examiner, to measure your muscle strength. The idea behind the test is that if you have an allergic response, you will find it difficult to raise your arm. However, there is little published evidence on the technique and in one study the results did not stand up against a double-blind test.

Auricular cardiac reflex method

This measures the strongest pulse at the wrist – in amplitude, not speed. The practitioner rests his or her thumb over the artery at the wrist so that the pulse is just past the tip of the thumb. A bright light is shone on the back of the hand so that the point of maximum amplitude comes directly under the thumb – this is known as a positive reflex. A filter containing an allergenic substance is then held over the patient's skin; if the reflex lasts for more than twelve beats, it's said to be a sign of allergy.

Hair analysis

Your hair is analyzed for the presence of toxic metals (such as lead, mercury and cadmium) or low levels of certain minerals (selenium, zinc, chromium, manganese and magnesium). Although hair analysis can indicate exposure to heavy metals (and subsequent heavy metal poisoning), it has not been validated as a method of diagnosing allergy.

Leukocytotoxic test

Your white blood cells are mixed with a suspected allergen and are then measured in different ways to see if they have changed. The theory is that if you are sensitive to an allergen, your white blood cells will change visibly under a microscope, possibly even swelling and breaking open. However, there is a high number of false positive or negative reactions, and the American Academy of Allergy says that there is no evidence of the test being effective for the diagnosis of food or inhalant allergy.

Neutralization/provocation testing

This is also known as the Miller technique. A specific dose of neutralized allergen drops are placed under the tongue or injected into the skin. If symptoms occur, the test is considered positive and various concentrations are given until a dose is found that "neutralizes" the symptoms. Various other chemicals, hormones, food extracts, and other natural substances may be prescribed as "neutralizing" agents. However, in double-blind tests, the results were the same for allergens and salt-water solution, so conventional medicine does not recognize the test as valid.

Vega testing

This is an electrical test, described also as "bio-energetic regulatory technique". The machine measures the conductivity of electromagnetic fields produced by the sufferer. You will hold electrodes, or they may be connected to acupuncture points. Different solutions are then put in a metal tray. The machine is calibrated by putting a glass container of a toxic substance into the tray, which causes a reduction in electrical conductivity. Other substances are then placed in the tray; if they give a similar reading to the toxic substance, it is reported as an allergic or sensitive reaction.

However, there have been no valid clinical trials and the BMA recommends that Vega testing should be avoided, because the elimination tests often prescribed as a result of Vega testing should only be prescribed by a qualified nutritionist or dietician.

The allergies you don't suspect

There may be occasions when you have vague or generalized symptoms, such as breathing problems or fatigue, and your symptoms do not seem to fit into the category of specific allergies. It may be that you have an allergy to something you use very frequently – such as household cleaners – or even to mercury, if you have fillings in your teeth. However, chemical sensitivity and sensitivity to amalgam (mercury fillings) are controversial areas which are still undergoing a great deal of research.

It's worth switching chemical cleaners to more natural alternatives for a few weeks, to see if your symptoms improve. Keep a symptom diary so that you can show your GP and ask for the relevant allergy tests (such as to chlorine, formaldehyde, perfume, solvent and isocyanates) if there is a distinct change.

5

Treatments

PREVENTION

Avoidance of allergen

Allergen avoidance is often the first step in the management of conditions such as asthma, in conjunction with drug treatment.

Creating an allergen-free environment

Bedding

Bedding contains very high levels of dust mites – up to 2 million in one mattress – because the sweat and body heat produced at night create a favourable environment for mites, and skin and hair shed overnight gives them food. Replacing old mattresses and using dust-proof bedding covers can help remove dust mites. The covers need to encase the mattress, duvet and pillows entirely, and they need to be house dust mite impermeable but water vapour and air permeable, allowing moisture to escape. Your usual bedding is then used on top of the covers as normal (preferably washed at temperatures greater than 56°C, to kill mites), but the dust-proof covers should be wiped down regularly to remove skin scales and mites from the surface.

Reducing dust levels

Even with bagless vacuum cleaners, dust will still settle in carpets – home to mites, giving them food and a surface they can "stick" to – so removing carpets in favour of smooth flooring such as wood or tiling (particularly in bedrooms) can help. Vacuum regularly and use cupboards rather than shelves for storage – dust gathers on ledges and clutter. Replacing cloth upholstery can also help, as can using washable curtains (again washed at temperatures greater than 56°C) and vertical or roller blinds rather than ones with horizontal slats where dust can gather.

Reducing humidity

Dust mites like humidity, and studies have shown that reducing humidity in the home will reduce mite allergen levels and improve asthma.

Centrally heated houses with double-glazing often have internal condensation, and older houses can have rising damp. Your house may also have penetrating damp caused by overflowing gutters and blocked drainpipes.

Once you've dealt with the dampness aspects, you can reduce humidity by improving the ventilation and improving air exchange – that is, moving air away from humid rooms (such as kitchens and bathrooms) – and introduce non-humid air into other rooms. Ways of doing this include:

- keeping windows open and doors to other rooms closed when running a bath or cooking (particularly if your bathroom is en-suite, as your bedroom will be exposed to more water vapour)
- using an extractor fan
- having a ventilation system and heat exchange unit fitted (this brings in filtered air from outside, warms it with air from the bathroom and kitchen, and circulates it throughout the home – but your house must have an airtight construction and the windows must be kept shut for it to work)

Reducing the numbers of mites

Killing mites with chemicals such as acaricidal benzyl benzoate doesn't work because the allergen is in their droppings, which remain on surface tops. However, you can reduce the number of mites and droppings by washing soft toys and furnishings; the temperature needs to be high enough to kill the mites (56°C and above), or you could try putting soft toys in the freezer once a week, which will kill the mites and stop the build-up of allergens.

PRESCRIPTION DRUGS

Adrenaline

Adrenaline is usually given by injection.

Uses

To treat angioedema and anaphylactic shock.

How it works
It narrows the blood vessels in the skin and intestine and stimulates heart activity.

Effectiveness
It acts within five minutes and lasts for up to four hours.

Side effects
• Dry mouth
• Palpitations
• Headache
• Blurred vision
• Restlessness

It may cause raised blood pressure if you are taking beta blockers or certain antidepressants (MAOI). If you are a diabetic, the effectiveness of your medication may be reduced by adrenaline.

Anticholinergic drugs
Acetylcholine is the hormone in the body's parasympathetic nervous system, concerned with calming the system down; its effects are called "cholinergic" and include narrowing the airways. Atropine (derived from deadly nightshade or belladonna) was used until the beginning of the twentieth century but the side effects were unpleasant; however, research showed that one change to the atropine molecule reduced the side effects and also helped enhance the perfomance of ß2 agonists. It's usually used as an inhalant and the most commonly prescribed forms are:
• atropine
• butethamate
• ipratropium bromide (Atrovent, Duovent, Ipratropium, Respontin, Steri-Neb) – this has fewer side effects than other anticholinergic drugs
• oxitropium bromide (Oxyvent)

Uses
To treat wheezing in asthma, particularly in cases of irritant substances such as cigarette smoke, ozone and sulphur dioxide.

How they work
Anticholinergic drugs block the receptors in the body for

acetylcholine, and therefore prevent the action of the hormone, which stops the airways narrowing.

Effectiveness
Anticholinergic drugs take up to an hour and a half to take effect, and last for up to six hours. They are less effective than ß2 agonists, especially if your asthma is caused by an allergy, but may be more effective if you also have bronchitis.

Side effects
- Dry mouth (rare)
- Glaucoma – caused by an increase in pressure inside the eye when using a nebulizer
- Benign prostatic hyperplasia – a non-cancerous enlargement of the male prostate gland, causing incontinence and difficulty passing urine
- Flushing/dry skin
- Blurred vision
- Constipation

Antihistamines
Antihistamines come in tablet, capsule or liquid forms. They are available by prescription as well as over the counter from pharmacies. In an emergency, antihistamines can also be injected directly into the bloodstream.

The most commonly prescribed forms are:

Eye drops:
- antazoline (Ainistine-Privine) – allergic conjunctivitis

Injection:
- chlorpheniramine (Aller-chlor, Haymine, Piriton, Phenetron) – hay fever, perennial allergic rhinitis, anaphylactic shock

Nasal spray:
- azelastine (Rhinolast) – hay fever

Tablets or liquid (* = **available without prescription**)
- acrivastine (Semprex) – hay fever and urticaria
- astemizole (Hismanal*, Pollon-eze*) – hay fever and skin conditions
- azatadine (Optimine*) – hay fever, itching, stings and urticaria
- brompheniramine (Dimotane Plus) – hay fever, perennial allergic rhinitis
- cetirizine (Zirtek) – hay fever
- chlorpheniramine (Aller-chlor, Haymine, Piriton*, Phenetron)

– hay fever, perennial allergic rhinitis, anaphylactic shock
* clemastine (Tavegil*, Aller-eze*) – hay fever, perennial allergic rhinitis
* cyproheptadine (Periactin*) – itchy skin conditions
* dimethindine maleate (Feonostil Retard*, Vibrocil) – hay fever, urticaria
* hydroxyzine hydrochloride (Atarax, Ucerax) – itchy skin conditions, urticaria
* ketotifen (Zaditen) – perennial allergic rhinitis, allergic conjunctivitis, exercise-induced asthma
* loratadine (Clarityn*) – hay fever, perennial allergic rhinitis
* mebhydrolin (Fabahistin) – hay fever
* mequitazine (Primalan) – hay fever, perennial allergic rhinitis
* oxatomide (Tinset) – hay fever
* phenindamine (Thephorin*) – hay fever
* pheniramine (Daneral) – allergic reactions in general
* promethazine (Phenergan*) – allergies, nausea and vomiting
* terfenadine (Seldane*, Triludan*) – perennial allergic rhinitis, urticaria
* trimeprazine (Vallergan) – itching
* triprolidine (Actidil, Actifed, Pro-Actidil*) – allergic reactions in general

Uses
Treatment of:
* Allergic conjunctivitis
* Anaphylactic shock
* Asthma (mainly in Japan and for exercise-induced asthma)
* Hay fever (itching, sneezing, angioedema)
* Perennial allergic rhinitis
* Skin conditions
* Stings
* Urticaria

How they work
Antihistamines block the action of histamine released from the mast cells, so histamine can't act on the cells of the capillaries, nerve-endings or other cells that have histamine receptors. They attach to the histamine receptors so the histamine is left with nothing to attach to, so they work best if they're taken before you start suffering symptoms. Some of the newer antihistamines such as terfenadine also limit the release of histamine from mast cells.

Effectiveness

The newer, "second generation" antihistamines are very effective and do not have the side effects of the "first generation" antihistamines such as Piriton. They usually start working within an hour of being taken and the greatest effects are five to seven hours after taking them. Increasing the dose doesn't increase the effects and can be dangerous.

Don't take with alcohol or tranquillizers, as antihistamines react with them to suppress the central nervous system, making you feel groggy.

Check with your doctor before taking antihistamines if:

- you have thyroid disease, heart disease or high blood pressure, as some antihistamines may cause palpitations
- you have glaucoma
- you have an enlarged prostate gland
- you have epilepsy
- you have liver or kidney problems
- you are taking certain medications, including antidepressants, sleeping tablets, the antibiotic erythromycin, or drugs prescribed for fungal infections (such as ketoconazole or fluconazole)
- you have porphyria
- you have a stomach or duodenal ulcer
- you have Parkinson's disease
- you are planning to become pregnant
- you are pregnant or breastfeeding

Side effects

"First generation" antihistamines cross into the brain so they make you feel drowsy, affecting your ability to drive or operate machinery. Even if you don't feel drowsy, they will affect your ability to react quickly. You may also suffer from:

- blurred vision
- difficulty urinating
- digestive disturbance
- dry mouth
- rash

"Second generation" antihistamines don't cause drowsiness, but you may have the following side effects:

- appetite changes (increase or loss)
- constipation
- difficulty urinating
- digestive upsets

- dizziness
- dry eyes
- dry mouth
- headache
- impotence
- irregular heartbeat
- irritability (more likely in children)
- nasal irritation (from nasal sprays)
- nausea
- nervousness (more likely in children)
- nightmares (more likely in children)
- restlessness (more likely in children)
- skin rash
- slowed reaction time
- taste problems
- unusual jumpiness (more likely in children)
- weight gain

Beta$_2$ (ß$_2$) adrenoreceptor agonists

ß2 adrenoreceptor agonists (often called ß2 agonists) are a form of bronchodilator – a medication that opens the airways by relaxing the muscles that tighten during an asthma attack. They tend to be used as the "first-line" treatment, on a "need to use" basis, so they're often used intermittently. They're usually used in the form of inhalers (a metered dose inhaler, dry powder inhaler or a nebulizer – *see* the section on *asthma* in the chapter on *allergic illnesses* for more details) but may also be prescribed as tablets or syrup.

The most commonly prescribed ß2 agonists are:

- bambuterol (Bambec)
- fenoterol (Berotec, Duovent)
- isoprenaline sulphate (Medihaler-Iso)
- orciprenaline sulphate (Alupent)
- pirbuterol (Exirel, Maxair)
- reproterol (Bronchodil)
- rimiterol (Pulmadil)
- salbutamol (Aerolin autohaler, Airomir, Asmasal, Asmaven, Combivent, Maxivent, Rimasal, Salamol, Salbulin, Salbuvent, Steri-Neb Salamol, Serevent, Ventolin, Ventodiscs)
- salmeterol (Serevent)

- terbutaline sulphate (Brethaire, Brethine, Bricanyl, Monovent)
- tolbuterol (Brelomax)
- tulobuterol (Brelomax, Respacal)

Uses
To treat wheezing in asthma

How they work
ß2 agonists have the same effect as adrenaline in that they stimulate the ß2 receptors in the smooth muscles in the walls of the airways, making the muscles relax and the tubes widen, but they don't give the unwanted side effects of adrenaline (i.e. raised blood pressure and increased heart rate).

Effectiveness
They act quickly (within about 15 minutes) and are very effective for occasional attacks of wheezing after contact with allergens or after exercise; they can act for up to six hours. However, your system may become tolerant to the drug. If your asthma appears to be getting worse, talk to your GP rather than increasing your dose, because you may need to switch to a different broncho-dilator. If you need to use it more than once a day or at night, your GP will prescribe a preventer inhaler as well – overusing a ß2 agonist can be dangerous or even fatal.

Side effects
You may suffer from increased sensitivity to triggers (the "rebound effect") immediately after the drug has worn off. ß2 agonists do not relieve the ongoing inflammation so they are not effective for severe asthma, which is treated by inhaled anti-allergic drugs – see entries for cromoglycate, nedocromil and steroids in this section. Other side effects include:
- abnormal heartbeat
- dizziness
- heart tremor
- headache
- muscle cramps (rare)
- nausea
- nervousness
- palpitations

Check with your doctor before taking bronchodilators if:
- you have thyroid disease, heart disease or high blood pressure, as some bronchodilators may cause palpitations
- you have glaucoma

Immune suppressants

Drugs such as cyclosporin suppress the immune system, to prevent the allergic reaction that causes your symptoms, and are only prescribed in very severe cases. It was originally used in transplant operations, to stop the donated organs being rejected.

Uses
- For severe eczema that doesn't respond to other treatment
- For psoriasis

Effectiveness
It's very effective.

Side effects
As it blocks the immune system, you won't have much resistance to infection. You'll need regular blood and urine tests to check that your kidneys have not been damaeed. Other side effects include:
- swollen gums
- increased hair growth
- nausea
- tremor

Corticosteroids

See entry for *Steroids* in this chapter.

Cromoglycate

Sodium cromoglycate (also known as cromolyn — trade names Aerocrom Syncroner, Intal and Nalcrom) is used as an inhalant (either though a metered-dose inhaler or a nebulizer) or nasal spray.

Uses

It is used to reduce inflammation in the lungs or nose, for example, in hay fever and asthma; in ointment form, it is also good for allergic conjunctivitis.

How it works

It is known as a "mast cell stabilizer" because it stops the mast cells and eosinophils releasing histamine. It is a preventative treatment, so it is not helpful once an asthma attack has started because it will not widen the airways.

Effectiveness

It does not work for everyone, and is more likely to work for children than for adults. It is particularly good for children who need long-term therapy.

On the whole, it is very effective, provided that you take it before you come into contact with the allergen. You also need to take it regularly – three or four times a day, at regular intervals. If you need to reduce it, you should do so slowly and under medical supervision; you may need to reintroduce steroids at the same time to keep your asthma under control.

Side effects

Side effects are rare and are more likely to affect young children. They include:
• headache
• rash
• upset stomach

Decongestants

Decongestants come in liquid (nasal spray) and tablet form. They are available by prescription as well as over the counter from pharmacies.

Uses

To relieve a blocked nose in hay fever and perennial allergic rhinitis.

How they work

Nasal drops or sprays containing ephedrine or xylometazoline (for example, Otrivine or Sudafed) constrict the vessels that supply blood to the lining of the nose. This makes the nasal tissue shrink and will relieve a blocked nose.

They are known as alpha-adrenergic blockers because they stop an adrenaline-type hormone locking on to receptor sites in the blood vessels, and they can also counteract the drowsiness caused by some antihistamines.

Effectiveness
They act rapidly and are very effective.

Side effects
Nasal decongestant sprays should only be used short-term (i.e. for a few days) because they can cause tissue damage from shutting off the blood supply to the nose, which will make your symptoms worse. They can also have a "rebound" effect, so that in repeated use they become less effective and nasal congestion becomes worse when the drugs wear off.

Tablets (usually pseudoephedrine, under the trade names Sudafed and Galpseud, and phenylpropanolamine) can affect other adrenaline receptors in your body and side effects often include:
• Irritability
• Nervousness
• Sleeplessness
• Raised blood pressure
• Headaches
• Rapid heart beat

Emollients

Uses
To soothe and moisturize itchy, scaly skin.

How they work
Creams work into the skin; ointments tend to be greasier and sit on the skin. Some emollients can also be added to bath water.

Effectiveness
There are several different types such as aqueous cream and E45. Because people's skins differ, you may find that something that works for a friend doesn't work for you, and vice versa.

Side effects
You may be allergic to the preservative contained in the emollient.

Nedocromil sodium

Uses
Nedocromil sodium (Tilade) is used as an inhalant to reduce inflammation in the lungs – for example in hay fever and asthma; in ointment form, it is also good for allergic conjunctivitis.

How it works
It works in the same way as cromoglycate. It is known as a "mast cell stabilizer" because it stops the mast cells and eosinophils releasing histamine.

Effectiveness
Very effective, provided that you take them before you come into contact with the allergen – you need to take them regularly. Particularly good for children over the age of six who need long-term therapy.

Side effects
• Cough
• Dry mouth

Nedocromil sodium should not be used in pregnancy.

Steroids

Uses
Eye drops: for allergic conjunctivitis. The most commonly prescribed steroids are:
• betamethasone (Betnesol, Vista-Methasone)
• clobetasone (Eumovate)
• fluorometholone (FML)
• dexamethasone (Maxidex)
• prednolisone (Minims, Pred Forte, Predsol)

Inhalant or injection: to reduce inflammation in the lungs (e.g. asthma). The most commonly prescribed steroids are:
• beclomethasone (Aerobec Autohaler, Beclazone, Becloforte, Beclovent, Becodisks, Becotide, Filair, Qvar, Vanceril)
• budesonide (Pulmicort)

- dexamethasone (Dalalone, Decadron, Hexadrol)
- fluticasone propionate (Flixotide, Flovent)

Nasal spray: to relieve a blocked nose (e.g. hay fever and perennial allergic rhinitis). The most commonly prescribed steroids are:
- beclomethasone (Beconase)
- betamethasone (Betnesol, Vista-Methasone)
- budesonide (Rhinocort)
- dexamethasone (Dexa-Rhinaspray)
- flunisolide (Syntaris)
- fluticasone propionate (Flixonase)

Ointment: most commonly prescribed for skin allergies such as contact dermatitis, eczema and angioedema.

Tablets: for asthma. The most commonly prescribed tablets are:
- prednisolone (Deltacortril Enteric, Deltasone, Deltastab, Hydeltrasole, Precortisyl, Prednalone, Prednesol, Prednisolone, Sintisone)
- triamcinoline (Azmacort, Kenacort, Kenalog, Ledercort)

They are generally given to people with more severe symptoms that do not respond to other medicines. These steroids are corticosteroids, based on the natural body hormone cortisol, and have no connection with anabolic steroids, used by bodybuilders. The risks of not taking a large enough dose are greater than the risks of side effects.

How they work
They do not block the release of histamines and the other complex chemicals from mast cells, but they are good at relieving inflammation by preventing the genes within the cells from making cytokines (the body's chemical messengers that influence the body's immune system).

Effectiveness
They work well but may have side effects in tablet form. Newer synthetic corticosteroids (such as budesonide and fluticasone propionate) are effective on the surface of the lungs, nose and skin, but are not absorbed into the bloodstream and therefore have fewer side effects.

For asthma, they reduce inflammation and mucus in the airways; they reduce the number of mast cells in the airway lining; and they can improve the action of $ß_2$ agonists.

Side effects
When artificial steroids are taken for long periods in tablet form, the body reduces the amount of steroids produced naturally. It's dangerous to stop taking them suddenly because your body won't be able to cope; you need to switch to a lower dose under medical supervision. If you're taking a long course (or have done so in the last two years), you need to carry a special warning card in case you're taken ill or have an accident. The card will tell doctors that you'll need extra steroids during treatment. If you take them with food, you're less likely to suffer from stomach upsets.

Side effects from short-term use in tablet form:
• Heartburn or indigestion
• Increased appetite
• Menstrual irregularities and cramps
• Weight gain (slight – usually related to the increased appetite!)

Side effects from long-term use in tablet form
• Acne
• Cataracts
• Diabetes
• Development of cataracts and glaucoma
• Easy bruising
• Facial reddening
• High blood pressure
• Increased hairiness (hirsutism)
• Raised blood sugar
• Stomach ulcers
• Susceptibility to new infections, such as thrush
• Weakened bones (osteoporosis) and skin
• Weight gain or fluid retention

In nasal spray/inhalant form
There are concerns about children's reduced rate of growth after heavy use; you may also bruise more easily, have an upset sense of taste or smell, and suffer nosebleeds or crusting of the nose. You may have a greater risk of developing cataracts, and should not use them if you have glaucoma or a family history of glaucoma.

There are fewer side effects from inhaled steroids, but you may suffer from a hoarse voice, a cough, a sore throat or thrush, a fungal infection of the mouth and throat. The risk of these side effects can be minimized by using a spacer device, which can reduce the amount of medication residue in the mouth and throat.

Ointments

These may cause dryness or loss of skin colour.

Using strong steroid ointments for a long period can cause skin to become thin, fragile and easily bruised, less elastic and prone to stretch marks

The doctor will work out the strength of steroid cream you need, which is either mild, moderately potent, potent or very potent. The prescription is based on how severe your eczema is, where it is, the size of the area affected, how old you are and if you are using any other treatment. For example, if you are using bandages to control eczema, your doctor will prescribe a weaker steroid because the bandaging makes the steroids more potent. Even if you are prescribed a potent steroid, use it as directed; if you don't use enough to control the flare-up, you may need even stronger steroids to control it.

It doesn't matter whether you use the steroid before or after an emollient, provided you leave at least fifteen minutes between the two treatments.

Check with your doctor if you:

• have had glaucoma
• have had a peptic ulcer
• are pregnant or breastfeeding

Sympathomimetics

These are usually used as nasal sprays or drops, and eye drops.

Uses

To treat symptoms of hay fever – blocked nose, watery eyes and blocked Eustachian tubes (ear problems)

How they work

Sympathomimetics copy the effect of adrenaline, which produces the body's "fight or flight" reaction. They make the capillaries (small blood vessels) contract, which reduces swelling, redness and pain; they have the opposite effect of histamine.

Effectiveness
They're very effective and work quickly.

Side effects
• Stinging and irritation
• Blurring of vision (eye drops only)
• Fast heartbeat
• Insomnia
• Irritability
• Headaches
• You may also suffer from "rebound congestion" (see discussion under *Decongestants*).

Check with your doctor before using them if:
• you have a heart condition, thyroid problems, high blood pressure, glaucoma or epilepsy
• you are taking antidepressants
• you are pregnant

Xanthine derivative drugs
These include caffeine, theophylline and theobromine. Strong coffee has been used to treat asthma for over a hundred years, but isn't very effective; theobromine is also not effective. Theophylline is more effective, and is usually made into a compound (usually an amine compound) so it becomes soluble in the body. The most commonly used theophylline compounds are:
• aminophylline (theophylline ethylene diamine)
• choline theophyllinate (Choledyl)
• diprophylline
• proxyphylline

They're usually taken in tablet (slow-release) form, with the dosage calculated according to your body weight. In severe cases, you may be given an injection.

Uses
To treat asthma

How they work

They relax the muscles in the walls of the airways, particularly when the muscles are tight. They also reduce fatigue in the respiratory muscles (particularly the diaphragm).

Effectiveness

Very effective but the dose has to be right. Too little and it won't work; too much, and there will be side effects. They are not suitable for people with panic disorders, and there are circumstances where blood levels of theophylline are increased, which could cause side effects, especially in people who:

- are overweight
- are older than 50
- are at risk of heart failure
- have liver disease
- are taking medications, particularly
  - allupurinol (Zyloric, Hamarin)
  - cimetidine (Tagamet)
  - ciprofloxacin antibiotics (Ciproxin)
  - erythromycin antibiotics
  - oral contraceptive
  - flu virus vaccination

Side effects

- Abdominal pain
- Convulsions
- Diarrhoea
- Headache
- Hyperactivity
- Insomnia
- Irregular heartbeat
- Loss of appetite
- Nausea
- Palpitations
- Personality changes
- Rapid pulse
- Tremor
- Vomiting

Important notes

- Do not chew theophylline tablets because too much medication will be released too quickly – they're meant to be slow-release and long-lasting.

• Theophylline should be taken on an empty stomach, as taking it with food (particularly hot food) will release the medication too quickly.

Zafirlukast

Uses
This is an anti-inflammatory for asthma, also known as a leukotriene receptor antagonist. It is taken twice a day in tablet form, and can be used as an inhaler.

How they work
It blocks the effect of leukotrienes, chemicals released during an immune response which tighten the airways. Leukotriene D4 affects more asthmatic people than any other, and causes inflammation, swelling and production of mucus; zafirlucast (Accolate) blocks the receptor for leukotriene D4.

Effectiveness
It is effective for exercise-induced and aspirin-induced asthma and works more quickly than steroids. If you take it regularly, it takes 2–4 hours to have an effect but lasts for up to 24 hours in total. It does not stop an asthma attack once it has started.

Side effects
Stomach upset

OTC MEDICATIONS THAT CAN HELP

Coal tar
Coal tar helps to soothe inflammation in cases of skin allergy; it is also antiseptic. However, it is very messy and can stain clothing. Don't use on broken skin. Shampoos containing coal tar can help scaliness on the scalp; let your hair dry naturally after using it, if possible.

Hydrocortisone cream
One per cent hydrocortisone cream is a very mild synthetic steroid which can treat mild to moderate outbreaks of eczema. It should

only be used twice a day for up to a week; if your eczema hasn't cleared in that time, see your doctor. Don't use it on broken or infected skin, or on your face; if you're pregnant or under ten years old, see a doctor.

OTHER NON-DRUG TREATMENTS

Ultra-violet light treatment

In cases of severe eczema, you may be prescribed a course of mixed UVA and UVB light treatment at hospital.

ALTERNATIVE THERAPIES THAT CAN HELP

With all alternative therapies, it's best to consult a qualified practitioner rather than trying to treat yourself with over-the-counter remedies. Your doctor may be able to recommend someone. *Appendix 3* contains a list of organizations that can put you in touch with a registered practitioner.

Acupuncture

Needles are inserted into various points of your body, known as "meridians" or energy pathways, with the aim of rebalancing the body. A mild electrical current may be applied to the needles, or they may be manipulated by hand. You can also use finger pressure on the acupuncture points instead; this is known as acupressure. Some practitioners use a technique called moxibustion, where herbs are burned and placed around the needles, or a stick of burning herbs (a moxa stick – usually made from ragwort) is held close to the acupuncture point.

Acupuncture can provide immediate relief of headaches. Try rubbing the highest spot of the muscle in the webbing between the thumb and index finger for a minute. This can also be effective for itching eyes and sneezing. Acupuncture is also effective against mild ashma.

Alexander technique

This involves working on the correct posture of your body. It can help asthma by increasing muscle strength and thus improving lung function.

Aromatherapy

Aromatherapy uses essential oils – concentrated oils distilled from plants and their bark, leaves, flowers and seeds. They can be made into ointments or oils to be used on the skin, in the bath or burned in a vaporizer and inhaled. Some oils are contraindicated for certain conditions (such as pregnancy or epilepsy) and it's best to do a skin test to check that you're not sensitive to the oils.

Chinese herbal medicine

Although it is known as "herbal" medicine, animal and mineral ingredients are also used as part of some of the remedies. The practitioner will mix the ingredients to suit the patient's condition, personality and yin/yang balance (i.e. the opposing forces in the body: hot and cold, male and female, dark and light, active and passive).

Research has shown that Chinese herbal medicines can be very effective; however, there have been reports of liver damage, so it should be avoided if you have a liver or kidney complaint, or if you're pregnant. The British Association of Dermatologists recommends that Chinese medicine should be used as part of a formal trial, and you should be monitored for side effects such as liver damage throughout the treatment.

Herbalism

Medicines used are made from whole plants and herbs rather than isolating a single active ingredient, as with traditional medicine. Medicines may be prescribed as pills, capsules, tinctures, teas (tisanes), ointments or creams. They sometimes work more slowly than conventional medicines, but you should expect an improvement to show in a couple of days for acute conditions, and within a couple of weeks for chronic conditions.

Homeopathy

Homeopathy has existed since the time of Hippocrates but was developed further by the German doctor Samuel Hahnemann in the early nineteenth century. It is based on the theory that "like cures like" – that is, substances that produce symptoms when given to a healthy person will restore health when given to someone who has those symptoms as part of an illness. The remedies are made from plants, herbs and minerals, and are repeatedly diluted and shaken – a process known as "potentization". Diagnosis is based on the individual, so two people with the same symptoms might be given different treatment.

Building up the immune system to help prevent allergies

This is also known as immunotherapy or desensitization. If you are pregnant or have a cold or fever, your GP will suggest waiting until after the birth or your illness has run its course.

How it works

Your GP will give you a series of injections of the allergen, starting with a very minute dose and increasing the dose with each injection, provided you did not react to the last one. The treatment is usually once or twice a week at first, and gradually reduces to once a month. It may need to be a lifelong treatment. For children and very sensitive patients, oral (sublingual) therapy may be available.

Effectiveness

It is only effective against hay fever, seasonal allergies and anaphylaxis caused by insect stings. It can't be used against food or drug allergies, asthma, perennial allergic rhinitis, digestive system problems or skin problems. It won't start working for at least three months.

Side effects

You may have a red, itchy, slightly swollen area at the injection site, which can be treated by applying a cold compress and taking a mild antihistamine.

"Systemic" reactions are rarer and more serious, and tend to occur within 20 minutes of the injection; they need immediate treatment, so if you suffer from any of the following symptoms, tell your GP immediately:

* sneezing
* itchy, watery eyes
* itching
* urticaria
* chest tightness or wheezing

Allergens that can be treated by desensitization injections

ANIMAL HAIR: cat, cow, dog, goat, guinea pig, hamster, horse, pig's bristles, rabbit, rat, sheep

FEATHERS: budgerigar, chicken, duck, goose, pigeon

GRAIN: barley flour, rye flour, wheat flour

MITES: dust mite (*Dermatophagoides pteronyssinus*), grain mite (*Dermatophagoides farinae*)

MOULDS AND FUNGI: *Alternaria alternata, Alternaria tenuis, Aspergillus fumigatus, Aspergillus niger, Aureobasidium pullulans, Botrytis cinerea, Candida albicans, Chaetomium globosum, Cladosporium cladosporioides, Cladosporium herbar., Curvularia lunata, Fusarium culmorum, Fusarium moniliforme, Helminthosporium halodes, Merulius lacrymans, Mucor mucedo, Neurospora sitophila, Penicillium brevicompactum, Penicillium notatum, Phoma betae, Pullularia pullulans, Rhizopus nigricans, Saccharomyces mellis, Serpula lacrymans, Ustilago tritici*

POLLENS: alder (*Olnus glutinosa*), ash (*Fraxinus excelsior*), aster (*Oster chinensis*), barley (*Hordeum vulgare*), beech (*Fagus sylvatica*), bent grass (*Agrostis stolonifera*), Bermuda grass (*Cynodon dactylon*), chrysanthemum (*Chrysanthemum koreanum*), cocksfoot (*Dactylis glomerata*), couch grass (*Agropyron repens*), dahlia (*Dahlia cultorum*), dandelion (*Taraxacum officinale*), elder (*Sambucus nigra*), elm (*Ulmus sp.*), English plantain (*Plantago lanceolata*), golden rod (*Solidago virgaurea*), goosefoot (*Chenopodium album*), hazel (*Corylus avellana*), hornbeam (*Carpinus betulus*), horse chestnut (*Aesculus hippocastanum*), lichen (*Tilia cordata*), lilac (*Syringa vulgaris*), linden (*Tilia cordata*), locust (black), (*Robinia pseudoacacia*), London plane (*Platanus acerifolia*), maize (*Zea mays*), maple (*Acer sp*), meadow fescue (*Fescue rubra*), meadow foxtail (*Alopecurus pratensis*), meadow grass (*Poa pratensis*), mugwort (*Artemisia vulgaris*), nettle (*Urtica dioica*), oak (*Quercus robur*), oat grass (*Arrhenatherum elatius*), oat (*Avena sativa*), olive (*Olea europea*), orchard grass (*Dactylis glomerata*), oxeye daisy (*Chrysanthemum leucanthemum*), pine (*Pinus sylvestris, contorta, strobus*), poplar (*Populus sp*), ragweed (*Ambrosia elatior* and *Ambrosia trifida*), rape (*Brassica napus* var. *napus*), red sorrel (*Rumex acetosella*), reed (*Phragmites communis*), rough pigweed (*Amaranthus retroflexus*), rye (*Secale cerale*), rye grass (*Lolium perenne*), silver birch (*Betula verrucosa*), sweet vernal (*Anthoxanthum odoratum*), syringa (*Philadelphus coronarius*), timothy grass (*Phleum pratense*), velvet grass (*Holcus lanatus*), wall pellitory (*Parietaria sp.*), wheat (*Triticum satium*), willow (*Salix sp*)

Allergens that can be treated by desensitization sublingual therapy

ANIMAL HAIR: cat, cow, dog, guinea pig, hamster, horse, rabbit, sheep

FEATHERS: budgerigar, chicken, duck, goose,

GRAIN: barley flour, rye flour, wheat flour

MITES: dust mite (*Dermatophagoides pteronyssinus*), grain mite (*Dermatophagoides farinae*)

MOULDS AND FUNGI: *Alternaria alternata, Alternaria tenuis, Aspergillus fumigatus, Botrytis cinerea, Chaetomium globosum, Cladosporium cladosporioides, Cladosporium herbar, Curvularia lunata, Fusarium moniliforme, Helminthosporium halodes, Mucor mucedo, Neurospora sitophila, Penicillium notatum, Phoma betae, Pullularia pullulans, Serpula lacrymans, Ustilago tritici*

POLLENS: alder (*Alnus glutinosa*), ash (*Fraxinus excelsior*), aster (*Aster chinensis*), barley (*Hordeum vulgare*), beech (*Fagus sylvatica*), bent grass (*Agrostis stolonifera*), Bermuda grass (*Cynodon dactylon*), chrysanthemum (*Chrysanthemum koreanum*), cocksfoot (*Dactylis glomerata*), couch grass (*Agropyron repens*), dandelion (*Taraxacum officinale*), elder (*Sambucus nigra*), elm (*Ulmus sp.*), English plantain (*Plantago lanceolata*), golden rod (*Solidago virgaurea*), goosefoot (*Chenopodium album*), hazel (*Corylus avellana*), hornbeam (*Carpinus betulus*), horse chestnut (*Aesculus hippocastanum*), lilac (*Syringa vulgaris*), lichen (*Tilia cordata*), linden (*Tilia cordata*), London plane (*Platanus acerifolia*), maize (*Zea mays*), maple (*Acer sp*), meadow fescue (*Fescue rubra*), meadow foxtail (*Alopecurus pratensis*), meadow grass (*Poa pratensis*), mugwort (*Artemisia vulgaris*), nettle (*Urtica dioica*), oak (*Quercus robur*), oat grass (*Arrhenatherum elatius*), oat (*Avena sativa*), olive (*Olea europea*), orchard grass (*Dactylis glomerata*), oxeye daisy (*Chrysanthemum leucanthemum*), pine (*Pinus sylvestris, contorta, strobus*), poplar (*Populus sp*), ragweed (*Ambrosia elatior* and *Ambrosia trifida*), rape (*Brassica napus* var. *napus*), red sorrel (*Rumex acetosella*), reed (*Phragmites communis*), rough pigweed (*Amaranthus retroflexus*), rye (*Secale cerale*), rye grass (*Lolium perenne*), silver birch (*Betula verrucosa*), sweet vernal (*Anthoxanthum odoratum*), syringa (*Philadelphus coronarius*), timothy grass (*Phleum pratense*), velvet grass (*Holcus lanatus*), wall pellitory (*Parietaria sp.*), wheat (*Triticum satium*), willow (*Salix sp*)

Detoxing

Detoxing – that is, removing the accumulated chemicals from your body (acquired by breathing them in, eating or drinking them) by fasting or chelation therapy – is thought to reduce the amount of stress on your immune system and therefore reduce your allergy symptoms. If you decide to undertake a detoxification programme, check with your GP first – particularly if you are pregnant, diabetic or taking medication – to ensure that you do not become deficient in vitamins or minerals.

A water or juice fast usually lasts for a weekend and involves drinking between four and eight pints of water on the Saturday and eating only raw fruit or salad on the Sunday; it's advisable to avoid exercise, other than some gentle walking. You may develop a headache, a furred tongue or feel nauseous or tired. These symptoms will be short-lived; rather than taking medication to resolve them, if you can't live with them, break the fast.

Chelation therapy uses an artificial amino acid called EDTA which is infused into a vein over a period of around 90 minutes; the treatment is repeated around twenty times over a three-month period. It was originally developed to treat people suffering from metal poisoning (e.g. lead poisoning) as the amino acid chelates (chemically binds) with the lead, allowing its elimination from the body.

Avoiding chemicals from refined foods, sugar, caffeine, alcohol and tobacco, plus drinking extra (purified) water and increasing your intake of fibre by eating more fruit and vegetables (preferably organic) can also help to detox your body.

6

Special cases

BABIES AND YOUNG CHILDREN

The most common allergies in babies and young children are eczema, asthma, allergic rhinitis (hay fever) and food allergies. Roughly one in ten children is allergic to foods; one in five suffers from eczema; and one in seven suffers from asthma.

A recent Swedish study showed that children with eczema are more likely to develop asthma and allergic rhinitis, and that a family history of eczema is associated with an increased risk of developing asthma, particularly if the child develops sensitivity to foods before the age of three.

Department of Health guidelines recommend that babies are only breast-fed or bottle-fed until four months old, and solid foods should be introduced gradually after certain ages to help avoid the development of food allergies. The recommendations are:

Age 4–6 months
- Vegetables
- Fruit (except citrus fruit)
- Rice
- Meat
- Chicken
- Pulses (e.g. lentils)

Age 6–12 months
- Wheat (including bread, biscuits, pasta)
- Fish
- Eggs
- Yoghurt
- Cheese
- Citrus fruit

Age 12 months plus
- Cow's milk

Age 3 years plus
• Peanuts and foods containing peanuts (especially if other members of the family have allergies)

Introduce the foods one at a time and watch the baby closely for a few days after each new addition. If the baby develops a rash or becomes wheezy, snuffly or colicky, stop giving the new food. And if there is a family history of allergy to fish, nuts, peanuts or wheat, don't give them to your child for the first year.

PREGNANCY AND ITS EFFECT ON YOUR SYMPTOMS

Asthma

Almost 7 per cent of women suffer from asthma. Although many of them will have a trouble-free pregnancy, it's a good idea to tell your GP before you start trying to conceive so that you can discuss the management of your condition. Asthma treatments are safe to use during pregnancy, though your GP may change your particular drug to one that's been rigorously tested. If your asthma is not well controlled during pregnancy, you are more likely to have a premature baby, or your baby may have a low birth weight; you're also more likely to suffer pre-eclampsia and high blood pressure.

Roughly a third of women – usually those with mild asthma – find that their symptoms improve in pregnancy; a third stay the same and a third get worse and need increased medication. If you feel a severe attack coming on during pregnancy, call an ambulance immediately – they'll have oxygen, which is important for helping your baby cope during the asthma attack.

Asthma symptoms are likely to be at their most severe between 29 and 36 weeks of pregnancy, and it tends to be better just before labour and delivery. During labour, your body produces extra steroid hormones (cortisone and adrenaline) which help to prevent attacks; however, if you start wheezing during labour, it's safe to use your reliever inhaler. Epidurals, gas and air and other methods of pain relief are quite safe but your medical carers need to know that you have asthma, in case you need to have an operation; as long as the anaesthetist is aware of the situation, there should be no problems.

Your asthma will usually return to "normal" (i.e. the same state as before you were pregnant) within three months of the birth.

Asthma drugs are generally safe for breast-feeding, because inhaled steroids do not enter the bloodstream so they won't pass through to the breast milk; however, theophylline may pass through the breast milk and make your baby irritable.

Eczema

As with asthma, your eczema symptoms may stay the same during pregnancy, they may improve or they may worsen. Because medication can pass through the placenta and affect the baby – particularly in the first three months – it's best to talk it through with your doctor, particularly if you need to use steroids; though weak topical steroids (such as 1 per cent hydrocortisone cream) are safe to use.

In most cases, you'll be advised to carry on with your usual skin care routine in pregnancy and use emollients regularly to keep your skin moisturized, especially around the stomach area to help prevent stretch marks.

If you use alternative therapies, make sure the practitioner is aware that you're pregnant.

Rhinitis

Because the volume of blood in your body increases by 25 per cent during pregnancy, and because pregnancy-associated hormones affect your nasal blood flow and mucus glands, you may find that rhinitis becomes worse during pregnancy. This doesn't mean that your allergy is worse – simply that the changes in your body make your symptoms temporarily worse. You should find that, after the birth, your allergic condition will go back to its pre-pregnancy state.

ALLERGIES IN THE UNBORN CHILD

Allergic conditions such as asthma, hay fever and eczema tend to run in families. If both parents have asthma, the child has almost a 60 per cent chance of developing asthma. If only one parent has asthma, the chances are lower but asthma is more likely to be passed on through the maternal rather than the paternal side.

Studies show that children of mothers who smoke are twice as likely to develop asthma and wheezing than children of mothers who don't smoke.

And a recent study funded by the British Lung Foundation and the National Asthma Campaign showed that pregnant women who suffer from allergies are more likely to have babies who develop allergies and asthma later in life. By the first twenty-two weeks of pregnancy, babies are able to recognize the common allergens their mothers are exposed to in the home, such as dust mites, and babies who develop allergic responses have an altered immune response which makes them more susceptible to allergies.

It's not known precisely how much allergenic material gets through to the baby or how it passes from the mother to the baby; this is currently under research. It's possible that the allergens pass through the placenta (as the maternal circulation is in close contact with the baby through the placenta – for example, egg proteins will be found in the mother's blood two hours after eating eggs, so they may pass through to the baby as well) or through the amniotic fluid/membrane. Immune cells responding to allergens have been found in cord blood and in amniotic fluid.

The study also found that mothers can influence whether their baby develops sensitization to allergies by controlling their own reactions to allergens, especially in the second and third trimesters of pregnancy. Allergen avoidance seems to be the key – see the section on *Avoidance of Allergens* in *Treatments*.

THE ELDERLY AND THOSE WITH WEAKENED IMMUNE SYSTEMS

Asthma

Symptom changes and late-onset asthma

Allergic reactions tend to start by middle age at the latest, but if you have had asthma from a young age, you may find that your symptoms change as you grow older; for example, you may find that shortness of breath is more of a problem. Or you may be diagnosed with asthma for the first time in later life – known as "late-onset asthma". Your GP may suggest keeping a record of your symptoms and peak flow meter readings for a few weeks; he or she may then give you a trial course of steroid tablets to see whether your symptoms and peak flow readings improve, and use the results of the trial to decide on the best medication for you.

Triggers

In older people, the symptoms of asthma are less likely to be triggered by allergies to house dust mites, animal hair and dander, or pollen. The most likely triggers include:

VIRAL INFECTIONS: including colds and flu

EXERCISE

EMOTION: laughing, depression

MEDICATION: beta-blockers, aspirin, ibuprofen

COLD AIR

PERFUMES

AIR POLLUTANTS such as cigarette smoke and chemical fumes

Using medication

If you have arthritis in your hands or cannot hold an inhaler, your GP may suggest using a Haleraid or Turboaid, which fits some spray-type inhalers and lets you release the medication by pressing with your palm. Your GP may also suggest a breath-activated inhaler which works by releasing the medication when you breathe in.

Asthma and other medical conditions

If you have other medical conditions, check with your GP whether your asthma or asthma treatments may affect them. For example, asthma may affect heart disease, and theophylline can increase blood pressure.

If you are taking steroids, your GP will check your eyes yearly for glaucoma, and your bones for osteoporosis.

See also the section on *Asthma* in *Allergic illnesses*.

Osteoporosis

Studies show that taking steroid tablets or high doses of inhaled steroids for a number of years may increase the risk of osteoporosis, a bone-thinning disease that affects one in three women after the menopause. The risks can be reduced by using a spacer to take inhaled steroids, and rinsing your mouth out after taking the steroid inhaler.

7

Allergic illnesses

Asthma
What is asthma?

Asthma is a condition that affects your airways – the small tubes that carry air in and out of your lungs – and causes difficulty breathing. The word "asthma" comes from the Greek, meaning "hard breathing" or panting.

If you have asthma, your airways are inflamed and sensitive, so they react badly when you have a cold, a viral infection or when you come into contact with an allergen that triggers your asthma, such as tobacco smoke, pollen or chemical fumes at work. The blood vessels in your lungs will swell and become leaky; fluid then seeps from the blood into the lung tissue, causing it to swell. This means that the airways inside your lungs become narrower and produce more sticky mucus, which clogs up the airways even more; the effect of the muscular contraction shuts off some of the smaller airways (bronchi) which, together with the increased mucus and inflammation, makes it harder to breathe and may also cause coughing and wheezing.

Eosinophils and neutrophils – types of white blood cells – migrate into the cells lining the smaller airways and release chemical mediators that damage the lining of the airways and cause more sticky mucus to be produced.

During an attack, breathing out takes longer, air gets trapped in the lungs and the effort of trying to empty the lungs causes more wheezing. Your chest will also look larger than usual because of the extra air.

You may find that sometimes your symptoms are milder than others; there may also be periods of days or even weeks when you have no symptoms at all. Some women find that their symptoms are worse just before or during a period, when levels of the hormones oestrogen and progesterone change.

The UK has one of the highest rates of asthma in the world; over 3 million people in the UK suffer from asthma, including one in seven children and one in twenty-five adults. And although most attacks are mild, over 2,000 people a year die from asthma, so if you suspect that your symptoms may be worsening, you should always check with your GP: if your condition deteriorates gradually, you may have an unexpected severe attack which could be life-threatening.

Asthma often runs in families, and smoking during pregnancy almost doubles the chances of the child developing asthma. Allergic rhinitis, or "hay fever", is also a risk factor in developing asthma, as nearly four-fifths of people who suffer from asthma also suffer from allergic rhinitis. Other factors that may increase your chances of developing asthma include:

- being born at a time of year when the pollen count is high
- being brought up in a house where there were pets
- certain foods (mainly cow's milk and eggs) being introduced to your diet at an early age

Occupational asthma

You may also develop asthma for the first time as a result of exposure to allergens in your workplace, for example through inhaling fumes, gases, dust or other potentially harmful substances. If you already suffer from asthma, your condition may be worsened by this. You may find that your symptoms occur shortly after you start work, and improve or even disappear during days off. The three main causes of occupational asthma are:

- *direct irritants* – such as hydrochloric acid or ammonia; you may start wheezing soon after exposure, although the immune system is not affected, so it is an irritant reaction rather than a true allergic reaction
- *long-term exposure* – such as to enzymes in washing powder or chemical molecules; the body's immune system develops allergic antibodies after a period of months or even years of exposure
- *accumulation of naturally occurring chemicals in the body* – such as histamine or acetylcholine within the lung, which in turn leads to asthma – for example, insecticide sprays can cause a build-up of acetylcholine

If you realize that you're exposed to an occupational asthma allergen within about six months, and manage to avoid the allergen after that, your asthma should clear up. However, if your exposure continues for more than six months, your asthma will be permanent, even if you change jobs.

What are the symptoms?

Not everyone has all the symptoms of asthma. They include:

Breathing problems
- Shortness of breath or difficulty in breathing, particularly in breathing out
- Rapid breathing or hyperventilation
- Wheezing
- Coughing, particularly at night or after exercise; it's usually a dry cough, though some yellow sputum may be produced – the discoloration is caused by eosinophils, cells released during an allergic attack
- A feeling of tightness in the chest, when the airways narrow
- A feeling of tightness in the throat, if the larger airways are affected

Nose problems
- A runny nose
- Nasal congestion
- Sinusitis

Eye problems
- Eye irritation

Heart problems
- Increased heart rate

Symptoms are often worse at night; this is because levels of the hormone adrenaline drop, and it doesn't fulfil its usual function of relaxing the muscles of the lung airways. The level of the body's corticosteroids also drops at night, impairing their function of reducing inflammation. It's worth talking to your GP about it because there are drugs available to alleviate it.

Around a third of women find that their asthma gets worse just before or during their period; this may be connected to changes in the body's levels of the hormones progesterone and oestrogen. Again, it's worth talking to your GP about it because he or she may be able to prescribe a different type of preventer medication or hormone treatment.

In severe asthma, because the amount of oxygen in the blood is low, you may find that there is a bluish discoloration in your face, particularly around the mouth; this is known as cyanosis. It may go with a condition called "silent chest" where there is no wheezing, because the airways are very tight and air cannot get into or out of the chest. This needs medical help immediately.

Childhood asthma

Roughly a third of children with asthma grow out of it by the time they are adults, and others find that their symptoms become milder. Under the age of twelve, boys are more than twice as likely to suffer than girls.

Up to 80 per cent of children with asthma develop the symptoms before age five, so parents are likely to notice various signs, such as:

• your child has less stamina during play than his or her peers
• your child tries to limit or avoid physical activities, to prevent coughing or wheezing
• noisy breathing (normal breathing is quiet)
• recurrent or constant coughing spells, particularly at night
• wheezing and coughing between colds, especially after exercise, when excited, or after exposure to cigarette smoke and allergens such as dust, pollens and pets.

Asthma is actually more common than bronchitis, but is often misdiagnosed as bronchitis because children have small, narrow airways that are more easily blocked and bronchitis or a cold can produce enough mucus in the airways to trigger wheezing. It's also difficult to diagnose in under-fives as they can't use peak flow meters or describe their symptoms to you

Asthma tends to be episodic in children; the most common triggers are viral infections and exercise. Children are often sick during an asthma attack, because the lungs fill up too much with air and this puts pressure on the stomach.

Because very young children find it hard to manage metered dose inhalers, your child may be offered syrup instead of an inhaler. If your child is given a long course of steroids (three weeks or more), you need to be particularly vigilant about asthma triggers, because he or she is more vulnerable to a severe attack for up to a year after the steroid course has finished.

Asthma and school

If your child has asthma, you need to tell the class teacher and the school, to make sure that your child has easy access to any medication and that the teacher can remind your child to take medication, for example before exercise (particularly if it's outdoors and the air is cold), art activities or a science class, where fumes from chemical experiments (such as sulphur dioxide), glues or pet allergens may affect your child.

Asthma and sinusitis

If you have asthma, you may also suffer from sinusitis, which will make your asthma symptoms worse. The main symptoms are:

- nose problems – blocked, stuffy, post-nasal drip
- cough
- pain in the face – usually around the cheeks and eyes, and often worse when you bend forward
- sore throat
- loss of smell and taste
- headache and earache

Sinusitis may come on after a cold or it may be in response to an allergen such as occupational allergens, pets or cigarette smoke.

Triggers that provoke asthma

There may be more than one "trigger" or situation that provokes your asthma. The most common ones include:

AIRBORNE ALLERGENS: pollen (tree, grass and ragweed), animal fur, feathers, animal dander, animal saliva and urine (particularly that of dogs, cats and horses), house dust mite; cockroaches, moulds

AIRBORNE PARTICLES: flour, chalk dust, wood dust, coal dust, talcum powder, grains, coffee and flour

AIR POLLUTANTS: cigarette smoke, wood smoke, chemicals in the air (such as fly sprays and air fresheners), sulphur dioxide (given off by some food and drink; also produced by industrial areas, coal-fired power stations and coking plants), diesel particulates (particularly in bus and coach stations, and near main roads heavily used by diesel vehicles) and ozone (poor air quality – caused by sunlight acting on nitrogen oxide given off from car exhausts and industrial smoke effluent)

ALCOHOL: this can be worsened if you are also diabetic and take the drug chlorpropamide

ARTIFICIAL FIBRES

COLDS, FLU, SINUSITIS OR VIRAL INFECTIONS – the symptoms of asthma may last for up to six weeks after the cold has gone, and there are also more asthma attacks during the autumn, when colds are more prevalent

COSMETICS: citronella oil

DRINK: tea

DYES

EMOTIONAL UPSET AND EXCITEMENT: particularly in small children

EXERCISE – particularly in winter, when cold, dry air enters the mouth and changes the fluid lining the airways in the lung; some people find that they only suffer severe exercise-induced asthma when they eat certain foods before exercising (celery is a particular culprit, though it's not clear why!)

FOOD – particularly in children's asthma; the most likely foods to affect asthma include cow's milk, eggs, wheat, cheese, yeast, nuts, fish, pork and corn; others include apple, asparagus, avocado, bamboo shoots, barley, buckwheat, carrot, celery, chick pea, currants, lentil, melon, onion, pea, peanuts, potato, soya, strawberry, yeast

FOOD ADDITIVES

COLOURS: E102 (Tartrazine); E104 (Quinoline yellow); 107 (Yellow 2G); E120 (Cochineal or carminic acid); E122 (Carmoisine); E123 (Amaranth); E124 (Brilliant scarlet 4R or Ponceau); E132 (Indigo carmine); E133 (Brilliant blue FCF); E154 (Brown FK); E155 (Chocolate brown HT)

PRESERVATIVES (though only 5–15% of asthmatics are sulphite-sensitive): E210 (Benzoic acid); E211 (Sodium benzoate); E212 (Potassium benzoate); E213 (Calcium benzoate); E214 (Ethyl 4-hydroxybenzoate); E216 (Propyl4-hydroxybenzoate); E217 (Propyl4-hydroxybenzoate sodium salt); E218 (Methyl paraben); E219 (Methyl 4-hydroxybenzoate); E220 (Sulphur dioxide); E221 (Sodium sulphite); E222 (Sodium bisulphite); E223 (Sodium metabisulphite); E224 (Potassium meta-bisulphite); E226 (Calcium sulphite); E227 (Calcium hydrogen sulphite); E249 (Potassium nitrite); E250 (Sodium nitrite); E251 (Sodium nitrate)

ANTIOXIDANTS: E310 (Propyl gallate); E311 (Octyl gallate); E312 (Dodecyl gallate)

FLAVOUR ENHANCERS: E621 (Monosodium glutamate (MSG); E622 (Monopotassium glutamate); E623 (Calcium glutamate); E627 (Sodium guanylate); E631 (Sodium 5'-inosinate); E635 (Sodium 5'-ribonucleotide)

HERBS/SPICES: aniseed, coriander, cumin, garlic, mace, mint, oregano, rosemary, tarragon

INSECT STINGS

LATEX

MEDICATION particularly
- aspirin (menthol and mint aromas are chemically similar to aspirin and may also provoke a reaction, for example in toothpaste or cough sweets)
- other non-steroidal anti-inflammatory drugs (such as ibuprofen)
- beta-blockers (used to treat heart disease, high blood pressure or migraine headaches); these may also be contained in eye drops used to treat glaucoma
- contraceptive pills containing oestrogen
- hormone replacement therapy (HRT)

OCCUPATIONAL EXPOSURE TO ALLERGENS, VAPOURS, DUST, GASES OR FUMES: isocyanates (found in paints and varnishes, particularly polyurethane and gloss paints), epoxy resin, amines, chemicals (acrylate, anhydrides, castor oil, chloramine-T, epoxy resin, formaldehyde, isocyanates, persulphate), dyes, enzymes, metals (chromium, cobalt, nickel, platinum salts, vanadium salts), mushroom compost, paint, PVC, soldering fumes, solvents (alcohol solvents, aromatic hydrocarbons, chlorinated hydrocarbons, esters, glycols, glycol ethers, halogenated solvents, ketone solvents), wood pulp, wood dust

PLANTS

SALICYLATES

STRONG SMELLS, such as perfumes, household cleaners, cooking fumes (especially from frying), paints, varnishes, strong-smelling flowers

TEMPERATURE AND HUMIDITY CHANGES

Medical treatments available

Most asthma medication is delivered using an inhaler, which delivers very small amounts of the medication directly into the lungs. The two main types of asthma medication are relievers and preventers.

Reliever inhaler

This is usually blue. It opens up the airways, which causes the muscles to relax so that you can breathe more easily. It should only be used when the symptoms of asthma appear. If you need to use it more than three times a week, it's likely that the amount of inflammation in your airways needs a stronger treatment, called a preventer.

Preventer inhaler

This is usually a brown, white, red or orange inhaler containing corticosteroids. It calms the inflammation in your airways and stops the blood vessels dilating and becoming leaky, so you're less likely to react badly when you come across an asthma trigger. It needs to be taken regularly (every day) and you should not stop taking it when your symptoms die down and you feel better – if you do, next time you come across your particular "trigger", you will have another asthma attack. If you forget a dose, take it as soon as you remember.

If you wash your mouth out afterwards and spit the water out, it will reduce the side effects.

Types of inhalers

- **Metered dose inhaler:** The metered dose inhaler is available for all asthma medications. With this inhaler, the drug is dissolved in organic solvent and sealed in a small canister under pressure. As you breathe in, you press the canister into the plastic casing and inhale the drug, holding your breath for about ten seconds. You then breathe out and wait another thirty seconds before taking another dose of the drug.

- **Autohaler:** The autohaler is available for salbutamol, beclmethasone, sodium cromoglycate and oxitropium. With this inhaler, the pressurized aerosol is completely encased, with a lever at the top. When you set the lever and breathe in, the aerosol is automatically triggered and dispenses the drug. You need to keep breathing or the medicine will be lost in your mouth rather than going into your airways.

- **Spacer devices:** Spacer devices avoid the medicine either being lost in the mouth if you don't breathe in properly (as a reaction to the coldness of the medication), or depositing medicine at the back of the throat – it doesn't matter so much with bronchodilators, but steroids can make your throat dry. A spacer device works by enveloping the cloud of medication and giving you time to breathe it in. You put the inhaler into the end of the spacer, put the mouthpiece in your mouth, press the canister, take a slow, deep breath in, and hold it for about ten seconds. As with the metered dose inhaler or autohaler, you then wait another thirty seconds before taking a second dose. Spacer devices also tend to be used for children, who find it hard to manage inhalers.

In an emergency, you can make a spacer out of a plastic (not polystyrene) cup: cut a cross in the bottom of the cup and put the mouthpiece of the inhaler in it, then put the open part of the cup over your mouth, fire the inhaler and breathe in. You can also use a paper bag in the same way: cut a small hole in the bottom and fit the mouthpiece of the inhaler in it, and bunch the open end of the bag against your mouth, fire the inhaler and breathe in.

- **Dry powder inhaler:** The dry powder inhaler works with capsules of medicine. You put the capsule into the inhaler, then suck in a deep breath; the capsule of drugs is punctured and forms a cloud of powder which you then breathe in.
- **Nebulizer:** Nebulizers turn liquid drugs into a fine mist that can be breathed in through a mouthpiece or mask. It tends to be used with people who have "brittle asthma" (and need larger doses of drugs), small children with severe asthma (because it's an easier way for them to take the drugs) and in an emergency if you have a severe asthma attack.

Treating an asthma attack

Take your reliever medication. If it doesn't work, try to stay calm and try again in five or ten minutes. Keep sitting upright, propped up with pillows if need be, and loosen any tight clothing around your neck, such as a tie or buttons. If there is no improvement in fifteen minutes, call a doctor immediately.

Staying calm is particularly important; if a child has an asthma attack, hold his or her hand for reassurance, but don't put your arm round the child's shoulders, as it makes it harder for the child to breathe.

To cope with an attack:

- Stay calm – if you panic, you will hyperventilate (breathing quickly, using just the upper part of your chest), which will make the attack worse
- Focus on the outbreath – if you breathe out as fully as you can, the inbreath will be easier
- Breathe slowly – this will help bring the attack under control
- Open a window – fresh air (as long as it isn't too cold) will help
- Drink lots of water – during an asthma attack, fluid is lost through the surface of the airways and you can become dehydrated
- Stand or sit up rather than lying down – it makes it easier to breathe

Signs of deterioration in asthma

There is often a deterioration in the condition for a while before an attack. Your condition is deteriorating if:
- Bronchodilator drugs don't seem to have an effect
- You need to use your inhaler more often
- You have persistent wheezing
- You have nasal discharge
- You notice pallor and listlessness in children

It's a good idea to check with your GP; if you leave it, you may find that:
- You wheeze loudly and constantly
- You're tired easily
- You're using a bronchodilator almost hourly

From there on, if your condition worsens, you will need emergency treatment.

In an emergency

If an asthma sufferer has any of the following symptoms, call a doctor immediately:
- Blueness around the lips or tongue (cyanosis)
- Confusion, drowsiness or exhaustion from the attack
- Severe breathing difficulties
- Difficulty in speaking – particularly if he or she can't finish a sentence without gasping for breath
- Rapid pulse and breathing
- He or she can't rise from a chair

Symptoms in a young child that indicate a severe attack needing medical attention include:
- Only being able to say one or two words between breaths
- Tongue, lips or fingernails are blue
- Nostrils are flared
- Hollows between the ribs
- Fast pulse rate (over 100 beats per minute)
- Wheezing, particularly if this stops – this is "silent chest", where the airways are too narrow for air to pass through them

The doctor will want to know:
- What steroids have been taken, if any
- If a nebulizer has been used
- If the drug theophylline has been used

This is to avoid any overdose of medication. The doctor will check your pulse, blood pressure and peak flow reading. He or she may also take a blood test to check oxygen and carbon dioxide levels in the blood, and a chest X-ray may also be taken to check that there has been no damage to your lungs. In severe cases, you may need oxygen and a ventilator, or you may be given steroid injections and bronchodilator drugs with a nebulizer.

Self-help tips

Besides taking your medication regularly, you can help yourself by getting to know the things that trigger your asthma and avoiding them where possible. You only need to avoid the triggers if they affect you – for example, if you are not allergic to dust mites, you don't need to buy expensive anti-mite products or change the way you furnish/clean your home.

Avoiding air pollutants
- Avoid smoking in the house
- Avoid walking or cycling on busy roads – ozone is concentrated at ground level and nitrogen oxides from car fumes can also make asthma worse
- Keep the house well ventilated to reduce fumes
- Ventilate the area when painting
- Keep car windows closed if you pull up behind a lorry or a bus, as more particles will be emitted from the vehicle as it sets off
- Breathe through your nose if you're in polluted air

Avoiding colds and viral infections
- Vitamin C supplements can reduce the number and severity of colds
- Wear a scarf over your face to avoid breathing cold air
- Avoid smoky rooms in the winter
- Have a flu jab in the autumn
- Avoid people who have colds and flu
- Don't hug or kiss people in the winter months

Avoiding dust mites and dust
- Reduce humidity in the house
  - Open a door or window to ventilate bathrooms and kitchen during bathing, washing and cooking
  - Keep doors to other rooms closed to stop moisture spreading through the house

  - Dry clothes outdoors only (unless you have a dryer which is vented outside)
  - Air bedding before you make beds
- Reduce dust
  - Use cupboards rather than shelves for storage, and avoid clutter
  - Damp-dust (i.e. use a damp or oiled cloth to clean surfaces – dry dusting releases dust mite droppings into the air) and use a mask when dusting
  - Ask someone else to do the tasks that stir up a lot of dust, e.g. vacuuming, dusting, turning over mattresses
  - Reduce the number of carpets and soft furnishings in the home
  - Vacuum regularly with a cleaner that keeps the allergens in, such as a HEPA (High Efficiency Particulate Arresting) air filtered vacuum cleaner – using a filter removes 99 per cent of the allergens blown back through vacuum cleaner exhausts
  - Avoid hot air heating systems and fan heaters because they make more allergens airborne
  - Avoid padded items in the bedroom such as headboards, cushions, ottomans, draught excluders, padded coat-hangers
  - Replace curtains with blinds or easily washable fabric – avoid plush fabrics and velvet

Bedding
- Shake blankets, pillows, quilts and duvets outside as often as possible
- Wash bedding, curtains and soft toys at temperatures over 56°C to kill mites
- Use dust-proof bedding covers – wipe them with a damp cloth and let them dry every time you change the bed
- Replace old mattresses, carpets and soft furnishings – dust mites can colonize a new mattress within four months, so use anti-mite coverings on a new mattress
- Replace feather pillows, duvets and eiderdowns and woollen blankets with synthetic ones
- Replace pillows every three months
- Air and dry beds and bedding

Flooring and fabrics
- Use wooden or tiled flooring rather than carpets, where possible
- Choose canvas, cane or leather rather than fabric for soft furnishings

Children
- Freeze soft toys once a week for at least six hours to kill mites
- Store toys in cupboards and wipe with a damp cloth to avoid dust
- Avoid using fabric books and soft blocks
- If children with asthma have to sleep in bunk beds, put them in the top one

Avoiding medication problems
- If you're sensitive to aspirin, check labels of any cold medication for menthol, as you may also react to it

Avoiding moulds
- Use hard floorings in bathrooms and kitchens – damp carpets are the perfect environment for mould growth
- Improve ventilation, use fan extractors in kitchens and bathrooms, and use a dehumidifier to keep the humidity below 50 per cent
- Wipe window-frames regularly to prevent mould growth; wiping surfaces with vinegar can help to reduce mould growth
- Reduce the number of house-plants, as mould can grow on soil
- Remove fallen leaves and grass clippings from the garden; avoid compost heaps and bark chip mulch

Avoiding occupational asthma triggers
- Talk to your employers about ways of avoiding your triggers. Try:
- moving the hazard to another part of the workplace
- using protective equipment such as masks
- improving ventilation in the workplace

Avoiding pet allergens
- Consider rehoming your pet (though their dander will linger in the air and furnishings for several months after they leave); or keep your pet outdoors wherever possible
- Wash your pet once a week
- Wash your hands after handling your pet
- Keep pets out of your bedroom

Avoiding pollens
See under *Hay fever*, below

Avoiding strong smells

- Don't use air fresheners or insect sprays
- Use a fan extractor to remove cooking smells
- Use unperfumed cosmetics, bath products and household cleaning products
- Avoid using heavily scented flowers, either in the garden or as cut flowers for the home – the most likely ones to affect asthmatics include:
  - broom
  - buddleia
  - carnations
  - chrysanthemums
  - daffodils
  - elder
  - honeysuckle
  - hycacinth
  - lavender
  - lilac
  - lilies
  - lily of the valley
  - marigolds
  - mimosa
  - pinks
  - privet
  - sweet peas
  - stocks
  - wallflowers
- Using artificial Christmas trees and wreaths rather than natural ones can also help.

  If you can't avoid the smell, holding your nose may help; using your reliever inhaler before exposure will reduce your symptoms, although it won't block the reaction.

Humidify the air

- Breathing in moist air can help during an attack

Weight control

- If you are overweight, your asthma may be worse because the extra fat layers will make it harder for your lungs to expand fully; try to maintain your recommended weight range.

Alternative therapies that can help

Aromatherapy

Some aromatherapy oils, such as lavender – particularly combined with massage – can help to relax you. Eucalyptus and peppermint are good for inhaling; camomile is antispasmodic and is good as a chest rub. However, if you are sensitive to strong smells, you may react to the oils.

Buteyko Method

This is a type of breathing that can help if you have a tendency to hyperventilate – that is, breathe in too much air, so the carbon dioxide levels in your blood are erratic and upset the nerve cells.

Homeopathy

- Calcarea phosphorica – for bronchial asthma
- Kalium phosphoricum – for nervous asthma or asthma with laboured breathing
- Kalium sulphuricum – for asthma accompanied by bronchitis

Relaxation techniques

Stress can worsen the symptoms of asthma; relaxation techniques can help reduce stress and improve the symptoms of asthma. Yoga is particularly good as it also teaches breathing exercises.

Hypersensitivity pneumonitis

What is hypersensitivity pneumonitis?

This is an allergic lung disease, caused by repeated and prolonged exposure to dust. It is also known as extrinsic allergic alveolitis.

What are the symptoms?

Symptoms may include cough, breathing problems, fever, headaches, nausea and sweating.

Allergens that provoke hypersensitivity pneumonitis

ANIMAL PROTEINS
CONTAMINATED SEWAGE
CHEESE (contamination by mites – *Acarus siro*)
DETERGENTS (enzymes)
DRUGS (amidarone)
DUCK (FEATHERS)

DUST: coffee dust, corn, flour (wheat), fur/hair, malt dust, wood/sawdust

EPOXY RESIN

GRAIN (contamination by weevils – *Sitophilus grainarius*)

ISOCYANATES (spray paint/varnish)

MOULDS: aspergillus; bird droppings; birds (chickens, duck, parakeets, pigeons, turkeys; cheese (*Aspergillus clavatus, Penicillium caseii, Penicillium roqueforti*), compost (*Aspergillus fumigatus*), cork dust, hay or grain (*Aspergillus flavus, Cladosporium, Penicillium*), house dust (contaminated with *Trichosporon cutaneum*); malt (*Aspergillus clavatus*); mushroom compost; sugar cane; typesetting water; wood

RAT URINE (present in rivers, especially in cities)

Diagnosis
Your GP may do some lung function tests, blood tests and chest X-rays.

Medical treatments available
As *Asthma*, above

Self-help tips
• Avoidance is key!
• Check storage at work to avoid mould growth
• Make sure the working area is properly ventilated; dust masks should be used for emergencies (for example, when ventilation systems are being repaired or maintained)

Contact dermatitis
What is contact dermatitis?
Dermatitis basically means "skin irritation". At one point, it was thought that dermatitis and eczema were completely different diseases, but contact dermatitis is actually a form of eczema. It develops when your body's immune system reacts against something that's in contact with your skin – either an allergen or an irritant.

In allergic dermatitis, the allergic reaction often develops over a period of time through repeated contact with the substance – for example, to nickel, which is often found in earrings and buckles. The reaction can occur up to 48 hours after contact with the allergen, and can last for up to 28 days. It's relatively common, with one in fifty people affected by it.

Irritant dermatitis usually appears on the hands and is caused by frequent contact with everyday substances – such as detergents and chemicals – which are irritating to the skin. The reaction usually occurs within minutes of contact with the irritant, and it's more common in adults than in children. It may occur after just one exposure to a strong or caustic substance, but it's more likely to develop over a period of time. You're more likely to suffer if you have a job where your hands are frequently wet or exposed to an irritant – such as hairdressing, catering, cleaning, housework, mechanical engineering and nursing. Figures from the Health and Safety Executive show that occupational dermatitis (irritant contact dermatitis caused by sensitivity to substances at work) accounts for up to a third of all working days lost by British industry. You're also more likely to suffer if you also have eczema, and if you have fair skin and red hair.

Under EU directives, from January 1997 all ingredients must be listed on cosmetics and toiletries throughout Europe, so you should be able to avoid trigger substances. If in doubt, hypo-allergenic ranges of cosmetics and toiletries are less likely to contain potential allergens.

What are the symptoms?
• Chapping, soreness and redness
• Itchy blisters on the skin

Allergens that provoke contact dermatitis
ADHESIVES

AIRBORNE PARTICLES

BATTERIES

BLEACH

CEMENT

CHEMICALS: acid, adhesives, alkalis, ammonia, antimony, benzoyl peroxide, butyl alcohol, chlorocresol, epoxy resin, ethylene diamine, formaldehyde, isocyanates, paraphenylenediamine (PPDA) mercaptobenzothiazole, phenylenediamines

CLAY

CLEANING MATERIALS: detergent, disinfectant

COSMETICS (including preservatives in cosmetics and creams): aluminium chloride, camphor oil, cinnamic aldehyde, cinnamon oil, citronella oil, deodorants, depilatories, douche preparations, eye liner, eye shadow, face powder, foundation, hair products, hand cream, lip balm, lipstick, mascara, moisturizer, mouthwash, nail varnish, perfume, shampoo, shaving products, skin care products, soap, suncream, toothpaste

DYES

ENZYMES: benzophenones

FOODS: bamboo shoots, beef, buckwheat, carrot, cashew nuts, chicken, chicory, citrus fruit, egg, endive, fish, flour, kiwi fruit, lemon, lettuce, lime, mustard, onion, orange, parsnip, pea, peanuts, pear, peppers, potato, radish, rice, rye, soya, strawberry, swede, wheat

FOOD ADDITIVES: food additives

– COLOURS: E104 (Quinoline yellow)

– PRESERVATIVES: E214 (Ethyl 4-Hydroxybenzoate); E215 (Ethyl 4-Hydroxybenzoate sodium salt); E216 (Propyl4-hydroxy-benzoate); E218 (Methyl paraben); E219 (Methyl 4-hydroxybenzoate); E282 (Calcium propionate)

HERBS/SPICES: allspice, caraway, cardamom, cayenne pepper, cinnamon, clove, cumin, curry powder, garlic, ginger, nutmeg, oregano, paprika, parsley, pepper, rosemary, turmeric

INSECTICIDES

LATEX

LEATHER GOODS (including leather additives)

MEDICATION: antifungals, antihistamines, antimitotic compounds, antiseptic, arnica, benzocaine, penicillin

METALS: beryllium, chromium, chromate, cobalt, copper sulphate, gold, iron, lead, mercury, nickel (1 in 10 women suffers from allergy to nickel, particularly earrings), palladium, platinum salts, potassium dichromate, selenium, silver, tellurium, zinc

PAINT AND PAINT THINNER

PARABENS

PLANTS – plants in the *rhus* family (poison ivy, poison oak or poison sumac) which contain a chemical called urushiol; other plants (giant hogweed, cow parsley and rue)

PLASTIC

SANITARY PRODUCTS

SCENT/FLAVOURING: balsam of Peru, menthol

SESAME

SOLVENTS: alcohol solvents, aromatic hydrocarbons, chlorinated hydrocarbons, esters, glycols, glycol ethers, halogenated solvents, ketone solvents

TALC

THURIAMS

TURPENTINE

WOOD DUST

WOOL

Medical treatments available

For irritant contact dermatitis, because the reaction is non-allergenic, treatment is usually aimed at relieving the symptoms and preventing further damage to the affected skin.

For allergic dermatitis, cold soaks and compresses can help in the early, itchy blistered stage of the rash. If the rash is limited to a small area of the skin, your GP may prescribe topical corticosteroid creams to offer relief. If the rash affects a large area, your GP may prescribe oral corticosteroids, which must be taken for the entire duration of the reaction.

Self-help tips

To stop the reaction repeating, you need to prevent contact with anything that you know causes a rash or irritates your skin (i.e. wear gloves and use barrier creams) and keep your skin moisturized.

Hand washing
- Use soap without scent or colour (glycerine-based), or preferably a substitute such as aqueous cream
- Rinse thoroughly, particularly under rings
- Dry (dab and do not rub) carefully between the fingers

Bathing
- Avoid highly scented bath products
- Sodium bicarbonate in a warm bath can help skin irritation

Detergents
- Measure quantities according to the manufacturer's instructions so the solution isn't too strong
- Avoid detergents labelled as "biological" or containing enzymes
- Wear plastic gloves when using shampoo or applying hair dyes and lotions

Housework
- Wear protective gloves with a cotton lining for washing up
- Avoid touching any polishes, solvents or stain removers (including white spirit and turpentine)

Gardening
- Use thick gardening gloves to avoid contact with soil, fertilizers, plant irritants and pesticides

Food
- Use gloves when peeling or squeezing citrus fruit, and handling raw vegetables, meat and fish

Rings
- Don't wear them when doing housework or washing hands (soap will remain under them)
- Clean them frequently with a brush
- Leave them in an ammonia solution overnight (1 tbs to 500 ml of water) and rinse thoroughly

Alternative therapies that can help
Aromatherapy
- Geranium oil can help to ease itching

Bach flower remedies
- Crab apple diluted in water can help to ease itching
- Rescue cream can also help

Homeopathy
- Calcarea carbonica – for cracked and itching skin (6c)
- Graphites cream – for dermatitis

Eczema
What is eczema?
Eczema – also known as atopic dermatitis – is a group of skin conditions which can affect all age groups, though it tends to start in very young children; it's rare for eczema to start for the first time in people over forty. It comes from the Greek, meaning "to boil over", which describes the hot, inflamed skin condition. In the UK, nearly 20 per cent of all school-age children have eczema, though roughly 70 per cent of children grow out of it by their mid-teens. One in twelve adults also suffers from eczema. Although it can sometimes look unpleasant, eczema is not contagious.

It tends to run in families (known as "atopy") and symptoms often start before a child is two years old, starting with the face and tummy, then moving into the backs of knees and elbows. It's the most common skin problem in young children, and can be very mild, just affecting one or two small areas, or it may cover the whole body. By the age of four, some children will grow out of eczema.

Eczema is also linked with asthma – half of all babies who suffer from eczema also develop asthma – and with hay fever.

It's often worse in cold weather or humid conditions, and is made worse by stress or anger.

The main types of eczema

Asteatotic eczema, or eczema craquelé

This is a type of eczema that tends to affect older people, whose skin is thinner and drier (i.e. produces less sebum). It usually starts on the shins and the skin looks "crackled", like the varnish on a very old painting. Humidifying the air and avoiding sitting close to an open fire can help.

Atopic eczema

This is the commonest form of eczema; it is also associated with asthma and hay fever, and it is thought to be a hereditary condition. Research has shown that there is a gene on chromosome 11 that causes abnormal antibody receptors to form on cells.

What happens is that the immune system reacts excessively to an allergen in the environment that is harmless to a "normal" person, so the body releases IgE, which then attaches to the allergen and the mast cells, causing the mast cells to leak histamine and other chemicals.

The natural oils of the skin are produced in smaller amounts, so the skin becomes dry and sheds more cells than usual, and more fluid than usual is lost from the deeper layers of the skin. Inflammation makes the small capillaries in the skin open wider (known in medical terms as vasodilation), to allow more blood to flow through; this makes the skin red and hot. The dryness and the extra heat make the skin itch, and scratching only makes it worse, causing the skin to crack and allowing infection to enter. The inflammation also makes the walls of the blood vessels "leaky", so fluid seeps from the blood into the skin; the fluid makes its way to the surface of the skin and forms blisters, known as "vesicles". These vesicles are the most characteristic feature of atopic eczema.

Atopic eczema usually affects the cheeks, forehead and scalp, then spreads to the wrists and hands, bends of the elbows and knees, and possibly the ankles and backs of the feet. In very young children, the rash is very inflamed and tends to ooze (known as exudation); the fluid that oozes from the rash contains the clotting agents present in blood, so it forms a crust or scab. As the child gets older, the oozing and crusting diminish and are replaced by drier, scaly skin. If it doesn't clear up completely by the age of five, it tends to improve in adolescence.

In adults, it tends to be less severe, and affects the bends of the elbows, behind the knees and the back of the neck. It is also often linked with urticaria or hives, and women sometimes suffer from dermatitis of the nipples.

Dermatitis herpetiformis

This is a very itchy (burning and stinging) skin rash with red raised patches around 1cm in diameter containing small blisters; it usually occurs on the elbows, back of the neck and scalp, upper back, buttocks and knees. It's caused by sensitivity to gluten (a protein found in wheat, rye, barley and oats) and is more common in men than in women. It's most likely to start when you're between 15 and 40 years old.

Discoid or nummular eczema

This type of eczema usually affects adults, particularly those who had atopic eczema as babies. It appears suddenly as coin-shaped areas of red skin, normally on your trunk or lower legs, which can become itchy, weep fluid and then be infected by bacteria. It looks similar to ringworm, so your doctor may need to perform some tests to check whether the problem is ringworm or eczema. The patches can vary in size from around 4cm to 10cm; they are often slightly swollen.

It tends to be worse in winter, in conditions of low humidity or dry air. Using moisturizing creams and humidifying the air in the home can help.

It may be caused by an allergy to bacteria, and your GP may prescribe antibiotics.

Hand eczema

This is also known as vesicular or pompholyx eczema. Itchy blisters up to 2.5cm across develop on the hands, usually on the palms but also on the sides of the fingers; they may also appear on the soles of the feet. It's usually caused by a contact allergy to detergents – see the section on *Contact dermatitis* – and is often worse in hot weather. The blisters may burst and become infected, so you may need antibiotics to clear up the infection; the skin may also become very dry and cracked.

Irritant eczema

This is where the skin reacts to an irritant or an allergen. See the section on *Contact dermatitis*.

Neurodermatitis, or lichen simplex

This is where skin becomes thickened, itchy and discoloured; it often affects the neck, wrist, arm, elbow or ankle, and is caused by rubbing or scratching the skin repeatedly. It's more common in women than in men, and is treated by antihistamines and steroid creams.

Photosensitive or chronic actinic eczema

This is a form of eczema caused by a reaction to sunlight. It's more likely to affect men than women, and tends to be worse in the spring and summer. Skin that's exposed to the sun (usually the face, neck, back of the hands and arms) is affected by a red rash which becomes itchy, sore and may weep. The rash can also spread to skin that hasn't been exposed to the sun.

It can also occur as a result of taking medication, such as antihistamines and anti-arthritis drugs, and using soap with antibacterial ingredients.

Using a sunscreen against UVA and UVB rays can help.

Seborrhoeic eczema

In babies, this is also known as "cradle cap". It is common in babies under a year old, and the exact cause is unknown. It starts on the scalp and spreads quickly, but it is not sore or itchy; it clears up in a few months, particularly with the help of moisturizing creams and bath oils and leaving the baby's nappy off as often as possible.

In adults, it is most likely to affect you if you're aged between twenty and forty, and it is believed to be caused by a yeast growth. It starts on your scalp as mild dandruff but the red, scaly, itchy rash may also spread to areas of your skin that contain a lot of sebaceous (oil-secreting) glands, such as your face, chest and back. Sweating may make it worse or cause secondary infection.

Using a medicated shampoo containing selenium sulphide, zinc pyrithione or an antiseptic may help.

Skin-to-skin contact dermatitis

If you are very overweight, you may have folds of skin which rub together – particularly under your breasts, in your groin or in your armpits. This chafing, called intertrigo, can cause dermatitis, particularly if you sweat a lot. There may also be a secondary infection, particularly thrush. The best way of sorting out the problem is to lose weight to stop the folds of skin occurring.

Varicose or statis eczema
This type of eczema usually affects your lower legs, particularly around your ankles, and is caused by poor circulation in the lower legs. The skin becomes irritated, inflamed, fragile and easily damaged, and the legs may also swell. It's more likely to affect you if you're middle-aged or older, if you're female, if you're overweight, and if you have varicose veins or have suffered from deep vein thrombosis. If it's untreated, your skin may become ulcerated. It's thought to be caused by circulation problems in the legs. Wearing support stockings or compression bandages helps; in severe cases, varicose veins can be surgically removed or sealed with a laser.

What are the symptoms?
- Dry skin, sometimes leading to scaliness
- Itchiness (pruritis)
- Redness and inflammation of the skin
- A "bubbly" rash
- "Infected" eczema (where the you've scratched the skin and it splits, becoming more prone to infection, then cracks and weeps)
- Flaky skin (particularly on the scalp)
- *For dermatitis herpetiformis*: a red itchy rash, abdominal discomfort, mild coeliac disease and anaemia (when the stomach is affected so that vitamin B12 is not absorbed properly)
- Thickened skin (after repeated rubbing and scratching) with a dry, wrinkled appearance

Allergens that provoke eczema
AIRBORNE ALLERGENS: house dust mite droppings, pet dander (skin flakes), pollen, mould
CHEMICALS: persulphate
DRY ENVIRONMENT
EMOTIONAL STRESS
FOOD (usually in children's eczema): the main culprits are eggs, milk, wheat, fish, chocolate, nuts, yeast, citrus fruits, food additives (particularly azo dyes, benzoates and sulphites), peas,

beans, soya, lentils, tomato, currants, berries; others which can cause eczema include avocado, barley, carrot, celery, cheese, flour, grapes, peanuts, plum, potato, rice, shellfish, soya,

GLUTEN (for dermatitis herpetiformis)

GRAIN MITES

HERBS/SPICES: allspice, cardamom, clove, coriander, garlic, ginger, mace, pepper

IRRITANTS such as wool, pet hair, pet saliva, feathers, biological washing powders, fragrance in skin creams and fabric softeners, creams containing Parabens

MEDICATION: particularly aspirin, beta blockers and antihistamine cream

OVERHEATING OR SWEATING

WEATHER: eczema is often worse in cold weather

How is it diagnosed?

Atopic eczema is usually diagnosed on skin examination, so the majority of sufferers do not need further tests.

For dermatitis herpetiformis, a biopsy or removal of a piece of skin will show IgA deposits in the skin.

Complications

Secondary infection

This is the most important complication, when germs are able to pass through the damaged skin into the deeper layers of the skin and grow in a warm, moist environment. The most common germs affecting eczematous skin include:

- Staphylococci (causing impetigo or boils – the skin will be inflamed, with increased oozing and crusting; it tends to be on the face, but your lymph nodes in your armpits, groin, back of the knees and elbows may also be tender and enlarged)
- Herpes simplex virus (causing cold sores) – this causes eczema herpeticum, a blistery rash which forms on top on the eczematous rash; the blisters often have a central depression and are filled with pus, and the skin on the top is fragile and easily rubbed away, leading to weeping and crusting. It often starts on the face and spreads to the rest of the body; it may clear up of its own accord (usually after the fifth day) or it can be treated by acyclovir (Zovirax)
- Human papillomavirus (warts)
- Fungi (athlete's foot and ringworm)

• *Mollusum contagiosum* virus (small lumps with a dimpled centre)

Kaposi's varicelliform eruption
This is also called eczema herpeticum, and occurs when the eczema patches are infected by a virus – usually the herpes simplex virus or coxsackie virus. It looks like chickenpox (varicella); the blisters filled with blood can cover the whole of the skin, and the virus may also affect the brain and spinal cord. There may also be a high fever.

It is treated with acyclovir (Zorvirax), though severe cases can be fatal.

The best way of avoiding it is to ensure that if you (or a child) have eczema, don't allow anyone with a cold sore to kiss you.

Medical treatments available
Emollients
These reduce water loss and prevent the dryness normally associated with eczema. They are applied directly to the skin, used as soap substitutes or added to the bath. You'll need to test a small amount on the skin, first, in case you're sensitive to some of the ingredients.

Topical corticosteroids
If you suffer from flare-ups (where the skin becomes inflamed) you'll need a corticosteroid to reduce the inflammation and itchiness and bring your eczema back under control. The strength of the cream prescribed by your doctor will depend on your age, how severe and widespread your condition is, and which part of the body is affected.

Oral steroids
In severe cases, if topical corticosteroids do not work, your GP or consultant dermatologist may prescribe oral steroids. If you are taking steroids, your GP will advise you to carry a card stating this, as the steroids could affect emergency treatment if you're involved in an accident.

Wet wrapping
This is used to soothe itchy, dry skin – a "wet wrap" or a tar paste bandage is applied to the affected area over emollients and steroid creams, which helps your skin absorb the medication, and a dry tubular bandage is placed on top to protect your clothes. It also

prevents scratching, so it's more likely to be used for children. It's usually used at night, but can be used during the day if needed.

Antihistamine
Sedating antihistamines, such as trimeprazine and hydroxyzine, are used to reduce itching, which tends to be worse in bed and interfere with sleep. They are available in tablet or syrup form. Some of the newer antihistamines will not cause drowsiness.

Antibiotics
If you have infected eczema, you may need a course of antibiotics to clear up the secondary infection, either in the form of a cream or as a tablet (such as flucloxacillin), together with a topical steroid. Your GP will take a swab which will be used to grow a culture of the organisms; this will show which particular germ is causing the problem and which antibiotic will clear it up – your GP is likely to prescribe erythromycin or cephalexin. You need to finish the course, even if the infection clears up quickly, to avoid antibiotic-resistant bacteria developing. If it doesn't clear up, you may have resistant staophylococci in your nose; your GP will take another swab to check this, and then prescribe either an ointment to be used in your nose or oral antibiotics.

Anti-fungal cream
For infected seborrhoeic eczema

A gluten-free diet
For dermatitis herpetiformis – it may take up to 2 years for the rash to go; in the meantime, sulphone cream will help keep the rash under control.

Ultra-violet light treatment:
In cases of severe eczema, your dermatologist may refer you for phototherapy. There are three different types of treatment:
- UVB – taken twice a week for at least six weeks
- narrowband UVB – this is more likely to be given in a short course
- PUVA (psoralen ultra violet A) – where a psoralen (a chemical compound found in plants that sensitizes the skin to ultra-violet light) is either taken by mouth or used as a bath two hours before UVA treatment.

Eczema often recurs after the treatment has stopped; as there is an increased risk of skin cancer with excessive ultraviolet treatment, some dermatologists are concerned about its use.

Immune suppressants

If your eczema is severe and does not respond to standard treatments or even oral steroids, your dermatologist may prescribe a short course of a medicine which suppresses the immune system, such as cyclosporin A or azathioprine, to prevent the allergic reaction that causes your eczema. You will need regular blood tests to make sure that the drugs are not adversely affecting your kidneys, liver or blood.

Self-help tips

Reducing the itch

- Use cotton clothing and bedding to keep the skin cool and allow it to breathe – wool and synthetic fabrics such as polyester or nylon can irritate
- Keep children's nails short and distract them to stop scratching
- Cold compresses may help
- Avoid tight-fitting clothes
- Avoid sports that make you sweat a lot
- Press the itchy area rather than scratching

Leisure and school

- Use emollients to protect your skin before swimming, then wash off the chlorine afterwards and apply more emollient
- Use an emollient on your small child's skin before he plays with sand, water, finger paints or play dough; wash his skin well afterwards and reapply the emollient
- At school, ask for your child to sit in a cool corner, away from radiators and sunny windows
- Use protective clothing as a barrier against glues, paints, clays, chemicals and detergents

Reducing the effect of the house dust mite

See section on *Asthma*, above

Avoiding moulds

See section on *Asthma*, above

Avoiding pet allergens
See section on *Asthma*, above

Avoiding pollen
See section on *Hay fever* in this chapter, plus
• Shower and wash your hair before applying emollient creams

Cleaning and washing
• Keep baths lukewarm rather than hot, and stay in for only a short time – excessive bathing (especially with hot water) will affect the skin's natural sebaceous oil (sebum) and make our skin dry out. Adding colloidal oatmeal to your bath can help moisturize your skin and reduce inflammation.
• Wash new clothes before you wear them, to remove any excess dye or chemical
• Use non-biological, unperfumed washing powders and cleansers and make sure detergents are rinsed out thoroughly
• Avoid using fabric softeners – the perfume can cause a flare-up
• Consider fitting a water softener if you live in an area of hard water – salts in hard water can make your skin dry

Housework and gardening
• Use rubber gloves with cotton linings for housework and food preparation
• Wear thick gardening gloves

Relaxation
• Stress can make eczema worse; relaxation techniques can help.

Swimming
• Try to find an non-chlorinated pool (chlorine can sting)
• Before entering the water, apply a thick coat of emollient to prevent stinging
• Rinse off all chlorine afterwards in the shower and apply more emollient to soothe the skin

Alternative therapies that can help
Aromatherapy
• Recommended essential oils: chamomile, fennel, geranium (for weeping eczema), hyssop, juniper (for weeping eczema), lavender, sandalwood
• For massage (clear skin only): calendula oil as a base for dry skins; otherwise, a bland carrier oil such as sweet almond.

Dilute 1 drop essential oil to 5ml carrier oil.
- Cold compress: use 6 drops of oil in 500ml cold water, dip a cloth into it and wring it out, then lay the cloth on the affected area until it has reached body temperature.

Evening primrose oil
- Capsules, taken for 2–3 months, help a small number of people with atopic eczema.

Herbalism
- Aloe vera
- Calendula ointment
- Camomile infusion (bathe with)
- Heartsease – use an ointment for weeping eczema

Homeopathy
- Calcarea carbonica – for cracked and itching skin (6c)
- Graphites – for eczema with weepy and cracked skin (6c)
- Hepar sulphuris – for eczema (6c)
- Natrum muriaticum – for eczema (6c)
- Graphites cream – for dermatitis
- Rhus toxicodendron – for eczema (6c)
- Sulphur – for eczema (6c)

Relaxation

Chinese herbal medicine
The formula varies for each patient. You should have regular blood tests, as some Chinese herbal treatments have caused liver damage.

Bach flower remedies
- Rescue Remedy cream can help

COELIAC DISEASE
What is coeliac disease?
Coeliac disease occurs when the body reacts to the protein gliadin, which is found in gluten, a substance in grains such as wheat, barley and rye. The protein damages the lining of the small intestine, which becomes inflamed and means that the gut can't absorb adequate nutrients from food. Coeliac disease is also

known as gluten sensitive enteropathy (intestinal damage), idiopathic steatorrhea, primary malabsorptive disease or non-tropical sprue.

Although it was once thought that coeliac disease was a childhood problem, symptoms can occur at any age, and recent Coeliac Society statistics show that most sufferers are diagnosed between 30 and 45 years.

Roughly 1 in 1500 people in the UK suffer from coeliac disease, and the condition runs in families – studies show that roughly 10 per cent of a coeliac's immediate relatives have the potential to develop the disease. It affects women slightly more than men. You're also more likely to suffer from coeliac disease if you have diabetes and need to take insulin.

You may also find that you're lactose intolerant if you have coeliac disease, because when the villi in the intestine lining are damaged, they can't produce the enzyme lactase, which helps the body absorb lactose (the sugar in dairy products). However, if you follow a gluten-free diet, the gut will heal within around six months, and you will be able to eat food containing lactose again.

What are the symptoms?

In *babies*, following the introduction of solids that contain gluten:
- pale, bulky, offensive-smelling stools
- becoming miserable and lethargic
- generally failing to thrive

In *children*:
- weight loss or failure to thrive
- small stature
- abdominal distension, possibly with pain
- vomiting
- diarrhoea
- tiredness
- lethargy
- inability to concentrate
- breathlessness

In *adults*, as above plus:
- a history of abdominal or intestinal upsets
- anaemia
- abdominal discomfort
- bloating
- constipation

- depression
- iron deficiency
- mouth ulcers
- weight loss
- wind
- skin changes – scaliness, bruising (due to deficiency of vitamin K), dermatitis herpetiformis

Because nutrients are not being absorbed, you may also have problems with bones, such as deformity, pain or liability to fracture.

Allergens that provoke coeliac disease
GLUTEN

WHEAT

RYE

BARLEY

OATS

How is it diagnosed?
A gastroenterologist will take a biopsy, or a small amount of material from the surface of the small intestine: the operation is also known as an endoscopy or a jejunal biopsy. The operation itself takes about ten or fifteen minutes, but you will need to have a local anaesthetic, which may make you drowsy afterwards.

The biopsy is done by putting an endoscope (a flexible telescope) through the mouth into the stomach and upper intestine, which allows the specialist to inspect the lining; a sample is taken by sucking a small piece of the intestinal lining into the tube, and a small knife cuts off the tissue and closes the hole. You may be given a mild sedative beforehand. If you have sensitivity to gluten, the biopsy will show that the villi (projections) in the lining of your intestine have become flattened.

If the test is positive, you will be put on a gluten-free diet, and your specialist will monitor the results for the first six months. If you show no improvement (and have stuck to the diet rigidly), there may be other food intolerance involved, or the problem may not be coeliac disease.

A CAP-RAST or ELISA blood test may also show a reaction to gluten.

Other blood tests will show if you are deficient in iron, folic acid or minerals.

Medical treatments available

A strict gluten-free diet is the only way to relieve symptoms; this should be followed for life, to avoid serious complications such as infertility in women, osteoporosis, and narrowing of the intestine. You should be able to tolerate rice, millet and maize; the Coeliac Society have a list of gluten-free foods.

Self-help tips

- Check labels for the presence of wheat flour, particularly processed foods where it's used as a processing aid, a binder, a filler or as a carrier for flavourings and spices
- Avoid tinned fruit and vegetables, cheeses that contain preservatives (e.g. spreads and dips), tinned or breaded meats, alcohol made from grain (beers, spirits, liqueurs), tinned soups, sweets, sauces and desserts – check that they're gluten-free
- Replace breads and flours based on wheat starch with products made from naturally gluten-free foods such as potato, rice or soya

FOOD ALLERGIES

What are food allergies?

Food allergies occur when the body cannot tolerate certain foods.

This may be:
- a normal reaction to consuming too much of a particular food (e.g. an increased heart rate after too much coffee)
- the body's reaction to an irritant food (food intolerance or sensitivity) where the IgE antibodies react with food protein
- the body being deficient in the enzymes needed to digest certain foods
  - lactase, used to digest milk
  - aldehyde dehydrogenase, used to digest alchohol
  - phenylketonuria (PKU), lacking the enzyme needed to metabolize the amino acid phenylalanine (needed for growth and development)
- false food allergy, where chemical components in food bind to the mast cells, which then release the same chemical messengers in the same way that IgE works – usually caused by lectins (found in beans, peanuts, pulses and wheat) and peptides (found in chocolate, egg white, fish, pork, shellfish,

strawberries and tomatoes); other foods that may trigger a similar reaction include buckwheat, mango, mustard, papaya, raw pineapple and sunflower seeds
- a true allergenic response, where the body produces IgE – usually in response to a protein (up to 90 per cent of allergic reactions are caused by the "big eight" of milk, eggs, peanuts, wheat, soya, fish, shellfish and nuts; the most severe reactions are caused by peanuts, nuts, fish and shellfish).

The rule of thumb is that if your symptoms are immediate, it's likely to be an allergy; if your symptoms take longer (for example, hours) to appear and involve larger amounts of foods, it's more likely to be an intolerance.

Food allergies are more common in young children – it's thought that 5 per cent of children suffer from them – or if you have other allergies such as hay fever and eczema; food allergies can trigger other allergies, such as asthma, or make them worse. According to the Food Allergy Network, around 40 per cent of Americans believe that they are allergic to food, whereas the real figure is around 1 per cent and the rest is either intolerance or sensitivity.

The effects of an allergic reaction can last from several minutes to hours, depending on how much of the food/drink has been consumed and the intensity of your allergy or intolerance. An allergy to a specific food or drink is usually lifelong, although some children grow out of allergies to milk, egg or soya.

If you are taking beta-blockers and have a food allergy, you are more at risk of anaphylactic shock.

You may also suffer from exercise-induced anaphylaxis – where exercising and eating certain foods leads to severe urticaria, wheezing and anaphylactic shock. The foods that are most often implicated are celery, carrots, apples, shellfish and chicken.

What are the symptoms?
The symptoms of sensitivity, intolerance or enzyme deficiency include:

Gastro-intestinal symptoms
- Bloating
- Constipation
- Crohn's disease
- Diarrhoea (often watery)

- IBS
- Indigestion
- Nausea
- Stomach cramps
- Stomach ulcer
- Vomiting

Headache
- Headache
- Migraine

Joint/muscular problems
- Joint pain
- Muscular aches
- Rheumatoid arthritis (exacerbating rather than causing)

Mouth symptoms
- Mouth ulcers (often recurrent)
- "Oral allergy syndrome" – itching of palate and swelling of lips and tongue

Nasal/ear symptoms
- Glue ear
- Rhinitis

Psychological symptoms
- Anxiety
- Depression
- Fatigue
- Hyperactivity (children)

Skin symptoms
- Angioedema (swollen lips, face, tongue)
- Flushed face
- Urticaria
- Water retention (oedema)

The symptoms of a true allergic reaction (i.e. one that involves IgE antibodies) include:
- eczema
- rash around the mouth
- diarrhoea
- stomach cramps

- tingling of lips
- rapid swelling of the lips
- swelling of the tongue
- severe and violent vomiting, if the food has been eaten
- widespread urticaria, if the food has been absorbed into the bloodstream
- wheezing (particularly in children)
- sharp drop in blood pressure
- abdominal pain and distension

How is it diagnosed?

Tests that can confirm food allergy/intolerance include:
- elimination
- food challenge
- intradermal test
- skin prick test
- CAP-RAST (Radio-Allergo-Sorbent Test)
- ELISA (Enzyme Linked Immuno-Sorbent Assay)
- ELISA/ACT (Enzyme Linked Immuno-Sorbent Assay/ Activated Cell Test

Prognosis

Children often grow out of food allergy; you may become less sensitive to certain foods over time. However, you should always undertake any tests under medical supervision, in case of analphylactic shock.

The elimination diet

The elimination diet is a way of confirming the diagnosis. Your diet will include a very restricted number of foods, based on those that are least likely to cause an allergic reaction, for example:

- one meat (such as chicken or lamb)
- one fruit (such as pears)
- one vegetable (such as carrots)
- one starch (such as rice or potato)
- one fat (milk-free margarine or a specific vegetable oil)

If your system can accept these foods, other foods will be added one at a time, so it's easy to see the source of the problem if you start to develop symptoms. The additional food is reintroduced for two or three days in a row before another food is reintroduced, because reactions often take two or three days to show up.

If you react to a newly reintroduced food, note your reaction, stop eating that food, and leave it a couple of days to let the reaction run its course before you reintroduce another food.

Common foods used include:

- *Meat*: bacon, beef, chicken, ham, lamb, turkey
- *Legumes and pulses*: kidney beans, lentils, soy
- *Fruit*: apricots, blueberries, cherries, pears, pineapple, plums, prunes
- *Vegetables*: artichokes, asparagus, carrots, celery, lettuce, sweet potato
- *Starch*: potato, rice
- *Fat*: olive oil, milk-free margarine
- *Other*: arrowroot, salt, sugar, white vinegar
- *Beverages*: ginger ale, soy milk, water

Allergens that provoke food allergies

The "big eight" are milk, eggs, peanuts, wheat, soya, fish, shellfish and nuts. Other foods include fruit, vegetables, other grains, legumes, herbs, spices, meat, poultry and food additives (particularly colours from azo dyes and "coal tar dyes" – see list under *Asthma*, above)

Medical treatments available

If you have accidentally eaten something that you are allergic to and your symptoms are not part of an anaphylactic reaction, the following medication can help:

- antihistamines – for gastrointestinal symptoms, urticaria, sneezing and a runny nose
- bronchodilators – for wheezing: can relieve asthma symptoms
- corticosteroids – to reduce inflammation

Self-help tips

After an attack:

- drink clear liquids (such as water, juice or tea) frequently during the day
- reduce your normal activities until the symptoms stop
- if you feel sick, suck an ice-cube
- stick to a bland diet for a couple of days after symptoms subside (cereal, rice, custard, baked potatoes)
- avoid fruit, alcohol and spicy foods for a few more days after returning to your normal diet

Other problems that can be caused by food allergies

Hay fever
See section on *Hay fever* below

Hyperactivity
This is also known as attention deficit disorder (ADD), when children over the age of four find it difficult to concentrate and always seem to be on the go, sleep less than other children, fidget, have no sense of danger, and are often impulsive or reckless. Foods containing salicylates and food additives (particularly the "azo dyes") may have an effect – see the section on *Hyperactivity* in the chapter on *Symptoms* for more details.

Migraine
Migraine affects around one in ten people. It is also known as a "vascular headache" because it affects the blood vessels. Before a migraine, the vessels around the brain narrow, then widen again to a much greater size than usual – this is when the headache occurs. There are several different types of migraine:

- Migraine without aura – this is a severe, often one-sided throbbing pain; it may be accompanied by nausea, vomiting, dizziness, sensitivity to light, flashing lights, sensitivity to noise and tingling in the limbs. Your face may also change colour – either it will flush (usually if you blush easily) or, more commonly, it will go very pale.
- Migraine with aura – as above, but there is an "aura" or warning signal that a migraine is about to occur. The aura lasts as the blood vessels constrict – anything between a couple of minutes and an hour – and may include flashing lights, double vision, or blind spots, with pins and needles or a feeling of weakness in the limbs, hands and feet

During an attack, you may feel very hot or cold, and be extremely sensitive to smells as well as light. The attack may last for anything between a couple of hours and two or three days, and you may find that the only thing that helps is lying down in a darkened room.

Migraine seems to affect three to four times as many women as men, and can start at any age, although it tends to start before the twenties. There may be a genetic link, as migraine sufferers often have relatives who have migraines.

Certain foods may cause migraines, though you may be sensitive to only one or two foods, and only in certain circumstances – for example, women may react to a food such as chocolate at a certain time in the menstrual cycle. The most likely triggers for migraine are:

ALCOHOL (particularly red wine, brandy and whisky)

AMINES including phenylethylamine, tyramine

DRINK: beer, wine

FOOD: aubergine, avocado, banana, beans, beef, broad beans, caffeine, cheese (particularly matured or blue), chocolate, citrus fruit, egg, fermented food, figs, fish, fish (pickled), game, nuts, onions, plum, pork, prune, sauerkraut, sausages, smoked foods, soy sauce, spinach, strawberry, tomato, vinegar and pickled foods, wheat, yeast

FOOD ADDITIVES: nitrites, nitrates, monosodium glutamate

FRIED FOOD

HERBS/SPICES: parsley

HISTAMINE

SEROTONIN

TOBACCO

Your GP may carry out tests to check that your migraines are not a symptom of a serious illness. Tests include:

- CAT scan (Computerized Tomography) – a precise and detailed X-ray scan of the brain to check for abcesses, tumours and malformation; it takes about twenty minutes
- ECG (Electrocardiogram) – measures the electrical activity of the heart and picks up abnormalities
- EEG (Electroencephalogram) – small metal electrodes are placed on your scalp to measure the pattern of electrical activity in the brain, known as "alpha rhythm" when the eyes are closed
- Lumbar puncture – this is done under a local anaesthetic; you lie on your side and a sample of cerebro-spinal fluid is taken through a fine needle introduced into your lower back; this is analyzed to check for diseases such as meningitis or a burst blood vessel on the surface of the brain (subarachnoid haemorrhage)

Your GP may offer you medication to treat individual attacks and prevent or reduce the severity and frequency of future attacks. These will include:

- painkillers (often aspirin, codeine, paracetamol, tolfenamic acid) – you may be sensitive to aspirin)

- anti-sickness drugs
- ergotamine – for severe but less frequent attacks; now less commonly prescribed
- 5-HT agonists such as Naratriptan, Rizatriptan, Sumatriptan – available as tablets, nasal sprays and injections – works with serotonin to regulate the width of the blood vessels – should not be used daily
- beta-blockers

Your GP may also suggest that you visit a specialist migraine clinic.

Ways of helping migraine
- Keep your blood sugar levels stable – eat breakfast, eat regularly and avoid sugary snacks
- Try a cold pack (e.g. frozen peas) or hot pack
- Hot and cold compresses
- Dark glasses
- Try to drink plenty of water during the attack to avoid dehydration
- Acupressure bands (for nausea)

Alternative therapies that can help
- **Acupuncture**
- **Alexander Technique**
- **Aromatherapy**: massage helps, particularly with essential oils of lovage, lavender, rosemary
- **Chiropractic**
- **Feverfew**: eat the chopped leaves in a sandwich
- **Homeopathy**
- **Hypnosis**
- **Osteopathy**
- **Reflexology**

Irritable Bowel Syndrome

IBS is a group of symptoms which persist without any serious underlying cause. It's very common: a third of people in the UK suffer occasional symptoms, according to the Digestive Disorders Foundation, and one in ten of those seek medical treatment. It tends to start in people aged between fifteen and forty, but may occur at any age. It's believed that IBS is caused by an abnormality of bowel contraction, which may be linked to problems in the nervous system that supplies the gut.

Symptoms

- Abdominal pain or spasm, often felt on the lower left side of the abdomen, which may be worse in the early hours of the morning; it's likely to be worse if you're constipated, and may be linked to menstruation in women
- Fullness and bloating, making clothes feel uncomfortable; your abdomen may feel tender and you may suffer from flatulence and rumbling
- Nausea, though not usually with vomiting
- Changes in bowel habit – often constipation, diarrhoea or an alternation between the two; you may find it difficult or uncomfortable to open your bowels, or feel that you're not completely empty after a bowel movement, and you may occasionally suffer from a feeling of urgency or even bowel incontinence. Diarrhoea is caused by the food moving too quickly through the system; with constipation, the food moves more slowly through the system and water absorption causes the faeces to become dry and hard. You may find increased urgency to go to the toilet
- *Proctalgia fulax* – this is a sharp pain, felt low down inside the rectum; it tends to pass within five minutes, and is not a common symptom (although IBS sufferers are more likely to experience it than non-sufferers)

Medical investigations

- Abdominal and (for women) gynaecological examination, to check that the problem is related to the gut and not endometriosis – a swab may also be taken for laboratory testing to check for bacteria
- Rectal examination
- Blood test (for anaemia)

If your GP is satisfied that there are no other likely causes, he may diagnose IBS. He may also send you to hospital for further tests to make sure that the problem isn't lactose intolerance, ulcers, diverticular or Crohn's disease.

Ways of helping IBS include

- Avoiding foods which make the symptoms worse – often rich or spicy foods, dairy products, citrus fruits, tea and coffee, bread and cereals
- Avoiding foods that cause gas – such as pulses, onions, cabbage, Brussels sprouts, dried fruit – and foods or drinks that allow

extra air into the stomach, such as chewing gum, sucking boiled sweets and drinking fizzy drinks
- Eating slowly
- Drinking herbal teas that have a calming effect on the digestive system, such as camomile, fennel, ginger and peppermint
- Increasing the amount of fibre in the diet
- Stress relief
- Eating little and often – large, infrequent meals tend to make it worse

Medical treatments
- *Abdominal pain*: anti-spasmodic drugs (alverine citrate, dichlomine, hyoscine butylbromide, mebeverine, propantheline) which reduce the strength of gut contraction
- *Diarrhoea*: loperamide (Imodium) or codeine phosphate, which slow down the passage of waste through the body and increase the absorption of water
- *Constipation*: extra fibre in the diet; bulking agents (e.g. Regulan) which increase the passage of waste through the body and retain more water, making faeces softer and easier to expel (though this can also produce more wind and bloating)
- *Wind*: reduce intake of gas-forming foods, avoid bulk-forming laxatives and check for lactose intolerance
- Corticosteroids, to bring the disease under control – budesonide, hydrocortisone, prednolisone
- Aminosalicylates, to prevent relapses of ulcerative colitis – balsalazide, mesalazine, olsalazine, sulphasalazine

Alternative therapies that can help
- **Acupuncture**
- **Aromatherapy**: fennel for constipation; neroli for diarrhoea and stomach cramps; peppermint for digestive problems
- **Bach flower remedy** (Rescue remedy – cherry plum, clematis, impatiens, rock rose and star of Bethlehem, all preserved in brandy – 4 drops in glass of water and sip slowly)
- **Evening primrose oil**: particularly if your symptoms vary with the menstrual cycle
- **Homeopathy**
- **Hypnotherapy**

Rheumatism/ rheumatoid arthritis
See *Rheumatoid arthritis*, below

HAY FEVER

What is hay fever?

Hay fever – also known as seasonal allergic rhinitis or pollenosis – is an allergy to airborne pollens and mould spores. It affects 15 to 20 per cent of the population in Britain. It tends to run in families and can affect people at any age, though children don't tend to suffer under the age of one as it takes time for the levels of IgE to build up. If you suffer from hay fever, you also have a one in ten chance of developing asthma, and if your child suffers from both asthma and hay fever, the allergen is usually the same for both conditions. Symptoms may be so mild that you merely sneeze during the pollen season and don't realize that you actually have hay fever, or they might be so severe that summertime becomes a complete misery for you.

In hay fever, when pollen grains enter the nose, they are trapped by a layer of sticky mucus. The cilia (fine hairs) on the cells lining the nose start to try to move them out, but the enzyme lysozyme in the body's tissues digests the outside of the pollen grains and releases the proteins that set off the allergic reaction. This normally happens within twenty minutes of exposure to the allergen.

The body reacts to the invading proteins by producing IgE antibodies which attach to the mast cells in the lining of the nose; the pollen protein then attaches to the mast cells, causing them to release histamine. Histamine makes the cells in the lining of the nose produce more mucus; it also affects the membranes of the eyes, making them produce more fluid and causing watery eyes. The blood vessels swell and the increased blood supply also makes watery fluid leak from them, causing the tissues to swell, blocking the nose. When the nose is blocked, the watery secretions may then drip down from the back of the nose into the throat – known as "post-nasal drip" or catarrh. Swelling of the mucous membranes in the nose and throat can also cause temporary blockage of the eustacian tubes (which equalize pressure on the ear drum), causing temporary deafness.

Histamine affects nerve endings, causing itching and a burning sensation, and also contracts the smooth muscles, including those in the airways.

As well as histamine, other chemicals are released from the mast cells. These include:

- proteases – enzymes that split proteins and damage small blood vessels
- prostaglandins – which stimulate nerve endings
- leukotrienes – which narrow the airways

What are the symptoms?
Not everyone has all the symptoms. Hay fever can cause:

Ear problems
- Temporary deafness
- Earache
- "Popping" in the ears

Eye problems
- Watering eyes
- Redness in eyes and eyelids
- Itching or gritty feeling in the eyes
- Swelling of the whites of the eyes

Headache
- Headache due to sinusitis (caused by swelling in the nose)

Nose problems
- Sneezing
- Runny or blocked nose
- Itching in the nose, throat, and deep in the ears – children often rub their noses upwards to relieve the itch, and the continual rubbing eventually causes a crease or ridge across the lower part of the nose, called an "allergic salute"
- Nose bleeds

Psychological problems
- Irritability
- Depression
- Tiredness

Respiratory problems
- Wheezing
- A feeling of tightness in the chest
- Coughing – often a dry cough that appears and disappears suddenly, with no apparent cause
- Constant clearing of the throat

Allergens that provoke hay fever
CHEMICALS: anhydrides, epoxy resin
COSMETICS: citronella oil
FOODS: grapes
FUNGI: moulds can release allergenic spores any time from May to

October. The most common mould pollens that affect people are *Aspergillus*, *Cladosporium* and *Alternaria*.

GRASS POLLENS: end of June to mid-July. The most common grass pollens that affect people are rye (*Lolium perennae*), cocksfoot (*Dactylis glomerata*) crested dog's tail (*Cynosurus cristatus*), Yorkshire fog grass (*Holcus lanatus*) and Timothy grass (*Phleum pratense*).

TREE POLLENS: generally in March and April. The most common tree pollens that affect people are ash, birch, elder, elm, maple, oak, pine and plane.

SCENT/FLAVOURING: peppermint oil

WEED POLLENS: August and September. The most common weed pollens that affect people are those from nettle dock, water dock and ragweed.

If you notice when your sneezing is at its worst, it can help to pinpoint your particular trigger.

Pollen tends to be released in the morning; it rises during the afternoon. In the countryside, the peak pollen count is usually between 3pm and 6pm; in towns, it's in the early evening, around 7.30pm, when the air cools enough to let the pollen drop again; and at the seaside, it's the evening when the wind changes and pollens that have been blown out to sea are brought back again.

Pollen counting is done by meteorologists at weather stations. A continuous jet of air is directed on to a specially prepared surface so that the pollen grains can stick to it. Because the volume of air is known (i.e. how long the air was directed on to the surface and the rate of airflow), when the pollen is counted under a microscope, the meteorologists can calculate the concentration of pollen in the air. Pollen counts are given in numbers of grains per cubic metre of air.

Weather conditions that cause the highest pollen counts are sunshine and rising temperatures, with no rain.

How is it diagnosed?
* Blood tests – ELISA and CAP-RAST
* Intradermal test (rare)
* Skin prick test

Medical treatments available
* *Antihistamines* – taken in tablet, capsule or liquid form or as nasal sprays. They help with nose and eye symptoms. The newer types of tablets (such as loratidine and cetirizine) don't

make you feel drowsy like the older versions, but you may need to experiment to find the one that suits you best. Don't take them with other sedative drugs (e.g. antidepressants or sleeping tablets) or alcohol. Best avoided if you're pregnant.

- *Decongestants* – sprays and drops – good at clearing a stuffed-up nose, but shouldn't be used for more than seven days at a time or you may get a rebound effect when you stop taking them. Don't use them if you are diabetic, have kidney, liver or heart problems, or suffer from high blood pressure.
- *Anti-allergy treatments* – used regularly, nasal sprays and eye drops or ointments containing sodium cromoglycate can help control symptoms, especially if they last more than a short time. Don't use them with contact lenses.
- *Corticosteroids* – using a steroidal nasal spray once or twice a day will reduce inflammation and help with both nose and eye symptoms. Check with your doctor rather than using over-the-counter sprays for under-12s or if you're pregnant or breastfeeding.

Self-help tips
Avoiding dust mites
- See under *Asthma*, above

Avoiding pollen
- Check pollen counts (often included in radio, TV and newspaper reports), and try to avoid going out when they're high; if you do have to go out, avoid grassy and leafy areas
- Remember that there's likely to be more pollen around first thing in the morning, in the early evening, on windy days and during thunderstorms
- Keep windows closed as much as possible to keep pollen out, especially in your bedroom
- Make the house a no-smoking zone – smoke may make the symptoms worse
- *Housework*: damp-dust; vacuum regularly with a bagless vacuum cleaner, particularly with a HEPA (high efficiency particulate) filter; replace your carpets with throw rugs (which trap pollen)
- *In the car*: keep car windows closed to keep pollen out; use HEPA pollen filters in your car
- *Gardening*: don't mow the lawn, rake up leaves or cut hay, and stay inside while it's being done; wear a hat when gardening to prevent pollen getting in your hair; don't use organic mulches

in the garden (e.g. tree bark and mushroom compost)

- *Washing*: don't hang washing out to dry, as pollens and moulds may collect in them
- *Clothing and personal hygiene*: wear wrap-around sunglasses to stop pollen getting in your eyes; wear a mask over your nose and mouth; shower and wash your hair every night to keep pollen from getting on your pillows and bedding.
- *Bedding*: cover bedding with a spare sheet to keep pollen from getting on your pillows and bedding – roll the sheet up carefully at night
- *Pets*: keep pets out of the house in the pollen season (they bring pollen in on their fur) or ask someone who is not allergic to pollen to brush them thoroughly before they come indoors

Relieving eye symptoms
- Lay a cool, damp facecloth over your eyes to relieve itching or bathe eyes in cool water
- If you wear contact lenses, consider changing to glasses – they'll protect your eyes against pollen as well as removing a potential source of irritation
- Don't rub your eyes

Relieving nose symptoms
- Smear petroleum jelly around your nose to prevent soreness – this also stops pollen going up your nose
- Try salt water nose drops
- Inhale steam, especially if you add a decongestant oil such as eucalyptus or menthol (stop if there's any irritation)

General
- Prepare a "hay fever kit" for outings of a damp face cloth, tissues, eye drops and any medication you use, and try eating local honey before the hay fever season begins, to help desensitize you to local pollen.

Alternative therapies that can help
Aromatherapy
- Lavender oil – dilute one drop to 5ml carrier oil and massage the side of the nose
- Steam inhalation can also help to relieve the symptoms, particularly if decongestant oils such as eucalyptus or peppermint are added to the warm water

Herbalism
- Buttercup Pol 'n' count – tablets contain garlic and echinacea; not suitable for children
- Gencydo – ointment containing boric acid, lemon juice and quince, to be applied inside the nostrils; also available as a nasal paint that can be diluted and used as a spray

Homeopathy
- Allium cepa – for hay fever (6c)
- Natrum muriaticum – for hay fever (6c)
- Pollenna – for hay fever; contains allium cepa, euphrasia officinalis, sabadilla officinarum
- Silica – for hay fever (6c)
- Weleda mixed pollens – for hay fever (30c); contains a wide range of pollens

PERENNIAL ALLERGIC RHINITIS

What is perennial allergic rhinitis?

Perennial allergic rhinitis has symptoms identical to those of hay fever, but it lasts all year round. It usually appears in sufferers before the age of 20, and may be diagnosed in babies a year old.

What are the symptoms?

See *Hay fever*, above

Allergens that provoke perennial allergic rhinitis

ALCOHOL
AMMONIUM PERSULPHATE (hairdressing chemical)
ANIMAL DANDER (skin flakes)
BIRD DROPPINGS
CAT SALIVA
CORK DUST
COTTON SEED
DUST LICE
ENZYMES
FLAX SEED
FLOUR (weevil-infested)
FOOD
FUR
HOUSE DUST MITES
INSECT PARTS
INSECT STINGS

LINT
MEDICATION (powdered form)
MOULDS – indoor; penicillum spores from cheese; spores from hay
MUSHROOM COMPOST
ORGANIC FIBRES
ORRIS ROOT
PYRETHRUM (insecticide)
SILVERFISH
VEGETABLE GUMS
WOOD PULP

Other problems caused by rhinitis

Allergic sinusitis

The sinuses are air-filled cavities in the skull; they are lined with membranes that link to the membranes in the nose. Rhinitis can cause inflammation in the sinus membranes, leading to headaches or an ache in the cheeks.

Glue ear (chronic secretory otitis media)

The nose is connected to the middle ear by the Eustachian tube, which equalizes pressure in the ears by draining fluid from them and letting air reach the ears. If the Eustachian tube becomes blocked with mucus from the nose, the air in the ear is replaced by a sticky mucus which sticks to the bones in the ear and causes deafness. It is particularly common in children, who may complain of itching in the ear or a feeling of the ears "popping".

Nasal polyps

If rhinitis is untreated for a long time, you may end up with nasal polyps, where the inflamed membranes have tiny grape-like protrusions. They are harmless but may make breathing difficult and you may also lose your sense of smell. If you are sensitive to aspirin, you may be more prone to nasal polyps.

Medical treatments available

- *Antihistamines* – taken in tablet, capsule or liquid form or as nasal sprays. They help with nose and eye symptoms. The newer types of tablets (such as loratidine and cetirizine) don't make you feel drowsy like the older versions, but you may need to experiment to find the one that suits you best. Don't take them with other sedative drugs (e.g. antidepressants or sleeping tablets) or alcohol. Best avoided if you're pregnant.
- *Decongestants* – sprays and drops – good at clearing a stuffed-up

nose, but shouldn't be used for more than seven days at a time or you may get a rebound effect when you stop taking them. Don't use them if you are diabetic, have kidney, liver or heart problems, or suffer from high blood pressure.

- *Anti-allergy treatments* – used regularly, nasal sprays and eye drops or ointments containing sodium cromoglycate can help control symptoms, especially if they last more than a short time. Don't use them with contact lenses.
- *Corticosteroids* – using a steroidal nasal spray once or twice a day will reduce inflammation and help with both nose and eye symptoms. Check with your doctor rather than using over-the-counter sprays for under-12s, or if you're pregnant or breastfeeding.
- *Immunotherapy treatment* – periodic injections given over a 3–5 year period which helps your immune system become more resistant to specific allergens

Self-help tips
- Mite avoidance – see *Asthma*, above
- Cat saliva and dander – wash the pet weekly with baby shampoo

Alternative therapies that can help
As *Hay fever*, above

PSORIASIS
What is psoriasis?
Psoriasis is a skin condition that is said to affect around 2–3 per cent of the world's population. Men tend to suffer from it more than women. It runs in families and the condition can come and go, though it usually develops either in the teens and twenties or in the fifties and sixties. If you have psoriasis, your skin cells, which normally take four weeks to grow from the bottom of the skin (or basal layer) to the top of the skin (or stratum corneum), grow much faster, reaching the top of the skin in only four or five days. These young skin cells are stickier than if they'd taken the normal amount of time to grow, and this stickiness causes the scaly appearance.

The blood vessels in your skin also become wider than normal, letting the blood flow through them more quickly; this causes the red appearance and also means that the patches of affected skin are more likely to bleed.

It is not contagious.

What are the symptoms?

Your skin has thick red patches, often oval in shape, which are covered by a silvery scale that flakes off quickly. It tends to appear mainly on the elbows, knees, scalp, trunk and back. It can look similar to eczema, and can therefore be difficult to diagnose; as a general rule, eczema tends to be itchy and psoriasis isn't, although some people with psoriasis find that the patches of skin are itchy.

The patch may start as a small reddened area that gradually increases in size. When it reaches around 5–8cm, it usually reaches a "stable phase" and stops growing.

Because the skin loses more water than normal, it becomes less pliable and cracks easily, particularly on the palms of the hands and the soles of the feet.

Types of psoriasis

Plaque-type psoriasis

The most common type – accounting for 96 per cent of cases – is plaque-type psoriasis, described above. It is also known as psoriasis vulgaris, or common psoriasis.

Erythrodermic psoriasis

This is an uncommon form of psoriasis, where the patches spread over the whole body, turning the skin red; the inflammation may cause you to lose a lot of water and body heat through the skin.

Flexural psoriasis

This is when the patches of psoriasis occur in the folds and creases of the body. It's also known as inverse psoriasis. It's more likely to affect you if you're over forty, and if you're overweight (and therefore have more folds of skin). The affected patches of skin will be moist rather than scaly, and can feel sore.

Guttate psoriasis

This is when the spots of psoriasis are very small and there are more of them; it tends to affect children more than adults, and often follows a sore throat, particularly streptococcal tonsillitis. They may clear up in a few weeks, or they may develop into larger patches.

Pustular psoriasis

This looks similar to ordinary psoriasis, but white blood cells cause pustules in the skin. It's more likely to occur on the palms of the hands and the soles of the feet.

This may occur on its own or as part of ordinary psoriasis. If your fingernails are affected, they may become pitted, giving the effect of a thimble; the nail may separate from the nail bed; and it may also change colour. If your toenails are affected, they may become thicker and look as if they have a fungal infection.

How is it diagnosed?

Usually, your GP will find it easy to diagnose psoriasis from the look of the affected skin and the fact that it doesn't itch. However, if your GP is unsure, he or she may scrape some skin cells off a patch and look at it through a microscope, to check that ringworm (a fungal infection that looks similar to both eczema and psoriasis) isn't responsible, or suggest patch testing, to check that it isn't eczema as the result of an allergy.

Allergens that provoke psoriasis

ALCOHOL
COFFEE
COLDS
COLD WEATHER
FOOD: citrus fruits, fatty foods, pineapple, tomatoes

Medical treatments available

- Ointments – including dithranol (brand names Alphodith, Anthranol, Antraderm, Dithrocream, Exolan) which is sometimes boosted by PUVA (psoralen ultra violet A) treatment – use petroleum jelly on normal skin around the affected area to prevent irritation by the ointment, wear plastic gloves during application, and don't apply to raw, blistered or oozing skin, or on the face, genital area or skin folds
- Tar treatments
- Corticosteroids
- PUVA treatment; this is where a psoralen (a chemical compound found in plants that sensitizes the skin to ultra-violet light) is either taken by mouth or used as a bath (30 minutes' immersion for smaller areas of skin) two hours before UVA treatment. Side effects include darkening of the skin (in all cases), an itching or stinging sensation (in up to 20 per cent

of cases), nausea, and redness of the skin. Most psoriasis sufferers find that the condition is greatly improved after 12–24 treatments.

Self-help tips
- Switch to non-biological detergents
- Aloe vera can help moisturize the skin
- Read labels on toiletries and cosmetics – avoid perfumes, lanolin
- Use natural fibres such as cotton or silk rather than synthetics for clothes and bed linen
- Wear gloves when doing housework – moisturize your hands first and use cotton gloves inside rubber gloves

Alternative therapies that can help
Aromatherapy
- Recommended essential oils: camomile, lavender. Use as a warm compress: use 6 drops of oil in 500ml hot water, dip a cloth into it and wring it out, then lay the cloth on the affected area until it has cooled to body temperature.

RHEUMATOID ARTHRITIS
What is rheumatoid arthritis?
Rheumatoid arthritis is a common disease which affects around 3 per cent of people in Britain, and can start at any age from childhood to the nineties, though the most common age for it to start is between thirty and fifty. It tends to affect women more than men and it isn't hereditary.

The disease causes the joints of the body to become inflamed. The blood flow to the join increases and causes redness and a feeling of warmth; cells and fluid build up in the synovium (the membrane that surrounds the joint) and cause swelling. The swelling causes the capsule of the joint to stretch, causing pain; the chemicals produced by the inflammation also irritate the nerve-endings, causing more pain.

What are the symptoms?
The symptoms include hot, swollen and tender joints, particularly the fingers, wrists, knees, toes and neck. Inflammation can lead to deformity and reduce your ability to use parts of the body; it may also cause thinning bones (due to decreased mobility).

Allergens that provoke rheumatoid arthritis

It is thought that certain foods exacerbate the symptoms, rather than cause them – particularly citrus fruit, red meat, dairy produce, tomatoes, potatoes, aubergines, tea, coffee and alcohol.

How is it diagnosed?

Your GP will make a clinical diagnosis – that is, he or she will examine you and ask you about your symptoms, and base a diagnosis on this information.

You may be offered a blood test; 80 per cent of people with arthritis are anaemic, and 80 per cent of people with rheumatism also have a protein in their blood which is produced by the immune system.

Your GP may also suggest having an X-ray, which can reveal any damage to the joints caused by inflammation. The feet tend to be affected first so, even if you haven't had a problem with your feet, your feet may be X-rayed.

Medical treatments available

- *Painkillers* – these tend to be used to top up other medication to help control the pain
- *Anti-rheumatic drugs* – these reduce the pain and stiffness by reducing the rheumatoid process, though they can take months to take effect and are a long-term treatment. They include sulphasalazine, gold, d-penicillamine (a distant relative of penicillin, but it is safe to take if you are allergic to penicillin), methotrexate
- *Anti-inflammatories*
- *Corticosteroids* – injected into the joint to relieve inflammation, injected into the muscle or vein to damp down a "flare-up", or taken by mouth
- *Cyclosporin*
- *Physiotherapy* (splints, exercises and manipulation to relieve pain)

Self-help tips

- Try to keep moving as much as you can; you need to reach a balance between resting to make the joints comfortable and using your joints enough to help retain movement and stop muscles wasting away. If a particular activity makes one or more joints become warm and swollen, or if you experience severe pain, then stop; otherwise, keep going!

- An elimination diet can help – the most likely foods to affect your condition include citrus fruit, red meat, dairy produce, tomatoes, potatoes, aubergines, tea, coffee and alcohol, although these vary from person to person.
- An epsom salts bath can also help – don't use soap in it
- Being overweight can put extra strain on your joints; maintaining your recommended weight can help.
- Essential fatty acids (EFAs) can also help because the body uses them to make prostaglandins and leukotrienes; the right balance of these is important to control inflammation. Omega-3 fatty acid is found in oily fish, especially mackerel, sardines, pilchards and salmon; eating oily fish three or four times a week can help with arthritis and rheumatism and also protect against heart disease.

Alternative therapies that can help
Acupuncture

Herbalism
- Evening primrose oil

Homeopathy

Osteopathy

URTICARIA

What is urticaria?
Urticaria is your skin's reaction to histamine in the upper layers of the skin. It is often due to a viral infection or a reaction to a drug, food or latex, and the reaction usually starts within less than an hour of exposure to the trigger.

It is estimated that at least 30 per cent of people will suffer from it at some point in their lives.

What are the symptoms?
The symptoms of urticaria are red, itchy, swollen areas of the skin; they vary in size and can appear anywhere on the body.

Types of urticaria
Dermographism
Caused by rubbing or chafing of the skin.

Cold-induced urticaria
Caused by exposure to low temperatures, e.g. swimming pools or ice cubes; the urticaria usually appears when the skin is warmed again, and is the most common form of urticaria in children.

Cholinergic urticaria
Caused by exercise, hot showers and/or anxiety; it's associated with sweating and the rash consists of tiny weals and reddened skin. It's more common in teenagers. Chemicals are also released from the nervous system, affecting the blood pressure and heart rate as well as the skin.

Aquagenic urticaria
Caused by contact with water, but not temperature related; it usually affects the neck, upper body and arms.

Pressure urticaria
Usually develops between two and six hours after exposure to pressure, for example tight clothing (belts, bra straps or socks), or the back/seat of a hard chair.

Solar urticaria
When the body is exposed to the sun; this may occur within a few minutes after exposure.

Allergens that provoke urticaria
AMINES: Chemicals: acetic acid, butyl alcohol, chloramphenicol, dimethyl sulphoxide, ethyl alcohol, formaldehyde, persulphate, phenol

COSMETICS: cetyl alcohol, cinnamic acid, cinnamic aldehyde

DRINK: beer, cider, tea, wine

ENZYMES: benzophenones

FOOD: apple, apricot, asparagus, aubergine, avocado, banana, barley, beans, beef, blackberries, blueberries, broad bean, buckwheat, caffeine, carrot, celery, cheese, cherries, chick pea, chocolate, cider vinegar, citrus fruit, corn, cucumbers, currants, dates, egg, fermented food, figs, fish, fish (pickled), game, gooseberries, grapes, kiwi fruit, lentil, lettuce, liquorice, malt, mango, melon, milk, mushrooms, mustard, nectarine, oats, orange, papaya, pea, peach, peanuts, peppers, pineapple, plum, pork, potato, prune, raisin, raspberry, sauerkraut, sausages, shellfish, soy sauce, soya, spinach, strawberry, tomato, wheat, wine vinegar, Worcestershire sauce, yeast

FOOD ADDITIVES: colours, preservatives, emulsifiers/stabilizers/ thickeners

HERBS/SPICES: aniseed, clove, cumin, curry powder, dill, fennel, mace, oregano, paprika, parsley, rosemary, tarragon, thyme, turmeric

ILLNESS OR INFECTION: colds (particularly in children), endocrine disorders, stress

INSECT STINGS

LATEX

MEDICATION: aspirin, other non-steroidal anti-inflammatory drugs (such as ibuprofen), high blood pressure medicines (ACE-inhibitors), painkillers containing codeine, penicillin, benzocaine, gentamycin, insulin, neomycin, streptomycin

POLLEN

SCENT/FLAVOURING: balsam of Peru, butyric acid, menthol

SALICYLATES

How is it diagnosed?
Your GP will make a clinical diagnosis based on your symptoms. He or she may also offer you a blood test or skin-prick test.

Medical treatments available
Some drugs or foods may take days to be eliminated from the body. In these cases, your GP may prescribe antihistamines to relieve your symptoms until the trigger food or drug is eliminated. In rare cases, if antihistamines do not work, your GP may prescribe an oral corticosteroid.

Self-help tips
• When the cause is identified, avoid the substance that causes it
• Read food labels
• Pressure urticaria – wear loose-fitting clothing
• Solar urticaria – wear protective clothing and apply sunscreen lotions when outdoors
• Avoid harsh soaps and frequent bathing to reduce the problem of dry skin, which can cause itching and scratching that can aggravate urticaria

Alternative therapies that can help
Herbalism
• Nelsons pyrethrum – liquid remedy for hives, bites and stings; also available as a spray. Contains arnica, calendula, echinacea, hypericum, ledum palustre, pyrethrum and rumex crispus.

8

A–Z of potential allergens

For more detailed information about symptoms and treatments, see the sections on *Symptoms* and *Treatments*.

ACE (angiotensin-converting enzyme) inhibitors

ACE inhibitors are drugs used to treat hypertension (high blood pressure) and heart failure. They allow the blood vessels to dilate by inhibiting the enzyme that produces angiotensin, which causes high blood pressure and constriction of the blood vessels.

Type of allergen: consumed

Symptoms, tests, treatments and self-help tips, see *Drugs*

Acetate

Acetate is a salt or ester of acetic acid. Its usual form is a synthetic textile fibre (made from partially hydrolyzed cellulose acetate) or a plastic-like film (made from cellulose triacetate).

Acetate is an irritant rather than a true allergen.

Type of allergen: inhalant

Likely sources of acetate: cosmetics – butyl acetate is used in nail varnish and perfume fragrance

Symptoms
Eye reactions: conjunctivitis

Tests
• Symptom diary

Treatments
Avoidance: in occupational situations, use protective equipment such as goggles to protect your eyes from the fumes.

Prescription medication: antihistamines, cromoglycate, nedocromil sodium, steroids, sympathomimetics

OTC remedies: antihistamines

Alternative remedies: herbalism, homeopathy

Self-help tips: for symptom relief see *Conjunctivitis* in the section on *Symptoms*

Acetic acid

Acetic acid is an organic acid ($C_2H_4O_2$), also known as ethanoic acid; it is usually associated with vinegar but also used to manufacture chemical products such as plastics. In manufacturing, it is made synthetically from alcohol and acetaldehyde.

Type of allergen: contact

Likely sources of acetic acid: plastics

Symptoms, tests, treatments and self-help tips, see *Chemicals*

Acetone

See *Solvents – ketone solvents*

Acetylene tetrachloride

See *Solvents – chlorinated hydrocarbons*

Acid

Acid is used in a variety of industrial processes. It can cause occupational asthma and dermatitis; if symptoms start soon after beginning work and improve at weekends or on holidays, occupational asthma or dermatitis should be suspected.

Type of allergen: inhalant, contact

Symptoms, tests, treatments and self-help tips, see *Chemicals*
See also *Acetic acid, Alpha-hydroxy acid, Cinnamic acid*

Acridine

Acridine is a fluorescing dye, used to stain DNA and RNA; it is often used to identify cancerous tumour cells.

Type of allergen: contact

Likely sources of acridine: chemical dyes, lipsticks

Symptoms, tests, treatments and self-help tips, see *Dyes*

Acrylate

Acrylate is a thickening agent. It can cause occupational asthma for adhesive handlers; if symptoms start soon after beginning work and improve at weekends or on holidays, occupational asthma should be suspected.

Type of allergen: inhalant

Likely sources of acrylate: waterproofing, waxy oils and nail varnishes

Symptoms
Respiratory reactions: asthma

Tests
• Symptom diary (including peak flow meter readings)

Treatments
Avoidance: in occupational situations, use protective equipment such as masks; improved ventilation can also help.

Prescription medication: anticholinergic drugs, antihistamines (exercise-induced), Beta2 (ß2) adrenoreceptor agonists, cromoglycate, nedocromil sodium, steroids, xanthine derivatives, zafirlukast

Alternative remedies: acupuncture (mild asthma only), Buteyko method, homeopathy, relaxation techniques, yoga

Self-help tips: for symptom relief, see *Asthma* in the section on *Symptoms*

Acrylic lacquer coatings and reducers
See *Solvents – aromatic hydrocarbons*

Acrylic sealant (window and door frames)
See *Volatile organic compounds*

Adhesives

Solvent-based adhesives can contain alcohols, ketones, hydro-carbons, plasticizers and free monomers.

Water-based adhesives can contain *formaldehyde* preservatives, amines, glycol ethers, alcohols, plasticizers and free monomers depending on the type of polymer used in the material.

Type of allergen: contact

Likely sources of adhesives
- *Solvent-based adhesives*: these materials are commonly used on laminates, tiles, parquet and vinyl flooring which can slow down the release of the volatile materials by absorption into wood or composite board sub-surfaces and/or by physically sealing them in.
- *Water-based adhesives:* as above, absorption into the surface and sealing of the adhesive can lead to long-term, slow release of some of these chemical volatiles.

Symptoms
Skin reactions: irritant contact dermatitis

Tests
- Skin patch

Treatments
Avoidance: use protective equipment such as gloves to protect your skin

Prescription medication: steroids, antihistamines

OTC remedies: coal tar, emollients, steroids

Alternative remedies: aromatherapy, Bach flower remedies, homeopathy

Self-help tips: for symptom relief, see *Contact dermatitis* in the section on *Symptoms*
See also *Acrylate, Benzene, Carpet, Chlorocresol* (preservative), *Colophony, Epoxy resin, Formaldehyde, Isocyanates, Latex, Nickel, Phenol, Solvents – esters, Volatile organic compounds*

Aerosols

The problem is likely to be with the hydrocarbon propellants used in spray cans.

Since the mid-1980s, the propellants of chlorinated hydrocarbon and chloro-fluorocarbon have been replaced in the main by hydrocarbon propellants such as pressurized carbon dioxide (CO_2). The type of propellant should be shown in the ingredient list on the side of the container.

Alternative products that won't cause a reaction: manual pump-sprayed products that do not contain any aerosol propellants
See also *Air freshener, Cleaning materials, Formaldehyde, Solvents – aromatic hydrocarbons, Solvents – halogenated solvents, Volatile organic compounds*

Aftershave
See *Benzocaine*

Airborne particles

These include chalk dust, coal dust, coffee, cork dust, cotton dust (which affects smokers more), flour, grains, powdered drugs, silk dust, soya bean dust, talcum powder, tea dust, tobacco dust, vegetable dust and wood dust.

Type of allergen: inhalant, contact

Symptoms
Eye reactions: allergic conjunctivitis

Respiratory reactions: asthma

Skin reactions: irritant dermatitis

Tests
- Blood test: CAP-RAST (castor bean, cotton seed green coffee bean, sunflower seed)
- Blood test: ELISA (castor bean, cotton seed, green coffee bean, isphagula, orris root, sunflower seed)
- Symptom diary (including peak flow meter readings)

Treatments
Avoidance
- Use protective equipment such as goggles, masks and gloves.

Prescription medication
- Conjunctivitis: antihistamines, cromoglycate, nedocromil sodium, steroids, sympathomimetics
- Asthma: anticholinergic drugs, antihistamines (exercise-induced), Beta2 (ß2) adrenoreceptor agonists, cromoglycate, nedocromil sodium, steroids, xanthine derivatives, zafirlukast
- Dermatitis: steroids, antihistamines

OTC remedies
- Conjunctivitis: antihistamines
- Dermatitis: coal tar, emollients, steroids

Alternative remedies
- Conjunctivitis: herbalism, homeopathy
- Asthma: acupuncture (mild asthma only), Buteyko method, homeopathy, relaxation techniques, yoga
- Dermatitis: aromatherapy, Bach flower remedies, homeopathy

Self-help tips: for symptom relief, see *Conjunctivitis, Asthma, Contact dermatitis* in the section on *Symptoms*

Air freshener
The problems are likely to be the propellant in the spray or the perfumes. See *Aerosols, Perfume*

Alternative products that won't cause a reaction
Use a bowl of bicarbonate of soda to remove odours.

Air pollutants

These include chemicals in the air, cigarette smoke, ozone (poor air quality) and wood smoke.

Type of allergen: inhalant

Symptoms

Mouth, nasal and ear reactions: rhinitis, sneezing

Respiratory reactions: asthma

Tests

- Symptom diary (including peak flow meter readings)
- Inhalation challenge

Treatments

Avoidance

- Use protective equipment such as masks where possible

Prescription medication

- Asthma: anticholinergic drugs, antihistamines (exercise-induced), Beta2 (ß2) adrenoreceptor agonists, cromoglycate, nedocromil sodium, steroids, xanthine derivatives, zafirlukast
- Rhinitis: antihistamines, decongestants, sodium cromoglycate, immunotherapy
- Sneezing: antihistamines, decongestants, sodium cromogylcate

OTC remedies

- Rhinitis: decongestants

Alternative remedies

- Rhinitis: aromatherapy
- Sneezing: acupuncture
- Asthma: acupuncture (mild asthma only), Buteyko method, homeopathy, relaxation techniques, yoga

Self-help tips

- Avoid smoking in the house
- Avoid walking or cycling on busy roads – ozone is concentrated at ground level and nitrogen oxides from car fumes can also make asthma worse
- Keep the house well ventilated to reduce fumes

- Breathe through your nose if you're in polluted air
- Keep car windows closed if you pull up behind a lorry or a bus, as more particles will be emitted from the vehicle as it sets off

Symptom relief, see *Asthma, Rhinitis, Sneezing* in the section on *Symptoms*
See also *Environmental pollutants, Fluoride*

Alcohol

Alcohol is oxidized into acetaldehyde in the body through the action of the enzyme alcohol dehydrogenase (ADH), and then oxidized again into acetic acid through the enzyme acetaldehyde dehydrogenase. The body finally converts acetic acid to carbon dioxide and it's breathed out.

It may be the alcohol itself that tightens your airways, or you may be affected by the congeners in the alcohol. Different types of alcohol (e.g. beer, wine, spirits) have different congeners, so if you can't drink wine you may be able to tolerate beer.

If your body has a low level of the enzyme aldehyde dehydrogenase, it will be unable to break down alcohol.

Type of allergen: inhalant, consumed

Symptoms
Gastrointestinal reactions: nausea, vomiting

Headache: migraine

Respiratory reactions: asthma

Skin reactions: flushing

Tests
- Symptom diary (including peak flow meter readings)
- Elimination diet
- Food challenge

Treatments
Avoidance
- Check labels on food and drink

Prescription medication
- Nausea: antihistamines
- Vomiting: anti-emetics
- Migraine: painkillers, anti-sickness drugs, ergotamine, 5-HT agonists, beta-blockers, sodium valproate, sumatryptan
- Asthma: anticholinergic drugs, antihistamines (exercise-induced), Beta2 (ß2) adrenoreceptor agonists, cromoglycate, nedocromil sodium, steroids, xanthine derivatives, zafirlukast

OTC remedies
- Nausea: antihistamines
- Vomiting: oral rehydration solution
- Migraine: aspirin, ibuprofen, paracetamol

Alternative remedies
- Nausea: aromatherapy, herbalism, homeopathy
- Vomiting: herbalism
- Migraine: acupuncture, Alexander technique, aromatherapy, chiropractic, herbalism, homeopathy, hypnosis, osteopathy, reflexology
- Asthma: acupuncture (mild asthma only), Buteyko method, homeopathy, relaxation techniques, yoga

Self-help tips: for symptom relief, see *Nausea, Vomiting, Migraine, Asthma* in the section on *Symptoms*

Alizarin

Alizarin is a red colour found originally in madder and produced artificially from anthracene.

Type of allergen: contact

Likely sources of alizarin: textile dyes

Symptoms, tests, treatments and self-help tips, see *Dyes*

Alkalase

Alkalase is used in the manufacturing of detergents.

Type of allergen: contact

Likely sources of alkalase: detergent

Symptoms, tests, treatments and self-help tips, see *Detergents*

Alkalis

Alkalis are caustic substances that are soluble in alcohol and water. They combine with fats and oils to form soap, and neutralize acids to form salts. Fixed alkalis include potash and soda; there are also vegetable alkalis, known as alkaloids, and volatile alkalis, such as ammonia.

Type of allergen: contact

Likely sources of alkalis: toilet bowl cleaners and detergents

Symptoms, tests, treatments and self-help tips, see *Chemicals*

Allspice

Allspice is a spice derived from the dried berries of the allspice tree. It is a contact allergen rather than an inhalant or consumed allergen.

Type of allergen: contact

Likely sources of allspice: processed meat; also used as a flavouring in foods

Symptoms, tests and treatments and self-help tips, see *Spices*
See also *Aromatherapy oils*

Allura red AC
See *Food additives – colourings*

Almond

Almond is from the tree *Prunus dulcis*. Two major allergens have been identified; one is heat-labile (i.e. it is only present in the raw state) and the other is heat-stable (i.e. it is not affected by heat and is therefore present in both raw and cooked states).

Type of allergen: contact, consumed

Symptoms, tests, treatments and self-help tips, see *Nuts*
See also Salicylates

You might also react to: apricots, cherries, peaches, plums

Alpha-amylase

Amylase is an enzyme that degrades starch, glycogen and other polysaccharides. It is found in both animals and plants.

Type of allergen: inhalant

Likely sources of alpha-amylase: pharmaceutical manufacturing

Symptoms, tests, treatments and self-help tips, see *Enzymes*

Alpha-hydroxy acids

The active ingredients of alpha-hydroxy acids or AHAs include lactic, glycolic and malic acids. As well as being an allergen, AHAs may thin the skin's protective layer, making it more susceptible to skin irritation or to allergic reactions.

Type of allergen: contact

Likely sources of alpha-hydroxy acids: skin products such as make-up or moisturizers

Symptoms
Skin reactions: angioedema, itching, irritation, tenderness

Tests
• Skin patch test

Treatments
Avoidance
• Check labels of all skin products

Prescription medication
• Angioedema: adrenaline, antihistamines, steroids
• Itching: antihistamines, emollients
• Skin irritation: emollients

OTC remedies
• Angioedema: antihistamines
• Itching: antihistamines, emollients
• Skin irritation: emollients

Alternative remedies
• Itching: aromatherapy, herbalism

Self-help tips: for symptom relief, see *Angioedema, Itching, Skin irritation* in the section on *Symptoms*

Alternative products that won't cause a reaction: look for hypoallergenic cosmetics which do not contain AHAs. See also *Cosmetics*

Aluminium chloride
Aluminium chloride is a white solid, A_lC_{l3}.

Type of allergen: contact

Likely sources of aluminium chloride: antiperspirants, antiseptics, deodorants

Symptoms
Skin reactions: contact dermatitis, rash

Tests
• Skin patch

Treatments

Avoidance: check labels carefully and don't use those containing aluminium chloride

Prescription medication: steroids, antihistamines

OTC remedies: coal tar, emollients, steroids

Alternative remedies: aromatherapy, Bach flower remedies, homeopathy

Self-help tips: for symptom relief, see *Contact dermatitis* in the section on *Symptoms*

Amaranth
See *Food additives – colourings*

Amethocaine
See *Anaesthetic, Drugs*

Amines

Vasoactive amines are organic compounds containing nitrogen; they are formed from ammonia, with between one and three of the hydrogen atoms replaced by hydrocarbon radicals. They include allylamine, amylamine, ethylamine, methylamine, phenylamine and propylamine and can cause occupational asthma for shellac and lacquer handlers. If symptoms start soon after beginning work and improve at weekends or on holidays, occupational asthma should be suspected.

Biogenic amines are formed when enzymes and bacteria break down amino acids in food, removing the acid group from amino acids and leaving just the amines – particularly cheese, chocolate and tuna. Some are found naturally in foods such as avocado, bananas, oranges, pineapple, plums, tomatoes and red wine; as fruit ripens and spoils, the level of amines increases. They may also be increased by processing, such as canning, pickling and juicing.

Amines include dopamine, histamine, norepinephrine, octopamine, phenylethylamine, serotonin, tyramine and tryptamine. They act as neurotransmitters which control various body processes; one example is serotonin triggering receptors in the brain that control the width of blood vessels. When the amine has done its job, the body uses the enzymes monoamine oxidase and aldehyde dehydrogenase to detoxify the amine and excrete it.

Type of allergen: inhalant, consumed

Likely sources of amines:
- Chemicals/industrial processing: shellac and lacquer
- Foods: avocado, bananas, cheese, chocolate, oranges, pineapple, plums, tomatoes, tuna and red wine

Symptoms

Gastrointestinal reactions: abdominal cramps, diarrhoea, nausea, vomiting

Headaches: headaches, migraine

Respiratory reactions: occupational asthma

Skin reactions: flushing, itching, urticaria

Tests
- Symptom diary (including peak flow meter readings)
- Elimination diet
- Food challenge

Treatments

Avoidance
- For sensitivity to amines in food, avoid the food that affects you and check labels carefully.
- For chemical/industrial processing, use protective equipment such as masks and gloves; improved ventilation may also help.

Prescription medication
- Abdominal pain and swelling: antacids, anti-spasmodic drugs
- Diarrhoea: antidiarrhoeal drugs
- Nausea: antihistamines
- Vomiting: anti-emetics
- Headache: painkillers, non-steroidal anti-inflammatories
- Headache: painkillers, anti-sickness drugs, ergotamine, 5-HT agonists, beta-blockers, sodium valproate, sumatryptan
- Asthma: anticholinergic drugs, antihistamines (exercise-

induced), Beta2 (ß2) adrenoreceptor agonists, cromoglycate, nedocromil sodium, steroids, xanthine derivatives, zafirlukast
- Itching: antihistamines, emollients
- Urticaria: antihistamines, emollients, steroids

OTC remedies
- Abdominal pain and swelling: antacids
- Diarrhoea: kaolin and morphine, calcium carbonate, pectin
- Nausea: antihistamines
- Vomiting: oral rehydration solution
- Itching: antihistamines, emollients
- Urticaria: calamine lotion, witch hazel

Alternative remedies
- Abdominal pain and swelling: aromatherapy, herbalism, homeopathy
- Diarrhoea: aromatherapy, herbalism, homeopathy
- Nausea: aromatherapy, herbalism, homeopathy
- Vomiting: herbalism
- Headache: acupuncture, aromatherapy, herbalism, homeopathy
- Migraine: acupuncture, Alexander technique, aromatherapy, chiropractic, herbalism, homeopathy, hypnosis, osteopathy, reflexology
- Asthma: acupuncture (mild asthma only), Buteyko method, homeopathy, relaxation techniques, yoga
- Itching: aromatherapy, herbalism
- Flushing: herbalism
- Urticaria: aromatherapy, herbalism, homeopathy

Self-help tips: for symptom relief see *Abdominal pain and swelling, Diarrhoea, Nausea, Vomiting, Headache, Migraine, Asthma, Flushing, Itching, Urticaria* in the section on *Symptoms*

Aminophenols
Aminophenols are produced when phenols are substituted by an amino group.
See *Hair care products*

Ammonia

Ammonia is the common name for the chemical NH_3, a colourless gas which is lighter than air and soluble in water. It is formed naturally by the metabolism of proteins in animals. It is an irritant and its effects on eyes and skin can be confused with an allergic reaction.

Type of allergen: inhalant, contact

Likely sources of ammonia
- *Chemicals/industry:* red dyes (ammonium dichromate), refrigerant gases, latex preservative, fertilizers (ammonium nitrate, ammonium phosphate and urea)
- *Cosmetics and personal care items:* deodorants, perfumes (ammonium dichromate), perm neutralizer (ammonium carbonate), hair bleaches, toothpaste
- *Household items:* cleaning materials, disinfectants

Symptoms, tests, treatments and self-help tips, see *Chemicals*

Ammonium acetate
See *Food additives – preservatives*

Ammonium carbonates
See *Food additives – anti-caking agents*

Amoxycillin

Amoxycillin is an *antibiotic*.

Type of allergen: consumed

Symptoms, tests, treatments and self-help tips, see *Drugs*

Ampicillin
See *Pencillin, Drugs*

Amyl acetate

Amyl acetate is used as a scent or flavouring in food and cosmetics.

Type of allergen: inhalant, contact

Symptoms
Headaches

Skin reactions: skin irritation

Tests
* Symptom diary
* Skin patch

Treatments
Avoidance
* Check labels of food and cosmetics, and replace with an alternative that does not contain amyl acetate.

Prescription medication
* Headache: painkillers, non-steroidal anti-inflammatories
* Skin irritation: emollients

OTC remedies
* Headache: as prescription medication
* Skin irritation: emollients

Alternative remedies
* Headache: acupuncture, aromatherapy, herbalism, homeopathy

Self-help tips: for symptom relief see *Headaches, Skin irritation* in the section on *Symptoms*
See also *Acetate, Solvents (esters)*

Amyl alcohol

Amyl alcohol is a solvent.

Likely sources of amyl alcohol: shellac thinner, paint and varnish remover, lacquer thinners

Type of allergen: inhalant

Symptoms
Eye reactions: conjunctivitis

Gastrointestinal reactions: nausea, vomiting

Respiratory reactions: breathing problems such as wheezing

Tests
• Inhalation challenge
• Symptom diary

Treatments
Avoidance
• Use protective equipment such as goggles, masks and gloves.

Prescription medication
• Conjunctivitis: antihistamines, cromoglycate, nedocromil sodium, steroids, sympathomimetics
• Nausea: antihistamines

OTC remedies
• Conjunctivitis: antihistamines
• Nausea: antihistamines
• Vomiting: oral rehydration solution

Alternative remedies
• Conjunctivitis: herbalism, homeopathy
• Nausea: aromatherapy, herbalism, homeopathy
• Vomiting: herbalism

Self-help tips: for symptom relief see *Conjunctivitis, Nausea, Vomiting, Breathing problems* in the section on *Symptoms*
See also *Solvents (alcohol solvents)*

Amylase
See *Enzymes*

Amylcinnamaldehyde
See *Perfumes*

Anaesthetic

Anaesthetics can cause allergic occupational dermatitis in pharmaceutical workers – particularly amethocaine, benzocaine, cinchocaine and procaine. You might also react to anaesthetics during an operation.

Type of allergen: contact

Symptoms, tests, treatments and self-help tips, see *Drugs*

Anaesthetic, local

See *Benzyl alcohol*

Anchovy

See *Fish*

Angelica

Angelica is a herb from the aromatic plant *Archangelica officinalis* or *Angelica archangelic*. It contains furanocoumarins, which can cause photosensitivity.

Type of allergen: contact

Likely sources of angelica
- Cosmetics: the roots and seeds are used in cosmetic products
- Foods: the leaf stalks are candied and used in confectionery; the roots and seeds are used as a tonic

Symptoms, tests, treatments and self-help tips, see *Herbs*

Angora

See *Animal hair*

Anhydrides

Anhydrides are chemical compounds that become acids in the presence of water, or a soluble base when the water is removed from the compound. Trimetallic anhydrides are particularly likely to cause problems such as occupational asthma. If symptoms start soon after beginning work and improve at weekends or on holidays, occupational asthma should be suspected.

Type of allergen: inhalant

Likely sources of anhydrides
• Industry: plastics, epoxy resins

Symptoms
Respiratory reactions: asthma (occupational), hay fever

Other reactions: coughing up blood, fever, muscle pain

Tests
• Symptom diary (including peak flow meter readings)
• CAP-RAST test (phthalic anhydride, trimetellic anhydride (TMA))
• Blood test: ELISA (trimetellic anhydride – TMA)

Treatments
Avoidance:
• Use protective equipment such as goggles and masks in occupational situations.

Prescription medication
• Hay fever: antihistamines, cromoglycate, decongestants, nedocromil sodium, steroids, sympathomimetics
• Fever: aspirin, ibuprofen, paracetamol
• Muscle pain: painkillers
• Asthma: anticholinergic drugs, antihistamines (exercise-induced), Beta2 (ß2) adrenoreceptor agonists, cromoglycate, nedocromil sodium, steroids, xanthine derivatives, zafirlukast

OTC remedies
• Hay fever: antihistamines, decongestants
• Fever: aspirin, ibuprofen, paracetamol
• Muscle pain: painkillers

Alternative remedies
• Hay fever: aromatherapy, herbalism, homeopathy
• Fever: herbalism, homeopathy

- Muscle pain: homeopathy
- Asthma: acupuncture (mild asthma only), Buteyko method, homeopathy, relaxation techniques, yoga

Self-help tips: for symptom relief see *Fever, Muscle pain, Asthma, Hay fever* in the section on *Symptoms*

Animal hair and epithelium

Strictly speaking, it is the dander (or flakes of skin) from the animal rather than the hair that causes problems. It can cause occupational asthma for animal handlers and breeders, laboratory workers, vets and pet owners. For those who work with animals, if symptoms start soon after beginning work and improve at weekends or on holidays, occupational asthma should be suspected.

Type of allergen: inhalant, contact

Symptoms
Mouth, nasal and ear reactions: rhinitis, sneezing

Respiratory reactions: asthma (including occupational), breathing problems

Skin reaction: angioedema

Tests
- Symptom diary (including peak flow meter readings)
- CAP-RAST test (budgerigar droppings, cat dander, chicken droppings, chinchilla epithelium, cow dander, deer epithelium, dog dander, dog epithelium, ferret epithelium, fox epithelium, gerbil epithelium, goat epithelium, guinea pig epithelium, hamster epithelium, horse dander, mink epithelium, mouse epithelium, pigeon droppings, rabbit epithelium, rat epithelium, reindeer epithelium, sheep epithelium, swine epithelium)
- ELISA test (angora epithelium, camel epithelium, cat hair, cat scurf, chinchilla, cow dander, deer hair/dander, dog dander, dog epithelium, ferret epithelium, fox epithelium, gerbil epithelium, goat epithelium, guinea pig epithelium, golden hamster epithelium, hare epithelium, horse dander, human hair, llama epithelium, mink hair, mouse epithelium, pig epithelium,

rabbit epithelium, rat epithelium, sheep epithelium)
- Skin prick test (cat, cow, dog, goat, guinea pig, hamster, mouse, pig's bristles, rabbit, rat)
- Intradermal test (camel, cat, cow, dog, goat, guinea pig, hamster, horse, mouse, rabbit, rat, sheep)
- Nasal challenge (cat, dog, guinea pig, horse)

Treatments
Avoidance
- Use protective equipment such as goggles and masks.

Prescription medication
- Rhinitis: antihistamines, decongestants, sodium cromoglycate, immunotherapy
- Sneezing: antihistamines, decongestants, sodium cromogylcate
- Asthma: anticholinergic drugs, antihistamines (exercise-induced), Beta2 (ß2) adrenoreceptor agonists, cromoglycate, nedocromil sodium, steroids, xanthine derivatives, zafirlukast
- Angioedema: adrenaline, antihistamines, steroids

OTC remedies
- Rhinitis: decongestants
- Angioedema: antihistamines

Alternative remedies
- Rhinitis: aromatherapy
- Sneezing: acupuncture
- Asthma: acupuncture (mild asthma only), Buteyko method, homeopathy, relaxation techniques, yoga

Self-help tips: for symptom relief see *Rhinitis, Sneezing, Asthma, Breathing problems, Angioedema* in the section on *Symptoms*
See also *Pets*

Animal proteins

Animal proteins can cause occupational asthma for animal handlers and breeders, laboratory workers and vets. If symptoms start soon after beginning work and improve at weekends or on holidays, occupational asthma should be suspected.

Type of allergen: inhalant

Symptoms
Respiratory reactions: asthma (occupational)

Tests
- Symptom diary (including peak flow meter readings)
- CAP-RAST (budgerigar serum, cat serum albumin, chicken serum, dog serum albumin, horse serum, mouse serum, rabbit serum, rat serum, swine serum albumin)
- ELISA (bovine serum, bovine serum albumin, budgerigar serum, canary serum, chicken serum, horse serum, mouse droppings, mouse epithelium protein, mouse serum, mouse urine, parrot serum, pigeon serum, rat droppings, rat epithelium protein, rat serum, rat urine)

Treatments
Avoidance: in occupational situations, use protective equipment such as goggles and masks. Improved ventilation may also help.

Prescription medication: anticholinergic drugs, antihistamines (exercise-induced), Beta2 (ß2) adrenoreceptor agonists, cromoglycate, nedocromil sodium, steroids, xanthine derivatives, zafirlukast

Alternative remedies: acupuncture (mild asthma only), Buteyko method, homeopathy, relaxation techniques, yoga

Self-help tips: for symptom relief see *Asthma* in the section on *Symptoms*

Animal urine

Animal urine can cause occupational asthma for animal handlers and breeders, laboratory workers, vets and pet owners. For those who work with animals, if symptoms start soon after beginning work and improve at weekends or on holidays, occupational asthma should be suspected.

Type of allergen: inhalant

Symptoms
Mouth, nasal and ear reactions: rhinitis, sneezing

Respiratory reactions: asthma (occupational), breathing problems

Tests
* Symptom diary (including peak flow meter readings)
* CAP-RAST (mouse urine, rabbit urine, rat urine, swine urine)

Treatments
Avoidance
* In occupational situations, use protective equipment such as goggles and masks. Improved ventilation may also help.

Prescription medication
* Rhinitis: antihistamines, decongestants, sodium cromoglycate, immunotherapy
* Sneezing: antihistamines, decongestants, sodium cromogylcate
* Asthma: anticholinergic drugs, antihistamines (exercise-induced), Beta2 (ß2) adrenoreceptor agonists, cromoglycate, nedocromil sodium, steroids, xanthine derivatives, zafirlukast

OTC remedies
* Rhinitis: *decongestants*

Alternative remedies
* Rhinitis: aromatherapy
* Sneezing: acupuncture
* Asthma: acupuncture (mild asthma only), Buteyko method, homeopathy, relaxation techniques, yoga

Self-help tips: for symptom relief see *Rhinitis, Sneezing, Asthma, Breathing problems* in the section on *Symptoms*
See also *Pets*

Anise
Anise is a spice made from the dried fruit of the anise *Pimpinella anisum*; the plant is part of the parsley family and looks similar to fennel. It has a flavour similar to liquorice. The volatile oil from the seeds contains anethole.

Type of allergen: contact

Likely sources of anise
- Cosmetics: perfumes
- Foods: as a flavouring in confectionery
- Medicines: a flavouring in medicines

Symptoms, tests, treatments and self-help tips, see *Spices*

You might also react to: caraway seed, carrot, celery, celery seed, coriander, cumin, dill, fennel, parsley, parsnip
See also *Aromatherapy oils*

Aniseed

Aniseed is the seed of the plant *Pimpinella anisum*. It contains *salicylates*, which have been linked to hyperactivity in children.

Type of allergen: inhalant, consumed

Symptoms, tests, treatments and self-help tips, see *Spices*

You might also react to: others in the *Umbelliferae* family, such as caraway, carrot, celery, celeriac, cumin, coriander, dill, fennel, parsley, parsnip
See also *Aromatherapy oils*

Annatto
See *Food additives – colourings*

Antibiotics

Antibiotics are drugs used to treat bacterial infections. They can cause dermatitis and occupational asthma, and you may also have allergic reactions if you take antibiotics (generally a rash). Antibiotics can cause occupational asthma in drug manufacturers, occupational allergic dermatitis in pharmaceutical workers (chloramphenicol, neomycin, penicillin, ampicillin, quinoline, sulphonamide), and can also cause allergic reaction when taken.

Antibiotics which can cause allergic reactions

- Amoxycillin (usually prescribed for treating ear, nose and throat infections, respiratory tract infections and cystitis)
- Cefaclor (usually prescribed for bacterial infections, particularly in the respiratory tract, sinuses, skin, middle ear and urinary tract)
- Cephalexin (usually prescribed for bronchitis, cystitis and skin infections)
- Nitrofurantoin (usually prescribed for urinary tract infections)
- Phenoxymethylpenicillin (usually prescribed for respiratory tract infections)
- Teicoplanin (usually prescribed for serious infections such as endocarditis, and infections caused by the bacteria *Staphylococcus aureus*)

Type of allergen: contact, inhaled, consumed, injected

Symptoms, tests, treatments and self-help tips, see *Drugs*

Anti-emetics

Anti-emetics are drugs used to suppress nausea and vomiting, either as a side-effect of medical treatment (such as cancer treatment) or in over-the-counter remedies for travel sickness.

Type of allergen: consumed

Anti-emetics which can cause problems: Tropesitron

Symptoms, tests, treatments and self-help tips, see *Drugs*

Antifreeze
See *Solvents – glycols*

Antifungal drugs

Antifungal drugs are used to treat fungal infections, such as thrush and athlete's foot.

Antifungal drugs which can cause reactions include

- Flucanozole is used to treat fungal infections in the mouth, respiratory tract, gastrointestinal tract, skin, head and feet; it may cause a rash.
- Nystatin is used to treat thrush; it may cause a rash, and also allergic occupational dermatitis in pharmaceutical workers.
- Terbinafine is used to treat infections of the nails, feet and head (it is an oral rather than a topical treatment); it may cause a rash, itching, and joint pain.

Type of allergen: contact, consumed

Symptoms, tests, treatments and self-help tips, see *Drugs*

Antihistamines

Antihistamines are used to treat the symptoms of allergic reactions.

Promethazine hydrochloride may cause allergic occupational dermatitis in pharmaceutical workers.

Type of allergen: contact, consumed

Symptoms, tests, treatments and self-help tips, see *Drugs*

Antimony

Antimony is a metal (chemical symbol Sb).

Type of allergen: contact

Likely sources of antimony: an alloy used in metalwork and soldering

Symptoms, tests, treatments and self-help tips, see *Metals*

Antiperspirants

See *Aluminium chloride, Cobalt, Formaldehyde*

Antiseptic

See *Aluminium chloride, Isopropanol, Solvents – alcohol solvents*

Antiseptic, topical
See *Benzyl alcohol, hexachlorophene*

Apple

Apples are the fruit from the tree *Malus*. They contain *salicylates*, which have been linked to hyperactivity in children. Apples contain more fructose than glucose; if your body has problems absorbing fructose, you could suffer from diarrhoea. You may find that it causes itching in your mouth during the pollen season (particularly birch).

The allergenic proteins in apples are not heat-stable so problems are more likely to occur after eating fresh fruit; the allergen levels vary with the ripeness of the apple and the variety.

Type of allergen: consumed

Symptoms, tests, treatments and self-help tips, see *Fruit*

You might also react to: pear, birch pollen, mugwort pollen, oak pollen

Apricot

Apricots are the fruit from the tree *Prunus armeniaca*. They contain *salicylates*, which have been linked to hyperactivity in children.

Type of allergen: consumed

Symptoms, tests, treatments and self-help tips, see *Fruit*

You might also react to: birch pollen, almonds, cherries, peaches, plums

Arnica

Arnica – also known as leopard's bane or mountain tobacco – is a herb from the plant *Arnica montana*, used for healing sprains, swellings and bruises.

Type of allergen: contact, consumed

209

Likely sources of arnica: herbal ointment, tablets

Symptoms, tests, treatments and self-help tips, see *Drugs*

Aromatherapy oils

You may find that any of the following essential oils cause an allergic skin reaction (usually a rash):

Allspice, aniseed, basil, bay, black pepper, cedarwood, celery seed, camomile, cinnamon, citronella, clary sage, clove, costus root, fennel, ginger, hops, juniper, lemon, lemongrass, lime, litsea cubeba, lovage, melissa, nutmeg, orange, parsley, peppermint, pine, sage, spearmint, tagetes, tea tree, thyme, ylang ylang

Type of allergen: contact

Symptoms, tests, treatments and self-help tips, see *Oils, cosmetic*

Arsenic

Arsenic is a grey metallic element, chemical symbol As.

Type of allergen: contact

Likely sources of arsenic: insecticides

Symptoms, tests, treatments and self-help tips, see *Metals*

Artichokes

Artichokes are the vegetable *Cynara scolymus*.

Type of allergen: consumed

Symptoms, tests, treatments and self-help tips, see *Vegetables*

You might also react to: chicory, dandelion, endive, lettuce, sunflower seeds, tarragon

Artificial fibres

Reactions to fibres may be from inhaling the fibres or fumes or by touching them.

Type of allergen: contact, inhaled

Likely sources of artificial fibres: nylon, polyester, polycotton

Symptoms
Headaches

Nasal reactions: itching, rhinitis

Respiratory reactions: asthma (including occupational), breathing problems

Skin reactions: itching

Tests
* Blood test: ELISA (acrylon, kapok, nylon, rayon, terylene)
* Symptom diary (including peak flow meter readings)

Treatments
Avoidance
* In occupational situations, use protective equipment such as gloves and masks. In domestic situations, check labels carefully.

Prescription medication
* Headache: painkillers, non-steroidal anti-inflammatories
* Rhinitis: antihistamines, decongestants, sodium cromoglycate, immunotherapy
* Asthma: anticholinergic drugs, antihistamines (exercise-induced), Beta$_2$ (β2) adrenoreceptor agonists, cromoglycate, nedocromil sodium, steroids, xanthine derivatives, zafirlukast
* Breathing problems: bronchodilators, corticosteroids
* Itching: antihistamines, emollients

OTC remedies
* Headache: as prescription medication
* Rhinitis: decongestants
* Itching: antihistamines, emollients

Alternative remedies
- Headache: acupuncture, aromatherapy, herbalism, homeopathy
- Rhinitis: aromatherapy
- Asthma: acupuncture (mild asthma only), Buteyko method, homeopathy, relaxation techniques, yoga
- Itching: aromatherapy, herbalism

Self-help tips: for symptom relief see *Headaches, Rhinitis, Asthma, Breathing problems, Itching* in the section on *Symptoms*

Alternative products that won't cause a reaction: Cotton, silk, linen

Asparagus

Asparagus is a vegetable from the *Liliacae* family. It contains *salicylates*, which have been linked to hyperactivity in children. It also contains carboxylic acid, which is a contact allergen.

Type of allergen: consumed, contact

You might also react to: other members of the *Liliacae* family, such as chives, garlic, leek, onion, shallot

Symptoms, tests, treatments and self-help tips, see *Vegetables*

Aspartame

Aspartame is the trademark name of an artificial sweetener and flavour enhancer, comprised of aspartic acid and phenylalanine, also known as Asp Phe Methyl Ester. Allergy to aspartame is controversial; the Ministry of Agriculture, Fisheries and Foods as at November 1999 believes that the sweetener is safe for all but those who suffer from phenylketonuria (PKU), who cannot metabolize phenylalanine effectively.

Type of allergen: consumed

Likely sources of aspartame: food and drink – "low-calorie" or "sugar-free" foods

Symptoms
Skin reaction: urticaria

Tests
* Symptom diary
* Elimination diet
* Food challenge

Treatments
Avoidance
* Check labels carefully.

Prescription medication
* Urticaria: antihistamines, emollients, steroids

OTC remedies
* Urticaria: calamine lotion, witch hazel

Alternative remedies
* Urticaria: aromatherapy, herbalism, homeopathy

Self-help tips: for symptom relief see *Urticaria* in the section on *Symptoms*

Asphalt
See *Colophony*

Asphalt sealant
See *Volatile organic compounds*

Aspirin
Aspirin, also known as acetyl salicylate, is a painkiller which also reduces fever and inflammation.

One in twenty asthma sufferers has a severe attack after taking aspirin, and women are more likely to be affected than men. Sensitivity to aspirin may be caused by low levels of the enzyme cyclo-oxygenase.

Type of allergen: consumed

Symptoms, tests and treatments, see *Drugs*

Self-help tips
- Tell your GP, dentist or other medical practitioner that you're sensitive to aspirin; if you're prescribed any new drug, remind your practitioner of your sensitivity to aspirin
- Read labels in any OTC medication and check with the pharmacist that it doesn't contain aspirin or NSAIDs before taking – particularly for medications treating headaches, colds, coughs, allergies, sinus problems, arthritis, rheumatism (joint pain), menstrual cramps, stomach acidity, backache, or urinary pain
- For symptom relief, see *Conjunctivitis, Heartburn, Rhinitis, Asthma*, in the section on *Symptoms*

Alternative products that won't cause a reaction
- Most sufferers should be able to use paracetamol, though 5 per cent of people sensitive to aspirin also react to paracetamol
- You may also be able to use non-acetylated salicylates

You might also react to:
- Non-steroidal anti-inflammatory drugs (NSAIDs) such as diclofenac, fenoprofen, ibuprofen, indomethacin, mefenamic acid, naproxen, paracetamol, phenylbutazone
- Codeine
- Food colours which are either azo dyes or "coal tar" dyes (originally made from coal tar, but now produced synthetically):
- E102 Tartrazine (note that some medication includes tartrazine)
- E104 Quinoline Yellow
- 107 Yellow 2G
- E120 Cochineal or carminic acid (red)
- E122 Carmoisine
- E123 Amaranth
- E124 Brilliant scarlet 4R (Ponceau)
- E129 (Allura red AC)
- E154 Brown FK
- E155 Chocolate brown HT
- Other food additives:
- E212 Potassium benzoate (preservative)
- E213 Calcium benzoate (preservative)

– E214 Ethyl 4-hydroxobenzoate (preservative)
– E215 Ethyl 4-hydroxobenzoate, sodium salt (preservative)
– E216 Propyl 4-hydroxobenzoate (preservative)
– E217 Propyl 4-hydroxobenzoate, sodium salt (preservative)
– E218 Methyl 4-hydroxobenzoate (preservative)
– E219 Methyl 4-hydroxobenzoate, sodium salt (preservative)
– E310 Propyl gallate (antioxidant)
– E311 Octyl gallate (antioxidant)
– E312 Dodecyl gallate (antioxidant)
– 621 Monosodium glutamate (flavour enhancer)
– 622 Monopotassium glutamate (flavour enhancer)
– E623 Calcium glutamate (flavour enhancer)
– 629 Sodium guanylate (flavour enhancer)
– 631 Inosine 5'-(disodium phosphate) (flavour enhancer)
– 635 sodium 5'-ribonucleotide (flavour enhancer)
• Foods containing salicylates (either as a food preservative or naturally occurring in the food) – fruit (apple, apricot, blackberry, blueberry, cherry, grape, orange, peach, plum, raisin, raspberry, strawberry), soft drinks, breakfast cereals, chewing gum, chocolate, liquorice, margarine, sandwich spreads
• Peppermint
• Mint
• Menthol
• Oil of wintergreen (methyl salicylate)

Aubergine

Aubergine is the fruit of the plant *Solanum melongena*; it is also known as eggplant.

Aubergines contain the amine *tyramine*, which causes the blood vessels to widen and may trigger migraines. It may also contain large quantities of *histamine*.

Type of allergen: consumed

Symptoms, tests, treatments and self-help tips, see *Vegetables*

You might also react to: other vegetables/plants in the night-shade family – cayenne, chilli, peppers (capsicum), paprika, potato, tobacco, tomato

Avocado

Avocado is the fruit of *Persea gratissima*. It is also known as the alligator pear.

When avocado is used in dips, sulphite compounds may form, which can trigger asthma.

Avocado also contains a protein similar to the one that causes an allergy to latex, so you may find that you react to avocado if you are allergic to latex.

Avocado contains the amine tyramine, which causes the blood vessels to widen and may trigger migraines.

Type of allergen: consumed, contact

Likely sources of avocado: dips such as guacamole; sunscreens (check the label for avocado oil)

Symptoms, tests, treatments and self-help tips, see *Fruit*

You might also react to: apple, bay leaves, cinnamon, latex

Azithromycin

See *Macrolides, Drugs*

Bacitracin

Bacitracin are organic compounds called cyclic peptides, produced by the bacteria *Bacillius licheniformis*, used as an antibiotic cream.

Type of allergen: contact

Symptoms, tests, treatments and self-help tips, see *Drugs*

Bacteria

Bacteria can cause allergy-type problems when they are inhaled; likely sources include humidifiers.

Type of allergen: inhaled

Symptoms
Headache

Mouth, nasal and ear reactions: rhinitis, sneezing

Other: fever

Tests
• Symptom diary

Treatments
Prescription medication
• Headache: painkillers, non-steroidal anti-inflammatories
• Rhinitis: antihistamines, decongestants, sodium cromoglycate, immunotherapy
• Sneezing: antihistamines, decongestants, sodium cromogylcate
• Fever: aspirin, ibuprofen, paracetamol

OTC remedies
• Headache: as prescription medication
• Rhinitis: decongestants
• Fever: aspirin, ibuprofen, paracetamol

Alternative remedies
• Headache: acupuncture, aromatherapy, herbalism, homeo-pathy
• Rhinitis: aromatherapy
• Sneezing: acupuncture
• Fever: herbalism, homeopathy

Self-help tips: if you use a humidifier, clean it regularly. Use distilled water as most tap water has some bacteria in it (even when chlorinated). For Symptom relief, see *Headache, Rhinitis, Sneezing, Fever* in the section on *Symptoms*

Balloons
See *Latex*

Balsam of Peru

This is produced from cutting the bark of a Latin American tree. It has a smell similar to cinnamon. It contains cinnamic acid.

Type of allergen: contact

Likely sources of Balsam of Peru: perfumes, cosmetics, medication and oil paints.

Symptoms, tests, treatments and self-help tips, see *Oils, cosmetic*

You might also react to: benzoin, citrus fruits (orange peel), clove, cinnamon, colophony/rosin, essential oils, eugenol, turpentine, wood tars

Bamboo shoots

Bamboo shoots are the young shoots of plants from the *Bambusiade* family, eaten as a vegetable.

Type of allergen: contact, consumed

Symptoms, tests, treatments and self-help tips, see *Vegetables*

Banana

The banana is the edible fruit of the plant *Musa sapientum*. It contains contain *salicylates* and the vasoactive amine *tyramine*. If you are taking certain antidepressants (called MAO inhibitors), you should avoid bananas as you may have a reaction. *Serotonin* in bananas can also cause migraine.

Type of allergen: consumed

Symptoms, tests, treatments and self-help tips, see *Fruit*

You might also react to: latex, pecan, ragweed pollen, plantain pollen

Barley

Barley – botanical name *Hordeum vulgare* – contains protein allergens associated with bakers' asthma. Barley also contains gluten and gliadin.

Type of allergen: inhalant, contact, consumed

Likely sources of barley: bran, flour

Symptoms, tests, treatments and self-help tips, see *Grain*

You might also react to: wheat

Barometers
See *Mercury, Metals*

Basil

Basil is the herb *Ocimum basilicum*; the leaves, flowers, oils and resins are used.

Type of allergen: contact

Symptoms, tests, treatments and self-help tips, see *Herbs*

You might also react to: birch and mugwort pollen, celery, mint, rosemary, sage
See also *Aromatherapy oils*

Bath products

These include oils, foams, gels, cubes, salts and "bath bombs". Perfumes and preservatives tend to cause most problems.

Type of allergen: contact

Symptoms, tests, treatments and self-help tips, see *Cosmetics*

Batteries
See *Mercury, Metals*

Bay leaf
Bay leaf is the herb *Laurus nobilis*.

Type of allergen: consumed

Symptoms, tests, treatments and self-help tips, see *Herbs*

You might also react to: avocado, cinnamon
See also *Aromatherapy oils*

Beans (pinto, white)
Beans are leguminous plants.

Type of allergen: consumed

Symptoms, tests, treatments and self-help tips, see *Vegetables*

Beans (red kidney)
The red kidney bean, *Phaseolus vulgaris*, is a legume. Albumin is the major allergen in red kidney beans; they also contain lectins, which can give gastric symptoms of "false food allergy".

Type of allergen: consumed

Symptoms, tests, treatments and self-help tips, see *Vegetables*

Bedding
See *Dust mite*

Bee and wasp stings

Bees are not aggressive and stings are rare. Wasps are aggressive and are the most common cause of insect sting allergy.

If you've ever been stung by a bee or wasp and had a large skin reaction (with redness/swelling over 10cm in diameter), you should ask your GP for allergy testing.

Roughly 80 per cent of people suffering from a large skin reaction suffer it with subsequent stings. The risk of anaphylactic shock with subsequent stings is less than 5 per cent.

Type of allergen: injected

Symptoms

Anaphylactic shock: this is likely to start between ten and thirty minutes after the sting.

Respiratory reactions: asthma, breathing difficulties, tightness in the chest

Skin reactions: angioedema, itching, swelling in areas other than the sting site, urticaria

Other reactions: hoarse voice, swollen tongue

Tests

- Skin test: skin prick (bee venom, wasp venom)
- Blood test: CAP–RAST (anisakis, ascaris), bee (*Bombus terrestris*), Berlin beetle (*Trogoderma angustum*), blood worm (*Chironomus thummi*), cockroach (*Blatella germanica*), echinococcus, fire ant (*Solenopsis invicta*), grain weevil (*Sitophilus granarius*), green nimitti (*Cladotanytarsus Lewisi*), hornet (white-faced, yellow and European), horse bot fly (*Gasterophilus intestinalis*), horse fly (*Tabanus sp*), Mediterranean flour moth (*Ephestia kuchniell*a), mosquito (*Aedes communis*), moth (*Bombyx mori*), wasp (common and paper)
- Blood test: ELISA, fire ant (*Solenopsis invicta*), ascaris, Berlin beetle (*Trogoderma angustum*), bumblebee, cockroach (*Blatella germanica*), echinococcus, fly, honeybee (*Apis mellifera*), hornet (*Vespa crabro*), white-faced hornet (*Dolichovespula maculata*), yellow hornet (*Dolichovespula arenaria*), horse fly (*Gasterophilus intestinalis*), midge (*Aedes spp*), red midge larva, schistosoma, common wasp (*Vespula vulgaris*), paper wasp (*Polistes spp*), water flea (*Daphnia cladocera*)

Treatments

Avoidance

- Insect repellents: use a commercial brand or eat raw garlic – insects don't like it

Prescription medication

- Anaphylactic shock: adrenaline, antihistamines, steroids; if you have a widespread reaction, feel dizzy, a rash appears away from the sting or you have difficulty breathing, use adrenaline immediately. If you don't have adrenaline, call an ambulance immediately.
- Swollen mouth, lips and tongue: ACE inhibitors
- Asthma: anticholinergic drugs, antihistamines (exercise-induced), Beta2 (ß2) adrenoreceptor agonists, cromoglycate, nedocromil sodium, steroids, xanthine derivatives, zafirlukast
- Breathing problems: bronchodilators, corticosteroids
- Angioedema: adrenaline, antihistamines, steroids
- Itching: antihistamines, emollients
- Urticaria: antihistamines, emollients, steroids

OTC remedies

- Angioedema: antihistamines
- Itching: antihistamines, emollients
- Urticaria: calamine lotion, witch hazel

Alternative remedies

- Asthma: acupuncture (mild asthma only), Buteyko method, homeopathy, relaxation techniques, yoga
- Itching: aromatherapy, herbalism
- Urticaria: aromatherapy, herbalism, homeopathy
- Hyposensitization – this is done in a specialist hospital centre; increasing concentrations and amount of the venom are injected under the skin for 15 weeks, then the highest dose is injected monthly for 3 years. It gives 90 per cent protection against anaphylactic shock.

Self-help tips

- Clothing: avoid wearing black, flowery, shiny or brightly coloured clothing, which attracts insects; wear shoes so you don't accidentally tread on a wasp or bee barefoot; wear long-sleeved tops and trousers to make your skin less vulnerable
- Gardening: wear gloves while gardening

- Avoid strong perfumes (including those in sunscreen products, hairspray, make-up and deodorant), which attract bees
- Avoid drinking/eating sweet things outside, which attract insects
- Don't panic or swat insects – move away quietly; if the insect lands on you, sit still as it will usually fly away again within a few seconds
- If you think there might be a nest near your house, ask your local council to remove it and make sure you're well out of the way while it's removed
- Remove the sting carefully
- For symptom relief, see *Asthma, Breathing problems, Angio-edema, Itching, Urticaria* in the section on *Symptoms*

Beef

Beef contains the vasoactive amine tyramine, which causes the blood vessels to widen and may trigger migraines. Those allergic to cow's milk may tolerate beef.

Type of allergen: contact, consumed

Symptoms, tests, treatments and self-help tips, see *Meat and poultry*

You might also react to: cedar, yeast (baker's and brewer's)

Beer

Beer contains the vasoactive amines tyramine and *phenyle-thylamine*, which causes the blood vessels to widen and may trigger migraines. It also contains oxalates, a derivative of oxalic acid.

Type of allergen: consumed

Symptoms
Gastrointestinal reactions: abdominal pain, diarrhoea, vomiting

Headache, migraine

Skin reactions: flushing, urticaria

Tests
- Elimination diet
- Food challenge
- Symptom diary

Treatment
Avoidance: check labels carefully

Prescription medication
- Diarrhoea: antidiarrhoeal drugs
- Vomiting: anti-emetics
- Headache: painkillers, non-steroidal anti-inflammatories
- Migraine: painkillers, anti-sickness drugs, ergotamine, 5-HT agonists, beta-blockers, sodium valproate, sumatryptan
- Urticaria: antihistamines, emollients, steroids

OTC remedies
- Diarrhoea: kaolin and morphine, calcium carbonate, pectin
- Vomiting: oral rehydration solution
- Headache: as prescription medication
- Migraine: aspirin, ibuprofen, paracetamol
- Urticaria: calamine lotion, witch hazel

Alternative remedies
- Diarrhoea: aromatherapy, herbalism, homeopathy
- Vomiting: herbalism
- Headache: acupuncture, aromatherapy, herbalism, homeopathy
- Migraine: acupuncture, Alexander technique, aromatherapy, chiropractic, herbalism, homeopathy, hypnosis, osteopathy, reflexology
- Flushing: herbalism
- Urticaria: aromatherapy, herbalism, homeopathy

Self-help tips: for symptom relief see *Abdominal pain, Diarrhoea, Vomiting, Headache, Migraine, Flushing, Urticaria* in the section on *Symptoms*
See also *Yeast*

Beetroot

Beetroot is the edible root of the vegetable *Beta vulgaris*. It contains oxalates, a derivative of oxalic acid. It is also used for food colouring.

Type of allergen: consumed

Symptoms, tests, treatments and self-help tips, see *Vegetables*

Benzene

Benzene is a colourless liquid, chemical symbol C_6H_6, which is used in the manufacturing of polymers, plastics, detergents, drugs and dyes. It is one of the aromatic hydrocarbons and was previously derived from coal tar, though is nowadays derived from petroleum. It is often used as a solvent.

Type of allergen: inhaled

Likely sources of benzene: cigarette smoke, detergents, dry-cleaning fluids, glue, ink, insecticides, lead substitute in unleaded petrol, paints, petrol, petroleum mixtures, resins, rubber, stain removers, wood varnishes and finishes

Symptoms
Gastrointestinal reactions: nausea, vomiting

Mouth, nasal and ear reactions: irritation of mucous membranes

Tests
- Inhalation challenge
- Symptom diary

Treatments
Avoidance
- Use protective equipment such as masks and goggles; improved ventilation may also help

Prescription medication
- Nausea: antihistamines
- Vomiting: anti-emetics
- Irritation of mucous membranes: painkillers

OTC remedies
- Nausea: antihistamines
- Vomiting: oral rehydration solution
- Irritation of mucous membranes: as prescription medication

Alternative remedies
- Nausea: aromatherapy, herbalism, homeopathy
- Vomiting: herbalism
- Irritation of mucous membranes: herbalism

Self-help tips: for symptom relief see *Nausea, Vomiting, Irritation of mucous membranes* in the section on *Symptoms*
See also *Solvents – aromatic hydrocarbons*

Benzocaine

Benzocaine is a local anaesthetic which stops the transmission of impulses along nerve fibres and at nerve endings

Type of allergen: contact

Likely sources of benzocaine: aftershave lotion, denture adhesives, sore throat lozenges, sunburn preparations, toiletries

Symptoms, tests, treatments and self-help tips, see *Drugs*

You might also react to: azo dyes (see *Dyes; Food additives – colourings*), butacaine, procaine, sulphonamides, tetracaine
See also *Anaesthetic*

Benzoic acid

See *Food additives – preservatives*
Note that it is also found naturally in anise, raspberries and tea.

Benzophenones

Benzophenones are *enzymes*.

Type of allergen: contact

Likely sources of benzophenones: hair spray, perfume, soap, sunscreens

Symptoms, tests, treatments and self-help tips, see *Enzymes*

Benzoyl peroxide

Benzoyl or benzenecarbonyl is a chemical compound radical, C_6H_5CO; it is the base of benzoic acid.

Type of allergen: contact

Likely sources of benzoyl peroxide: used as a bleach, drying agent and chemical hardener in cosmetics, fibreglass resin and food

Symptoms
Skin reactions: contact dermatitis, skin irritation (stinging, burning, peeling)

Tests
• Patch test
• Symptom diary

Treatments
Avoidance
• In occupational situations, use protective equipment such as gloves

Prescription medication
• Contact dermatitis: steroids, antihistamines
• Skin irritation/stinging: emollients

OTC remedies
• Contact dermatitis: coal tar, emollients, steroids
• Skin irritation: emollients

Alternative remedies
• Dermatitis: aromatherapy, Bach flower remedies, homeopathy

Self-help tips: for symptom relief see *Contact dermatitis, Skin irritation* in the section on *Symptoms*

Benzyl acetate

Benzyl acetate is an aromatic extract of jasmine.

Type of allergen: contact, inhaled

Likely sources of benzyl acetate: perfumes and soaps

Symptoms
Eye reactions: conjunctivitis

Respiratory reactions: wheezing

Skin reactions: skin irritation

Tests
• Skin patch
• Symptom diary

Treatments
Avoidance
• Check labels carefully

Prescription medication
• Conjunctivitis: antihistamines, cromoglycate, nedocromil sodium, steroids, sympathomimetics
• Skin irritation: emollients

OTC remedies
• Conjunctivitis: antihistamines
• Skin irritation: emollients

Alternative remedies
• Conjunctivitis: herbalism, homeopathy

Self-help tips: for symptom relief see *Conjunctivitis, Wheezing, Skin irritation* in the section on *Symptoms*

Benzyl alcohol

Benzyl alcohol is a liquid aromatic alcohol derived from plants (particularly cloves) and used as a *solvent*; it is also known as phenylmethanol.

Type of allergen: contact, inhaled

Likely sources of benzyl alcohol: local anaesthetic, preservative, solvent and topical antiseptic

Symptoms
Nasal reactions: irritated mucous membranes

Skin reactions: skin irritation

Tests
• Skin patch test
• Symptom diary

Treatments
Avoidance
• Check labels carefully

Prescription medication
• Irritation of mucous membranes: painkillers
• Skin irritation: emollients

OTC remedies
• Irritation of mucous membranes: painkillers
• Skin irritation: emollients

Alternative remedies
• Irritation of mucous membranes: herbalism

Self-help tips: for symptom relief see *Skin irritation, Irritation of mucous membranes* in the section on *Symptoms*

You might also react to: Balsam of Peru

Benzyl salicylate

Benzyl salicylate is a fixing agent.

Type of allergen: contact

Likely sources of benzyl salicylate: perfumes and sunscreens

Symptoms
Skin reactions: photoallergenic contact dermatitis, rash

Tests
- Skin patch test
- Photopatch test
- Symptom diary

Treatments
Avoidance
- Check labels carefully

Prescription medication
- Dermatitis: steroids, antihistamines
- Photoallergenic contact dermatitis: emollients, steroids

OTC remedies
- Dermatitis: coal tar, emollients, steroids

Alternative remedies
- Dermatitis: aromatherapy, Bach flower remedies, homeopathy

Self-help tips: for symptom relief see *Contact dermatitis, photoallergenic contact dermatiti*s in the section on *Symptoms*

Beryllium

Beryllium is a grey metallic element (symbol Be). It is used to make beryllium-copper alloys used in nuclear reactors; beryllium oxide is used in ceramics. Skin patch testing may lead to sensitization.

Type of allergen: contact

Likely sources of beryllium: ceramic manufacturing

Symptoms, tests, treatments and self-help tips, see *Metals*

Beta-blockers

Beta-blockers are a form of medication used to treat high blood pressure, heart disease and migraines. They block the transmission of chemical messages in the body at sites which contain beta receptors, slowing the heart rate and lowering blood pressure.

Type of allergen: consumed

Symptoms, tests, treatments and self-help tips, see *Drugs*

You might also react to: aspirin, codeine, NSAIDs (e.g. ibruprofen)

Bird droppings

Bird droppings can cause avian hypersensitivity pneumonitis, also known as "bird breeder's lung" or "bird fancier's disease".

Type of allergen: inhaled

Symptoms
Nasal reactions: rhinitis

Respiratory reactions: asthma

Tests
- Blood test: CAP-RAST
- Blood test: ELISA (budgerigar droppings, canary droppings, duck droppings, finch droppings, goose droppings, lovebird droppings, parrot droppings, pigeon droppings)
- Symptom diary (including peak flow meter readings)

Treatments

Avoidance

- In occupational situations, use protective equipment such as masks. Improved ventilation may also help.

Prescription medication

- Rhinitis: antihistamines, decongestants, sodium cromoglycate, immunotherapy
- Asthma: anticholinergic drugs, antihistamines (exercise-induced), Beta2 (ß2) adrenoreceptor agonists, cromoglycate, nedocromil sodium, steroids, xanthine derivatives, zafirlukast

OTC remedies

- Rhinitis: decongestants

Alternative remedies

- Rhinitis: aromatherapy
- Asthma: acupuncture (mild asthma only), Buteyko method, homeopathy, relaxation techniques, yoga

Self-help tips: for symptom relief see *Rhinitis, Asthma* in the section on *Symptoms*

Birds

See *Feathers*

Biscuits

See *Wheat*

Bites, insect

See also *Bee and wasp stings*

Reactions to the bites of flies, mosquitoes and fleas are likely to be responses to saliva.

Type of allergen: injected

Symptoms

Skin reactions: rash, itching

Tests

- Symptom diary

Treatments
Avoidance
- Insect repellents
- Treat carpets, soft furnishings, pet bedding by washing thoroughly using hot water and then treating with special sprays to kill the insect larvae

Prescription medication
- Itching: antihistamines, emollients

OTC remedies
- Itching: antihistamines, emollients

Alternative remedies
- Itching: aromatherapy, herbalism

Self-help tips: for symptom relief see *Itching* in the section on *Symptoms*
See also *Bee Stings, Wasp Stings*

Bithionol

Bithionol is a halogenated anti-infective agent used against worm infections.

Type of allergen: contact

Likely sources of bithionol: antiseptic soaps, cosmetics

Symptoms
Skin reactions: photoallergenic contact dermatitis

Tests
- Photopatch testing (the allergen is placed on two skin sites; one is exposed to sunlight after 48 hours, and then both areas are examined for a rash)
- Symptom diary

Treatments
Avoidance: use protective clothing such as gloves

Prescription medication: emollients, steroids

Self-help tips: for symptom relief see *Photoallergenic contact dermatitis* in the section on *Symptoms*

Bitter almond oil

Bitter almond oil is extracted from the seed of sweet almond.

Type of allergen: contact

Likely sources of bitter almond oil: eye creams, nail varnish remover, perfumes, soaps

Symptoms, tests, treatments and self-help tips, see *Oils, cosmetic*

Blackberry

Blackberries are the fruit of the bramble; the botanical name is *Rubus fruticosus*.

Blackberries contain *salicylates*, which have been linked to hyperactivity in children. They also contain oxalates, a derivative of oxalic acid.

Type of allergen: consumed

Symptoms, tests, treatments and self-help tips, see *Fruit*

You might also react to: raspberries, strawberries

Blackcurrant

Blackcurrant are the fruit of the shrub *Ribes nigrum*. They contain *salicylates,* which have been linked to hyperactivity in children.

Type of allergen: consumed

Symptoms, tests, treatments and self-help tips, see *Fruit*

Bleach
See *Chlorine, Chromate, Potassium dichromate*

Blockboard
See *Formaldehyde*

Blue mussel
See *Fish*

Blueberries

Blueberries are the berries of the *Vaccinium* species – usually *Vaccinium myrtillis*. They contain *salicylates*, which have been linked to hyperactivity in children

Type of allergen: consumed

Symptoms, tests, treatments and self-help tips, see *Fruit*

Blusher

Perfumes and preservatives tend to cause most problems.

Type of allergen: contact

Symptoms, tests, treatments and self-help tips, see *Cosmetics*

Body lotion/oil

Perfumes and preservatives tend to cause most problems.

Type of allergen: contact

Symptoms, tests, treatments and self-help tips, see *Cosmetics*

Boots, rubber
See *Latex, mercaptobenzothiazole, thiurams*

Brazil nut

Brazil nuts are from the tree *Bertholletia excelsa*.

Type of allergen: consumed, contact

Symptoms, tests, treatments and self-help tips, see *Nuts*

Bread
See *Wheat, Yeast*

Brilliant black
See *Food additives – colourings*

Brilliant blue
See *Food additives – colourings*

Broad beans

Broad beans contain the vasoactive amine tyramine, which causes the blood vessels to widen and may trigger migraines.

Type of allergen: consumed

Symptoms, tests, treatments and self-help tips, see *Vegetables*

Broccoli

Broccoli is a vegetable from the *brassica* family.

Type of allergen: contact, consumed

Symptoms, tests, treatments and self-help tips, see *Vegetables*

You might also react to: Brussels sprouts, cabbage, cauliflower, horseradish, mustard, radish, swede, turnip, watercress

Brown FK
See *Food additives – colourings*

Brussels sprouts
Brussels sprout is a vegetable from the *brassica* family.

Type of allergen: consumed, contact

Symptoms, tests, treatments and self-help tips, see *Vegetables*

You might also react to: broccoli, cabbage, cauliflower, horseradish, mustard, radish, swede, turnip, watercress

Buckles
See *Cobalt*

Buckwheat
Buckwheat is a member of the grass family: *Fagopyrum esculentum*. It is a major food allergen in Japan, due to the high consumption of Soba or buckwheat noodles; the allergen is glycoprotein.

Type of allergen: inhalant, contact, consumed

Likely sources of buckwheat: bread, pasta, noodles, pancakes

Symptoms, tests, treatments and self-help tips, see *Grain*

You might also react to: rhubarb, birch pollen

Budgerigars
See *Pets*

Bulgar wheat
See *Wheat*

237

Buttons
See *Cobalt*

Butyl acetate
See *Solvents – esters*

Butyl alcohol

Butyl alcohol is used in the manufacture of shampoos and as a solvent in fats, resins, shellac and waxes.

Type of allergen: contact, inhaled

Symptoms
Respiratory reactions: lung irritation

Skin reactions: contact dermatitis, contact urticaria

Tests
* Skin patch test
* Symptom diary (including peak flow meter readings)

Treatments
Avoidance
* In occupational situations, use protective equipment such as masks and gloves

Prescription medication
* Contact dermatitis: steroids, antihistamines
* Urticaria: antihistamines, emollients, steroids

OTC remedies
* Contact dermatitis: coal tar, emollients, steroids
* Urticaria: calamine lotion, witch hazel

Alternative remedies
* Contact dermatitis: aromatherapy, Bach flower remedies, homeopathy
* Urticaria: aromatherapy, herbalism, homeopathy

Self-help tips: for symptom relief see *Contact dermatitis, Urticaria* in the section on *Symptoms*

Butylated hydroxyanisole (BHA)
See *Food additives – antioxidants*

Butylated hydroxytoluene (BHT)
See *Food additives – antioxidants*

Butyric acid

Butyric acid – also known as butanoic acid – is a colourless water-soluble acid $C_3H_7CO_2H$, which smells like rancid butter. It is used to make esters for perfumes.

Type of allergen: contact

Symptoms
Skin reactions: contact urticaria

Tests
• Symptom diary

Treatments
Avoidance: in occupational situations, use protective equipment such as gloves

Prescription medication: antihistamines, emollients, steroids

OTC remedies: calamine lotion, witch hazel

Alternative remedies: aromatherapy, herbalism, homeopathy

Self-help tips: for symptom relief see *Urticaria* in the section on *Symptoms*

Cabbage

Cabbage is the vegetable *Brassica oleracea*.

Type of allergen: consumed

Symptoms, tests, treatments and self-help tips, see *Vegetables*

You might also react to: broccoli, Brussels-sprouts, cauli-flower, horseradish, mustard, radish, swede, turnip, watercress

Caffeine

Caffeine is a stimulant and diuretic; it is an alkaloid of coffee and tea, and is chemically related to the asthma drug theophylline.

Type of allergen: consumed

Likely sources of caffeine: chocolate, coffee, cola drinks, some painkillers, tea

Symptoms
Gastrointestinal reactions: heartburn

Headaches: migraine

Skin reactions: flushed face, urticaria

Other reactions: disturbed sleep, cystitis, fast heartbeat, shaking hands

Tests
- CAP-RAST (coffee, tea)
- Elimination diet
- Food challenge
- Symptom diary

Treatments
Avoidance
- Check labels carefully, check your diet with a dietitian to ensure that it is nutritionally sound, and cut down gradually as you may suffer withdrawal headaches

Prescription medication
- Heartburn: antacids, alginates
- Migraine: painkillers, anti-sickness drugs, ergotamine, 5-HT agonists, beta-blockers, sodium valproate, sumatryptan
- Cystitis: antibiotics (for infection)
- Urticaria: antihistamines, emollients, steroids

OTC remedies
- Heartburn: as prescription medication
- Migraine: aspirin, ibuprofen, paracetamol
- Cystitis: potassium citrate
- Sleep problems: various remedies (most of them include antihistamines)
- Urticaria: calamine lotion, witch hazel

Alternative remedies
- Heartburn: aromatherapy, homeopathy, herbalism
- Migraine: acupuncture, Alexander technique, aromatherapy, chiropractic, herbalism, homeopathy, hypnosis, osteopathy, reflexology
- Cystitis: aromatherapy, herbalism, homeopathy
- Sleep problems: aromatherapy, Bach flower remedies, herbalism, homeopathy, relaxation exercises, meditation
- Flushing: herbalism
- Urticaria: aromatherapy, herbalism, homeopathy

Self-help tips: for symptom relief see *Heartburn, Migraine, Cystitis, Palpitations, Sleep problems, Flushing, Urticaria* in the section on *Symptoms*

Cake
See *Grain, Wheat*

Calcium benzoate
See *Food additives – preservatives*

Calcium disodium
See *Food additives – emulsifiers, stabilizers and thickeners*

Calcium glutamate
See *Food additives – flavour enhancers*

Calcium hydrogen sulphite
See *Food additives – preservatives*

Calcium lactate
See *Food additives – emulsifiers, stabilizers and thickeners*

Calcium propionate

See *Food additives – preservatives*

Calcium sulphite

See *Food additives – preservatives*

Camomile

Camomile is the herb *Matricaria chamomilla*.

Type of allergen: consumed

Likely sources of camomile: herbal tea, herbal ointment, cosmetics, hair- and body-care products

Symptoms, tests, treatments and self-help tips, see *Herbs*

You might also react to: mugwort pollen, ragweed pollen

Camphor oil

Camphor oil is derived from the camphor tree *Cinnamomum camphora*. It is used as a plasticizer for cellulose nitrate, and for making lacquers.

Type of allergen: contact

Likely sources of camphor oil: insect repellent, skin creams

Symptoms
Skin reactions: contact dermatitis

Tests
• Skin patch test
• Symptom diary

Treatments
Avoidance
• In an occupational situation, use protective equipment such as gloves.

Prescription medication: steroids, antihistamines

OTC remedies: coal tar, emollients, steroids

Alternative remedies: aromatherapy, Bach flower remedies, homeopathy

Self-help tips: for symptom relief see *Contact dermatitis* in the section on *Symptoms*

Carambola

Carambola is the fruit *Averrhoa carambola*.

Type of allergen: consumed

Symptoms, tests, treatments and self-help tips, see *Fruit*

Caraway

Caraway is the herb *Carum carvi*, used as a seasoning. It is not thought to be a food allergen, but caraway oil is a contact allergen.

Type of allergen: contact, consumed

Likely sources of caraway: used in soaps, perfumes and mouthwashes

Symptoms, treatments and self-help tips, see *Spices*

You might also react to: others in the *Umbelliferae* family, such as aniseed, carrot, celery, celeriac, coriander, cumin, dill, fennel, parsley, parsnip
See also *Curry powder, Oils (cosmetic)*

Carbolic acid
See *Phenol*

Carbon paper

Carbon paper is thin carbon-coated paper used for making copies, particularly in typing.

Type of allergen: inhalant

Symptoms
Eye reactions: conjunctivitis

Tests
• Symptom diary

Treatments
Avoidance

Prescription medication: antihistamines, cromoglycate, nedocromil sodium, steroids, sympathomimetics

OTC remedies: antihistamines

Alternative remedies: herbalism, homeopathy

Self-help tips: for symptom relief see *Conjunctivitis* in the section on *Symptoms*

Carbon tetrachloride
See *Solvents – halogenated solvents*

Cardamom
Cardamom is the spice *Elettaria cardamomum*.

Type of allergen: contact, consumed

Symptoms, treatments and self-help tips, see *Spices*

You might also react to: ginger, turmeric

Carminic acid
See *Food additives – colourings; cosmetics*
Note that carmine might also be used in eye make-up and is linked to allergic conjunctivitis.

Carmoisine
See *Food additives – colourings*

Carob
Carob is the edible bean-shaped pods of the tree *Ceratonia siliqua*, often used as a substitute for chocolate.

Type of allergen: consumed

Symptoms
Mouth, nasal and ear reactions: rhinitis

Respiratory reactions: asthma

Tests
• Blood test: CAP-RAST
• Symptom diary (including peak flow meter readings)

Treatments
Avoidance

Prescription medication
• Rhinitis: antihistamines, decongestants, sodium cromoglycate, immunotherapy
• Asthma: anticholinergic drugs, antihistamines (exercise-induced), Beta2 (ß2) adrenoreceptor agonists, cromoglycate, nedocromil sodium, steroids, xanthine derivatives, zafirlukast

OTC remedies
• Rhinitis: decongestants

Alternative remedies
• Rhinitis: aromatherapy
• Asthma: acupuncture (mild asthma only), Buteyko method, homeopathy, relaxation techniques, yoga

Self-help tips: for symptom relief see *Rhinitis, Asthma* in the section on *Symptoms*

You might also react to: soya

Carp
See *Fish*

Carpets

Carpets are a source of allergy because:

- they harbour *dust mites*
- they can harbour *moulds* (e.g. in damp locations such as bathrooms)
- *artificial fibres* affect some people
- some carpets give off fumes (free residual formaldehyde or isocyanates, free vinyl acetate, chloride, butene, styrene in the foam backing), and hydrocarbon solvents from stain treatments, preservatives treatments and adhesives used to laminate the backing to the fibre)
- the *adhesive* used in the carpets can cause problems – particularly 4-phenylcyclohexene, (4-PC), which is a by-product of styrene-butadiene

Type of allergen: inhalant, contact

Symptoms
Eye reactions: conjunctivitis

Headache

Mouth, nasal and ear reactions: sore throat

Psychological problems: fatigue

Skin reactions: skin irritation

Other reactions: muscle pain

Tests
- Skin patch
- Symptom diary

Treatments
Avoidance
- Ventilate the room for 72 hours after a new carpet is laid

Prescription medication
- Conjunctivitis: antihistamines, cromoglycate, nedocromil sodium, steroids, sympathomimetics
- Headache: painkillers, non-steroidal anti-inflammatories
- Muscle pain: painkillers
- Skin irritation: emollients

OTC remedies
- Conjunctivitis: antihistamines
- Headache: as prescription medication
- Muscle pain: painkillers
- Skin irritation: emollients

Alternative remedies
- Conjunctivitis: herbalism, homeopathy
- Headache: acupuncture, aromatherapy, herbalism, homeopathy
- Muscle pain: homeopathy
- Fatigue: aromatherapy, Bach flower remedies, homeopathy

Self-help tips: for symptom relief see *Conjunctivitis, Headache, Muscle pain, Fatigue, Skin irritation* in the section on *Symptoms*

Alternative products that won't cause a reaction: change the carpet for hard flooring such as wood, tile or lino
See also: *Artificial fibres, Adhesives, Dust mites, Formaldehyde, Mould, Wool*

Carpet backings
See *Carpets, Volatile organic compounds*

Carpet cleaning fluids
See *Solvents – aliphatic hydrocarbons*

Carrageenan
Carrageenan is a polysaccharide found in seaweed (*Chondrus crispus*); it contains galactose. It is used as an emulsifier and thickener in foods.
Note that it can also be found in barium enemas.
See *Food additives – emulsifiers, stabilizers and thickeners*

Carrot

Carrots are the vegetable of the plant *Daucus carota sativa*. The protein is heat-labile, so cooked vegetables are less allergenic than raw. You may find that your reaction is more severe during the pollen season.

Type of allergen: contact, consumed

Symptoms, tests, treatments and self-help tips, see *Vegetables*

You might also react to: others in the *Umbelliferae* family (such as aniseed, caraway, celery, celeriac, cumin, coriander, dill, fennel, parsley, parsnip); also apples, birch pollen, mugwort pollen, potatoes

Casein

See *Milk*

Cashew nuts

Cashew nuts are from the tree *Anacardium occidentale*. The allergic reaction is caused by cardol in the nut shell.

Type of allergen: contact, consumed

Symptoms, tests, treatments and self-help tips, see *Nuts*

You might also react to: mango, pistachios

Cassia oil

Cassia oil is also known as oil of cinnamon.

Type of allergen: contact

Likely sources of Cassia oil: used in perfumes and toothpastes

Symptoms, tests, treatments and self-help tips, see *Oils, cosmetic*

Castor beans/oil

Castor oil is pressed from the castor bean *Ricinus communis*. It is used in the pharmaceutical industry and cosmetic production. Castor beans have been linked to occupational asthma. If symptoms start soon after beginning work and improve at weekends or on holidays, occupational asthma should be suspected.

Type of allergen: inhaled

Symptoms
Respiratory reactions: occupational asthma.

Tests
• Blood test: CAP-RAST test
• Symptom diary (including peak flow meter readings)

Treatments
Avoidance: in an occupational situation, use protective equipment such as masks. Improved ventilation may also help.

Prescription medication: anticholinergic drugs, antihistamines (exercise-induced), Beta2 (ß2) adrenoreceptor agonists, cromoglycate, nedocromil sodium, steroids, xanthine derivatives, zafirlukast

Alternative remedies: acupuncture (mild asthma only), Buteyko method, homeopathy, relaxation techniques, yoga

Self-help tips: for symptom relief see *Asthma* in the section on *Symptoms*

Catheters
See *Mercaptobenzothiazole*

Cats
See *Pets*

Cauliflower

Cauliflower is the vegetable *Brassica oleracea var. botrytis*.

Type of allergen: consumed

Symptoms, tests, treatments and self-help tips, see *Vegetables*

You might also react to: broccoli, Brussels sprouts, cabbage, horseradish, mustard, radish, swede, turnip, watercress

Caviar

See *Fish*

Cayenne pepper

Cayenne pepper is a spice derived from the ground, dried fruit of *Capsicum annuum*. It is also known as red pepper and Tabasco pepper. The problem is with capsaicin (the substance found in pepper that makes it hot).

Type of allergen: contact, consumed

Symptoms, treatments and self-help tips, see *Spices*

You might also react to: other vegetables/plants in the nightshade family: such as aubergine, chilli, peppers (capsicum), paprika, potato, tobacco, tomato
See also *Chilli pepper and curry powder*

Cedarwood oil

Cedarwood oil is distilled from the tree *Cedrus*.

Type of allergen: contact

Likely sources of cedarwood oil: insect repellents, perfumes and soaps

Symptoms, tests, treatments and self-help tips, see *Oils, cosmetic*

Cefaclor, Cefadroxil, Cefixime, Cefpoxidime, Cefprozil, Ceftibuten, Cefuroxime

See *Cephalosporin, Antibiotics, Drugs*

Celery

Celery is the vegetable *Apium graveolens*. The three main allergens in celery are Api g1 (celery protein), celery profilin and CCD.

Type of allergen: contact, consumed

Symptoms, tests, treatments and self-help tips, see *Vegetables*

You might also react to: others in the *Umbelliferae* family, such as aniseed, caraway, carrot, celeriac, cumin, coriander, dill, fennel, parsley, parsnip; also sage, birch, mugwort and grass pollens

Cement

See *Chromate, Chromium, Cobalt, Copper sulphate, Potassium dichromate, Solvents – ketone solvents*

Cephadrine, Cephalexin

See *Cephalosporin, Antibiotics, Drugs*

Cephalosporin

Cephalosporin is a broad-spectrum *antibiotic*, used for infections such as urinary tract infection and meningitis.

Roughly 10 per cent of people allergic to penicillin are also allergic to cephalosporin.

Cephalosporins include: cefaclor, cefadroxil, cefixime, cefpodoxime, cefprozil, ceftibuten, cefuroxime, cephalexin, cephradine.

Type of allergen: consumed

Symptoms, tests, treatments and self-help tips, see *Drugs*

Alternative products that won't cause a reaction:
antibiotics that are not mould-based, such as *tetracycline*

You might also react to: penicillin

Ceramics
See *Cobalt*

Cereals
See *Grain*

Cetyl alcohol

Cetyl alcohol is derived from spermaceti from the sperm whale.

Type of allergen: contact

Likely sources of cetyl alcohol: cosmetics

Symptoms
Skin reactions: urticaria

Tests
• Skin patch test
• Symptom diary

Treatments
Avoidance: check labels carefully
Prescription medication: antihistamines, emollients, steroids

OTC remedies: calamine lotion, witch hazel

Alternative remedies: aromatherapy, herbalism, homeopathy

Self-help tips: for symptom relief see *Urticaria* in the section on *Symptoms*

Cheese

Cheese may contain vasoactive *amines*, produced when bacteria start to break the food down; these are usually *tyramine, histamine* and *phenylethylamine*, and are found in higher concentrations in matured cheddar and blue cheese such as Stilton.

Cheese also contains *mites* and can cause problems for handlers and producers – usually eczema.

Casein is the most likely allergen in cheese (see *milk*) – the harder the cheese, the more casein it contains.

Type of allergen: consumed, contact

Symptoms
Anaphylactic shock: exercise-induced

Gastrointestinal reactions: people who are lactose-intolerant may have abdominal pain, bloating, diarrhoea, wind

Headache: migraine

Respiratory reactions: asthma, cough

Skin reactions: angioedema, eczema (occupational), flushed face, urticaria

Tests
- Blood test: CAP-RAST (cheddar and mould-type cheeses)
- Blood test: ELISA (parmesan, ewe's, goat's, cheddar, mould, Edam, Roquefort, Camembert, Swiss, Gouda, Leerdam)
- Skin prick test
- Elimination diet
- Food challenge
- Symptom diary (including peak flow meter readings)
- Exercise challenge

Treatments
Avoidance:
- Check labels carefully and check with a dietitian to ensure that your diet is still nutritionally sound
- In an occupational situation, use protective equipment such as gloves

Prescription medication
- Anaphylactic shock: adrenaline, antihistamines, steroids
- Abdominal pain and swelling: antacids, anti-spasmodic drugs
- Diarrhoea: antidiarrhoeal drugs

- Wind: antacids
- Headache: painkillers, non-steroidal anti-inflammatories
- Migraine: painkillers, anti-sickness drugs, ergotamine, 5-HT agonists, beta-blockers, sodium valproate, sumatryptan
- Asthma: anticholinergic drugs, antihistamines (exercise-induced), Beta2 (ß2) adrenoreceptor agonists, cromoglycate, nedocromil sodium, steroids, xanthine derivatives, zafirlukast
- Cough: antihistamines, bronchodilators, corticosteroids
- Angioedema: adrenaline, antihistamines, steroids
- Eczema: emollients, immune suppressants, steroids, UVA/UVB light treatment, wet wrapping, antihistamines
- Urticaria: antihistamines, emollients, steroids

OTC remedies
- Abdominal pain and swelling: antacids
- Diarrhoea: kaolin and morphine, calcium carbonate, pectin
- Wind: antacids
- Headache: as prescription medication
- Migraine: aspirin, ibuprofen, paracetamol
- Cough: demulcents, antitussives, expectorants
- Angioedema: antihistamines
- Eczema: emollients, hydrocortisone cream
- Urticaria: calamine lotion, witch hazel

Alternative remedies
- Abdominal pain and swelling: aromatherapy, herbalism, homeopathy
- Diarrhoea: aromatherapy, herbalism, homeopathy
- Wind: aromatherapy, herbalism, homeopathy
- Headache: acupuncture, aromatherapy, herbalism, homeopathy
- Migraine: acupuncture, Alexander technique, aromatherapy, chiropractic, herbalism, homeopathy, hypnosis, osteopathy, reflexology
- Asthma: acupuncture (mild asthma only), Buteyko method, homeopathy, relaxation techniques, yoga
- Cough: aromatherapy, homeopathy
- Eczema: aromatherapy, evening primrose oil, relaxation, herbalism, homeopathy, Chinese herbal medicine, Bach flower remedies
- Flushing: herbalism
- Urticaria: aromatherapy, herbalism, homeopathy

Self-help tips: for symptom relief see *Abdominal pain, Bloating, Diarrhoea, Wind, Headache, Migraine, Asthma, Cough, Angioedema, Eczema, Flushing, Urticaria* in the section on *Symptoms*

Alternative products that won't cause a reaction: if the *tyramine* in cheese causes your problems, you may be able to tolerate cottage cheese, quark, cream cheese and curd cheese, which do not contain tyramine.

Chemicals

There are four types of reaction to chemicals:

- true allergy, where chemicals trigger a reaction that involves IgE – this can be shown by blood tests or skin tests
- false chemical allergy, where chemical components bind to the mast cells, which then release the same chemical messengers in the same way that IgE works – the symptoms will be that of an allergy but tests will not show positive results
- irritant reactions – many chemicals have irritant or toxic properties but don't cause problems in low concentrations; high exposure rather than allergy causes the reaction. If you have a high exposure to them (e.g. you handle them at work), you may suffer from asthma, breathing problems, rashes and dizziness. Likely culprits are ammonia, chlorine, enzymes, isocyanates, nitrogen oxide, platinum salts, soldering flux and sulphur dioxide.
- chemical sensitivity, where very low levels of chemicals cause an adverse reaction involving IgE

Chemicals, cleaning: alkalis; ammonia; chloramine-T, chloramphenicol

Chemicals, industrial: acetic acid; ammonia; ethylene oxide; persulphate

Chemicals, other: Acid, chlorine

Symptoms
Anaphylactic shock (ethylene oxide)

Eye reactions: conjunctivitis (ammonia, chlorine)

Mouth, nasal and ear reactions: irritation of mucous membranes (chlorine); rhinitis (ethylene oxide)

Respiratory reactions: asthma (occupational) (acid, acrylate, chloramine-T, chloramphenicol, persulphate); breathing problems (chlorine, ethylene oxide)

Skin reactions: angioedema (persulphate); contact dermatitis, including occupational (acid, alkalis, ammonia); eczema (persulphate); urticaria (acetic acid, chloramphenicol, ethylene oxide, persulphate)

Tests
- Blood test: CAP-RAST (chloramine-T, ethylene oxide)
- Blood test: ELISA (ethylene oxide)
- Skin test: skin prick (chloramphenicol)
- Skin test: patch test (acetic acid, acid, alkalis, ammonia, chloramphenicol, persulphate)
- Inhalation challenge (chlorine)
- Symptom diary (including peak flow meter readings)

Treatments
Avoidance
- In occupational situations, use protective equipment such as gloves or masks; improved ventilation may also help.

Prescription medication
- Anaphylactic shock: adrenaline, antihistamines, steroids
- Conjunctivitis: antihistamines, cromoglycate, nedocromil sodium, steroids, sympathomimetics
- Irritation of mucous membranes: painkillers
- Rhinitis: antihistamines, decongestants, sodium cromoglycate, immunotherapy
- Asthma: anticholinergic drugs, antihistamines (exercise-induced), Beta2 (ß2) adrenoreceptor agonists, cromoglycate, nedocromil sodium, steroids, xanthine derivatives, zafirlukast
- Breathing problems: bronchodilators, corticosteroids
- Angioedema: adrenaline, antihistamines, steroids
- Dermatitis: steroids, antihistamines
- Eczema: emollients, immune suppressants, steroids, UVA/UVB light treatment, wet wrapping, antihistamines
- Urticaria: antihistamines, emollients, steroids

OTC remedies:
• Conjunctivitis: antihistamines
• Irritation of mucous membranes: painkillers
• Rhinitis: decongestants
• Cough: demulcents, antitussives, expectorants
• Dermatitis: coal tar, emollients, steroids
• Eczema: emollients, hydrocortisone cream
• Urticaria: calamine lotion, witch hazel

Alternative remedies
• Conjunctivitis: herbalism, homeopathy
• Irritation of mucous membranes: herbalism
• Rhinitis: aromatherapy
• Asthma: acupuncture (mild asthma only), Buteyko method, homeopathy, relaxation techniques, yoga
• Cough: aromatherapy, homeopathy
• Angioedema: antihistamines
• Contact dermatitis: aromatherapy, Bach flower remedies, homeopathy
• Eczema: aromatherapy, evening primrose oil, relaxation, herbalism, homeopathy, Chinese herbal medicine, Bach flower remedies
• Urticaria: aromatherapy, herbalism, homeopathy

Self-help tips: for symptom relief see *Conjunctivitis, Irritation of mucous membranes, Asthma, Breathing problems, Angioedema, Contact dermatitis, Eczema, Urticaria* in the section on *Symptoms*

Chemicals, engraving
See *Chromium*

Chemicals, photographic developing
See *Chromium*

Chemicals, printing
See *Chromium*

Cherry

Cherries are the soft stone fruit of the tree *Prunus*. They contain *salicylates*, which have been linked to hyperactivity in children.

Type of allergen: consumed

Symptoms, tests, treatments and self-help tips, see *Fruit*

You might also react to: birch pollen, pellitory pollen, almonds, apricots, peaches, plums

Chestnut

Chestnuts are the fruit of the tree *Castanea sativa*.

Type of allergen: consumed

Symptoms, treatments and self-help tips, see *Nuts*

You might also react to: latex

Chewing gum
See *Colophony*

Chick peas

Chick peas are the seeds of the leguminous plant *Cicer arietinum*.

Type of allergen: consumed

Symptoms, tests, treatments and self-help tips, see *Legumes*

You might also react to: beans, lentil, liquorice, pea, peanut, senna, soy

Chicken
See *Meat and poultry*

Chicken liver
See *Meat and poultry*

Chicory

Chicory is the dried, ground root of the chicory plant, *Cichorum intybus*.

Type of allergen: contact

Likely sources of chicory: low-caffeine coffee, alcoholic bitters, confectionery

Symptoms
Skin reactions: contact dermatitis (occupational)

Tests
• Symptom diary

Treatments
Avoidance: in an occupational situation, use protective equipment such as gloves

Prescription medication: steroids, antihistamines

OTC remedies: coal tar, emollients, steroids

Alternative remedies: aromatherapy, Bach flower remedies, homeopathy

Self-help tips: for symptom relief see *Contact dermatitis* in the section on *Symptoms*

You might also react to: artichoke, dandelion, endive, lettuce, sunflower seeds, tarragon

Chilli pepper

Chillis are the dried, hot-tasting pods of the capsicum plant, *Capsicum annuum*.

Type of allergen: contact, consumed

Symptoms, treatments and self-help tips, see *Spices*

You might also react to: other vegetables/plants in the night-shade family such as aubergine, cayenne, peppers (capsicum), paprika, potato, tobacco, tomato

Chipboard
See *Formaldehyde, phenol*

Chives
Chives are the herb *Allium schoenoprasum*.

Type of allergen: consumed

Symptoms, tests, treatments and self-help tips, see *Herbs*

You might also react to: asparagus, garlic, leek, onions, shallots

Chloramine-T
Chloramine-T is also known as sulphone chloramide. It is used to sterilize pipes and vessels in factories and can cause occupational asthma for cleaners. If symptoms start soon after beginning work and improve at weekends or on holidays, occupational asthma should be suspected.

Type of allergen: inhalant

Symptoms, tests, treatments and self-help tips, see *Chemicals*

Chloramphenicol
Chloramphenicol is a broad-spectrum antibiotic used for severe infections like typhoid.

Type of allergen: consumed

Symptoms, tests, treatments and self-help tips, see *Drugs*

Chlorine

Chlorine is a gas (chemical symbol Cl). It is used as a bleaching agent and disinfectant, and it is naturally present in the body. It is unlikely to be an allergen, although its irritant properties can affect the mucous membranes, causing eye irritation and wheezing. It is also used for water purification and for making plastics, especially PVC.

Type of allergen: inhalant

Likely sources of chlorine: bleach (liquid and powder), cleaners, disinfectants, sterilizers, tap water, swimming pools, bleached fabric and paper (including toilet paper, sanitary products and disposable nappies), fungicides

Symptoms, tests, treatments and self-help tips, see *Chemicals*

Chlorocresol

Chlorocresol is a preservative.

Type of allergen: contact, inhaled

Likely sources of chlorocresol: glues, gums, inks, leather goods, paints and textiles

Symptoms, tests, treatments and self-help tips, see *Preservatives*

Chloroform

Chloroform was once used as an anaesthetic. It has been banned for use in drugs and cosmetics in the USA.

Type of allergen: inhalant, contact

Likely sources of chloroform: cleaning products, paint thinners, paint stripper, plastic bonding, propellants, refrigerants

Symptoms

Respiratory reactions: wheezing

Skin reactions: skin irritation

Tests
- Skin patch
- Symptom diary

Treatments

Avoidance
- Use protective equipment such as masks and gloves.
- Improved ventilation may also help.

Prescription medication
- Wheezing: bronchodilator
- Skin irritation: emollients

OTC remedies
- Skin irritation: emollients

Self-help tips: for symptom relief see *Wheezing, Skin irritation* in the section on *Symptoms*
See also *Solvents – halogenated solvents, Solvents – chlorinated hydrocarbons*

Chlorsalicylamide

Chlorsalicylamide is an antibacterial agent.

Type of allergen: contact

Likely sources of chlorsalicylamide: fungicides

Symptoms
Skin reactions: photoallergenic contact dermatitis

Tests
- Photopatch testing: the allergen is placed on two skin sites; one is exposed to sunlight after 48 hours, and then both areas are examined for a rash
- Symptom diary

Treatments

Avoidance: use protective equipment such as gloves

Prescription medication: Photoallergenic contact dermatitis: emollients, steroids

Self-help tips: for symptom relief see *Photoallergenic contact dermatitis* in the section on *Symptoms*

Chocolate

A true allergy to chocolate is extremely rare. Chocolate contains the vasoactive amines phenylethylamine and tyramine, which can trigger migraine; it can also cause heartburn. It also contains oxalates, a derivative of oxalic acid.

Type of allergen: consumed

Symptoms

Gastrointestinal reactions: abdominal pain, diarrhoea, heartburn, vomiting

Headache: headache, migraine

Mouth, nasal and ear reactions: ears blocked

Skin reactions: flushing, urticaria

Tests

- Blood test: CAP-RAST
- Elimination diet
- Food challenge
- Symptom diary

Treatments

Avoidance

- Check labels carefully and check with a dietitian to ensure that your diet is still nutritionally sound

Prescription medication

- Abdominal pain and swelling: antacids, anti-spasmodic drugs
- Diarrhoea: antidiarrhoeal drugs
- Heartburn: antacids, alginates

- Vomiting: anti-emetics
- Headache: painkillers, non-steroidal anti-inflammatories
- Migraine: painkillers, anti-sickness drugs, ergotamine, 5-HT agonists, beta-blockers, sodium valproate, sumatryptan
- Ear problems: sympathomimetics
- Urticaria: antihistamines, emollients, steroids

OTC remedies
- Abdominal pain and swelling: antacids
- Diarrhoea: kaolin and morphine, calcium carbonate, pectin
- Heartburn: as prescription medication
- Vomiting: oral rehydration solution
- Headache: as prescription medication
- Migraine: aspirin, ibuprofen, paracetamol
- Ear problems: painkillers
- Urticaria: calamine lotion, witch hazel

Alternative remedies
- Abdominal pain and swelling: aromatherapy, herbalism, homeopathy
- Diarrhoea: aromatherapy, herbalism, homeopathy
- Heartburn: aromatherapy, homeopathy, herbalism
- Vomiting: herbalism
- Headache: acupuncture, aromatherapy, herbalism, homeopathy
- Migraine: Acupuncture, Alexander technique, aromatherapy, chiropractic, herbalism, homeopathy, hypnosis, osteopathy, reflexology
- Ear problems: aromatherapy, herbalism, homeopathy
- Flushing: herbalism
- Urticaria: aromatherapy, herbalism, homeopathy

Self-help tips: for symptom relief see *Abdomincal pain, Diarrhoea, Heartburn, Vomiting, Headache, Migraine, Ear problems, Flushing, Urticaria* in the section on *Symptoms*

Alternative products that might not cause a reaction: carob

Chocolate brown HT
See *Food additives – colourings*

Chromate

Chromate is a salt of the metal chromium.

Type of allergen: inhalant, contact

Likely sources of chromate: bleaches, cement, leather, matches, printing, tanning

Symptoms, tests, treatments and self-help tips, see *Metals*

Chromium

Chromium is a metallic element (symbol Cr). It is used in making alloy steels and in electroplating. It can cause occupational asthma for tanners, electroplaters and welders; if symptoms start soon after beginning work and improve at weekends or on holidays, occupational asthma should be suspected.

Type of allergen: inhalant, contact

Likely sources of chromium: chrome steel, stainless steel, chrome plating, cement, leather (including tanning materials), engraving and printing chemicals, paint, ink, foundry sand, solvents, wood preservatives, photographic developing chemicals, phosphate-containing detergents, shoe polishes, safety matches, green dyes used in felt, paper industry, glass polish/stain/glazing, magnetic tape, some textiles, and some cosmetics

For symptoms, tests and treatments, see *Metals*

Self-help tips
- Avoid leather unless it has been tanned with vegetable tannins rather than chromate
- Check labels of cosmetics and avoid those containing chromium salts, potassium dichromate, chromium, chrome, chromate, chromite

Chrysanthemums

See *Plants*

Chub mackerel
See *Fish*

Chymopapain

Chymopapain is a protein-digesting enzyme (or protease) occurring in the papaya plant *Carica papaya*.

Type of allergen: inhalant

Likely sources of chymopapain: meat tenderizers

Symptoms, tests, treatments and self-help tips, see *Enzymes*

Cider

Both cider and cider vinegar contains *salicylates*, which have been linked to hyperactivity in children.

Type of allergen: consumed

Symptoms
Psychological problems: hyperactivity

Respiratory reactions: wheezing

Skin reactions: angioedema, urticaria (this has been dismissed by some experts)

Tests
• Elimination diet
• Food challenge
• Symptom diary

Treatments
Avoidance
• Check labels carefully and check with a dietitian to ensure that your diet is still nutritionally sound

Prescription medication
• Hyperactivity: stimulant drugs

- Wheezing: bronchodilator
- Angioedema: adrenaline, antihistamines, steroids
- Urticaria: antihistamines, emollients, steroids

OTC remedies
- Angioedema: antihistamines
- Urticaria: calamine lotion, witch hazel

Alternative remedies
- Urticaria: aromatherapy, herbalism, homeopathy

Self-help tips: for symptom relief see *Hyperactivity, Wheezing, Angioedema, Urticaria* in the section on *Symptoms*
See also *Yeast*

Cider vinegar
See *Cider, Vinegar, cider*

Cigarette smoke
See *Tobacco*

Cigarettes
See *Formaldehyde*

Cinchocaine
See *Anaesthetic, Drugs*

Cinnamaldehyde
See *Cinnamic aldehyde, Perfumes*

Cinnamic acid
Cinnamic acid is a white crystalline carboxylic acid; its esters occur in some essential oils. See also *Aromatherapy oil*.

Type of allergen: contact

Symptoms
Skin reactions: contact urticaria

Tests
- Patch test
- Symptom diary

Treatments
Avoidance: check labels carefully

Prescription medication: antihistamines, emollients, steroids

OTC remedies: calamine lotion, witch hazel

Alternative remedies: aromatherapy, herbalism, homeopathy

Self-help tips for symptom relief see *Urticaria* in the section on *Symptoms*

Cinnamic alcohol
See *Perfumes*

Cinnamic aldehyde

Cinnamic aldehyde is also known as cinnamaldehyde. It is a yellow liquid used in perfumes and is also found in the spice cinnamon.

Type of allergen: contact

Symptoms
Skin reactions: contact urticaria, allergic contact dermatitis (occupational)

Treatments
- Patch test
- Symptom diary

Treatments
Avoidance
- Check labels carefully; in an occupational situation, use protective equipment such as gloves.

Prescription medication
- Contact dermatitis: steroids, antihistamines
- Urticaria: antihistamines, emollients, steroids

OTC remedies:
- Contact dermatitis: coal tar, emollients, steroids
- Urticaria: calamine lotion, witch hazel

Alternative remedies
- Contact dermatitis: aromatherapy, Bach flower remedies, homeopathy
- Urticaria: aromatherapy, herbalism, homeopathy

Self-help tips: for symptom relief see *Contact dermatitis, Urticaria* in the section on *Symptoms*

Cinnamon

Cinnamon is a spice made from the dried inner bark of the evergreen tree *Cinnamomum zeylanicum*.

Type of allergen: inhalant, contact, consumed

Symptoms, treatments and self-help tips, see *Spices*

You might also react to: avocado, bay leaf

Cinnamon bark

Oil extracted from the bark of cinnamon trees.

Type of allergen: contact

Likely sources of cinnamon bark: cosmetics

Symptoms, tests, treatments and self-help tips, see *Oils, cosmetic*

Cinnamon oil
See *Cassia oil*

Citronella oil

Citronella oil is derived from an Asian grass.

Type of allergen: contact

Likely sources of citronella oil: toiletries, insect repellent

Symptoms, tests, treatments and self-help tips, see *Oils, cosmetic*

Citrus fruits

Citrus fruits contain octopamine and are a source of *histamine*; they also contain synephrine (a vasoactive amine) and tyramine. There are higher levels of amine in the skin, so concentrated orange juice (where the whole orange, including the skin, is crushed to produce the concentrate) may affect you badly. Oranges also contain *salicylates*, which are linked to hyperactivity in children.

Type of allergen: contact, consumed

Symptoms, tests, treatments and self-help tips, see *Fruit*

Clam

See *Shellfish*

Clarithromycin

See *Macrolides, Drugs*

Clay

Clay can cause skin irritation for potters, kiln workers and craft workers.

Type of allergen: contact

Likely sources of clay: pottery and craft materials

Symptoms
Skin reactions: irritant contact dermatitis

Tests
* Skin patch test
* Symptom diary

Treatments
Avoidance: in an occupational situation, use protective equipment such as gloves

Prescription medication: steroids, antihistamines

OTC remedies: coal tar, emollients, steroids

Alternative remedies: aromatherapy, Bach flower remedies, homeopathy

Self-help tips: for symptom relief see *Contact dermatitis* in the section on *Symptoms*
See also *Cobalt*

Cleaning materials
Cleaning materials contain several different chemicals. A volatile carrier is used to allow the application of active materials or ingredients. For example, glass cleaners often include solvents such as isopropyl alcohol or methyl alcohol as well as soap, perfumes and water.

Symptoms, tests, treatments and self-help tips, see *Chemicals*
See also *Ammonia, Chlorine, Chloroform, Isocyanates, Isopropanol, Perfume, Solvents – alcohol solvents; Solvents – aliphatic hydro-Carbons, Turpentine, Volatile organic compounds*

Alternatives that might not cause a reaction:
* Glass cleaner – use a teaspoon of vinegar in 1.5 litres of hot water
* Furniture polish – use olive oil
* Fridge/freezer cleaners – use bicarbonate of soda in water

Clove oil

Clove oil is derived from the clove tree, *Eugenia caryophyllus*. The fragrance *eugenol* is derived from clove oil.

Type of allergen: contact, consumed

Likely sources of clove oil: antiseptic, flavourings

Symptoms, treatments and self-help tips, see *Spices*

Cloves

Cloves – *Eugenia caryophyllus* – contain *salicylates*, which have been linked to hyperactivity in children

Type of allergen: inhalant, contact, consumed

Symptoms, treatments and self-help tips, see *Spices*

Coatings

See *Solvents – glycol ether*

Cobalt

Cobalt is a metallic element (chemical symbol Co). It is used in nuclear weapons, alloys and pigments. Cobalt allergy often accompanies allergy to chromium and nickel.

Cobalt dichloride can cause occupational asthma for manufacturing workers in the following industries: polyester resins, car exhaust controls, electroplating, and rubber tyres. If symptoms start soon after beginning work and improve at weekends or on holidays, occupational asthma should be suspected.

Likely sources of cobalt: metal-plated objects such as buckles, buttons, zips and costume jewellery. It also is found in tools, kitchen utensils, instruments, pigments, cobalt blue paints, pottery, ceramics, printing ink, paper making, cutting oils, polyester manufacture, tattoos, and antiperspirants.

Cobalt salts (chloride and sulphate) are used as pigments in light brown hair dyes, cosmetics and adhesives.

Cobalt dichloride also can be found in metal alloys, cements, clay, glass, lubricating oils.

Type of allergen: inhalant, contact

Symptoms, tests and treatments, see *Metals*

Self-help tips
• Check labels and avoid anything including cobalt blue or cobaltous.
• Alternative products that may not cause a reaction: pewter, platinum, sterling silver

You might also react to: nickel
See also *Chrome*.

Cochineal
See *Food additives – colourings*

Cockroaches
The major antigens are in the insect's body parts; excreta and egg cases are less allergenic.

Type of allergen: inhalant

Symptoms
Anaphylactic shock

Mouth, nasal and ear reactions: rhinitis

Respiratory reactions: asthma

Tests
• Symptom diary (including peak flow meter readings)
• Blood tests

Treatments
Avoidance
• Use protective equipment such as masks where possible

Prescription medication
- Anaphylactic shock: adrenaline, antihistamines, steroids
- Rhinitis: antihistamines, decongestants, sodium cromoglycate, immunotherapy
- Asthma: anticholinergic drugs, antihistamines (exercise-induced), Beta2 (ß2) adrenoreceptor agonists, cromoglycate, nedocromil sodium, steroids, xanthine derivatives, zafirlukast

OTC remedies
- Rhinitis: decongestants

Alternative remedies
- Rhinitis: aromatherapy
- Asthma: acupuncture (mild asthma only), Buteyko method, homeopathy, relaxation techniques, yoga
- Immunotherapy

Self-help tips: for symptom relief see *Rhinitis, Asthma* in the section on *Symptoms*

Cocoa

Cocoa is the bean of the tree *Theobroma cacao*.

Type of allergen: inhalant (dust), consumed, contact

Symptoms
Gastrointestinal reactions: abdominal pain and swelling, diarrhoea

Headache: migraine

Mouth, nasal and ear reactions: rhinitis

Respiratory reactions: asthma

Skin reactions: angioedema, atopic dermatitis, contact dermatitis

Tests
- Skin prick test
- Blood test: CAP-RAST

- Elimination diet
- Food challenge
- Symptom diary (including peak flow meter readings)

Treatments
Avoidance
- Check labels carefully and check with a dietitian to ensure that your diet is still nutritionally sound; in occupational situations, use protective equipment such as gloves

Prescription medication
- Abdominal pain and swelling: antacids, anti-spasmodic drugs
- Diarrhoea: antidiarrhoeal drugs
- Migraine: painkillers, anti-sickness drugs, ergotamine, 5-HT agonists, beta-blockers, sodium valproate, sumatryptan
- Rhinitis: antihistamines, decongestants, sodium cromoglycate, immunotherapy
- Asthma: anticholinergic drugs, antihistamines (exercise-induced), Beta2 (ß2) adrenoreceptor agonists, cromoglycate, nedocromil sodium, steroids, xanthine derivatives, zafirlukast
- Angioedema: adrenaline, antihistamines, steroids
- Contact dermatitis: steroids, antihistamines

OTC remedies
- Abdominal pain and swelling: antacids
- Diarrhoea: kaolin and morphine, calcium carbonate, pectin
- Migraine: aspirin, ibuprofen, paracetamol
- Rhinitis: decongestants
- Angioedema: antihistamines
- Contact dermatitis: coal tar, emollients, steroids

Alternative remedies
- Abdominal pain and swelling: aromatherapy, herbalism, homeopathy
- Diarrhoea: aromatherapy, herbalism, homeopathy
- Migraine: acupuncture, Alexander technique, aromatherapy, chiropractic, herbalism, homeopathy, hypnosis, osteopathy, reflexology
- Rhinitis: aromatherapy
- Asthma: acupuncture (mild asthma only), Buteyko method, homeopathy, relaxation techniques, yoga
- Contact dermatitis: aromatherapy, Bach flower remedies, homeopathy

Self-help tips: for symptom relief see *Abdominal pain and swelling, Diarrhoea, Migraine, Rhinitis, Asthma, Angioedema, Contact dermatitis* in the section on *Symptoms*

Coconut

Coconut is the fruit of the tropical palm tree *Cocos nucifera.*

Type of allergen: consumed, contact

Symptoms, tests, treatments and self-help tips, see *Nuts*

You might also react to: dates

Coconut oil

Coconut oil is a saturated fat derived from coconut kernels.

Type of allergen: contact, consumed

Likely sources of coconut oil: soaps, toiletries, foods

Symptoms, tests, treatments and self-help tips, see *Oils, cosmetic*

Cod

See *Fish*

Codeine

Codeine $(C_{18}H_{21}NO_3)$ is an opioid painkiller related to morphine; it is also known as methylmorphine.

Type of allergen: consumed

For symptoms, tests and treatments, see *Drugs*

Self-help tips
- Tell your GP, dentist or other medical practitioner that you're sensitive to codeine
- Read labels in any OTC medication and check with the pharmacist before taking – particularly for medications treating headaches, colds, coughs, allergies, sinus problems, arthritis,

rheumatism (joint pain), menstrual cramps, stomach acidity, backache, or urinary pain

You might also react to: aspirin, non-steroidal anti-inflammatory drugs (NSAIDs), tartrazine (note that some medication includes tartrazine)

Coffee
See *Caffeine*

Coins
See *Copper sulphate*

Cold
See *Temperature*

Cologne
See *Perfume*

Colophony
Colophony, often called "rosin", is obtained from the sap of four species of pine trees. It is used in a wide variety of products for its ability to make things sticky. It causes occupational asthma where soldering fumes are inhaled. If symptoms start soon after beginning work and improve at weekends or on holidays, occupational asthma should be suspected.

Type of allergen: inhalant, contact

Likely sources of colophony: adhesives, paints, varnishes, asphalt products, soldering materials, polyethylene, linoleum; cosmetics and soaps; grease removers, waxes, polishes; matches, fireworks, chewing gums, postage stamps; printing inks and paper (environmentally friendly); topical veterinary medications (e.g. salves and hoof softeners)

Symptoms
Respiratory reactions: occupational asthma

Skin reactions: contact dermatitis, skin irritation

Tests
- Skin patch test
- Symptom diary (including peak flow meter readings)

Treatments
Avoidance
- In an occupational situation, use protective equipment such as masks. Improved ventilation may also help. Wear gloves when applying veterinary medications or when decorating.
- Check labels on products and avoid those that list: colophony, rosin, gum rosin, rosin gum, resina terebinthinae, W-W wood rosin, tall oil, abietic acid, methyl abietate alcohol, abietic alcohol, abietyl alcohol

Prescription medication
- Asthma: anticholinergic drugs, antihistamines (exercise-induced), Beta2 (ß2) adrenoreceptor agonists, cromoglycate, nedocromil sodium, steroids, xanthine derivatives, zafirlukast
- Contact dermatitis: steroids, antihistamines
- Skin irritation: emollients

OTC remedies
- Contact dermatitis: coal tar, emollients, steroids
- Skin irritation: emollients

Alternative remedies
- Asthma: acupuncture (mild asthma only), Buteyko method, homeopathy, relaxation techniques, yoga
- Contact dermatitis: aromatherapy, Bach flower remedies, homeopathy

Self-help tips: for symptom relief see *Asthma, Contact dermatitis, Skin irritation* in the section on *Symptoms*

You might also react to: wood tars, especially juniper tar (oil of cade); other evergreen trees in addition to pine trees; other plant materials including chrysanthemum; spices (nutmeg, paprika, mace, cloves); fragrances; essential oils

Conditioner (hair)
Perfumes and preservatives tend to cause most problems.

Type of allergen: contact

Symptoms, tests, treatments and self-help tips, see *Cosmetics*

Condoms
See *Latex, Thiurams*

Contact lens cleaning solution
Contact lens cleaning solution can cause conjunctivits in some people. Your optician can advise which solutions are less likely to cause a problem.

Type of allergen: contact

Symptoms
Eye reactions: conjunctivitis

Tests
• Symptom diary

Treatments
Avoidance

Prescription medication: antihistamines, cromoglycate, nedocromil sodium, steroids, sympathomimetics

OTC remedies: antihistamines

Alternative remedies: herbalism, homeopathy

Self-help tips: for symptom relief see *Conjunctivitis* in the section on *Symptoms*

Contraceptive creams
Some people are sensitive to the ingredients in contraceptive creams, which can cause skin rashes.

Type of allergen: contact

Symptoms, tests, treatments and self-help tips, see *Cosmetics*

Copper

Copper is a metallic element (symbol Cu).

Type of allergen: contact

Likely sources of copper: wiring

Symptoms, tests, treatments and self-help tips, see *Metals*

Copper sulphate

Copper sulphate is a blue crystalline solid, $CuSO_4$.

Type of allergen: contact

Likely sources of copper sulphate include: coins, dyes, electroplating, insecticides

Symptoms, tests, treatments and self-help tips, see *Metals*

Coriander

Coriander is the herb *Coriandrum sativum*. It is also known as cilantro and Italian parsley.

Type of allergen: contact, consumed

Symptoms, tests, treatments and self-help tips, see *Herbs*

You might also react to: others in the *Umbelliferae* family, such as aniseed, caraway, carrot, celery, celeriac, cumin, dill, fennel, parsley, parsnip
See also *Curry powder*

Coriander oil

Coriander oil is produced from the herb *Coriandrum sativum*.

Type of allergen: contact

Likely sources of coriander oil: cosmetics

Symptoms, tests, treatments and self-help tips, see *Oils, cosmetic*

Corn

Corn is more likely to give problems with intolerance rather than allergy. It is also known as maize.

Type of allergen: inhalant, contact, consumed

Likely sources of corn: corn on the cob, sweetcorn, breakfast cereals, soup and soup mixes, custard powder, gravy mixes, cornflour, polenta, ready meals and sauces

Symptoms, tests and treatments, see *Grain*

Self-help tips: check labels and avoid: baking powder, cereal starch, cornmeal, cornstarch, corn syrup, dextrimaltose, dextrin, dextrose (a sugar derived from maize), edible starch, food starch, glucose syrup (a sugar derived from maize), margarine, modified starch, popcorn, starch, vegetable gum, vegetable oil (usually a mixture containing maize oil), vegetable starch

You might also react to: other cereals – barley, millet, oats, rice, rye, wheat; bananas and pecans

Cosmetics

These include bath products, blusher, body lotion/oil, conditioner (hair), contraceptive creams, deodorants, depilatories, douche preparations, eye creams, eye liner, eye shadow, face powder, foundation, hair-care products (dye, gel, spray, wax), hand cream/lotion, lip balm, lipstick, mascara, moisturizer, mouthwash, nail varnish, perfume, sanitary products, shampoos, shaving products, skin-care products (creams, lubricants, preparations), soap, suncreams, toothpaste

Make-up, creams and lotions can contain many allergenic components, including alcohols, perfumes and preservatives.

To find out what may be causing you problems, first look at the part of your body that is affected, i.e.:

- armpits – this may be caused by deodorants and depilatories
- ears – this may be caused by perfume and cologne
- eyes – this may be caused by mascara, eyeliner and eyeshadow, moisturizer, cleanser, contact lens solutions or eye drops
- face – this may be caused by foundation, blusher, powder, shaving products and skin preparations
- feet – this may be caused by nail polish or remedies for athlete's foot
- groin area – this may be caused by scented sanitary pads or tampons, contraceptive creams or jellies, douche preparations, deodorants, vaginal medications
- hands – this may be caused by lotions, skin lubricants, nail polish and many topical medications (such as antibiotic, corticosteroid and anaesthetic creams); sunscreens containing PABA (para-aminobenzoic acid) are particularly likely to cause problems
- legs – this may be caused by depilatories (hair removers).
- mouth – this may be caused by toothpaste, mouthwash, lipstick, lip balms
- neck – this may be caused by perfume
- scalp – this may be caused by shampoo, conditioner, gel, wax, hairspray, hair dyes (paraphenylenediamine (PPDA))
- skin stinging – this may be caused by alpha-hydroxy acids, propylene glycol (used as a solvent and preservative) or perfume
- tummy – this may be caused by body lotion or oil, soap or bubble bath

Perfumes and preservatives tend to cause most problems.

Symptoms
Eye reactions
- Conjunctivitis – often perfume and preservatives in bath products, blusher, body lotion/oil, conditioner (hair), deodorant, depilatories, eye creams, eye liner, eye shadow, face powder, foundation, hair-care products (dye, gel, spray, wax), hand cream/lotion, lip balm, lipstick, mascara, moisturizer, mouthwash, nail varnish, perfume, shampoos, shaving products, skin-care products (creams, lubricants, preparations), soap, suncreams, toothpaste

Mouth, nasal and ear reactions
- *rhinitis* – perfume

Respiratory reactions: asthma, occupational: (hair-care products (dye, gel, spray, wax)

Skin reactions
- Angioedema – bath products, blusher, body lotion/oil, conditioner (hair), contraceptive creams, deodorant, depilatories, douches, eye creams, eye liner, eye shadow, face powder, foundation, hair-care products (dye, gel, spray, wax), hand cream/lotion, lip balm, lipstick, mascara, moisturizer, mouthwash, nail varnish, perfume, sanitary products, shampoos, shaving products, skin-care products (creams, lubricants, preparations), soap, suncreams, toothpaste
- Blisters – bath products, blusher, body lotion/oil, conditioner (hair), contraceptive creams, deodorant, depilatories, douches, eye creams, eye liner, eye shadow, face powder, foundation, hair-care products (dye, gel, spray, wax), hand cream/lotion, lip balm, lipstick, mascara, moisturizer, mouthwash, nail varnish, perfume, sanitary products, shampoos, shaving products, skin-care products (creams, lubricants, preparations), soap, suncreams, toothpaste).
- Contact dermatitis – bath products, blusher, body lotion/oil, conditioner (hair), contraceptive creams, deodorant, depilatories, douches, eye creams, eye liner, eye shadow, face powder, foundation, hair-care products (dye, gel, spray, wax), hand cream/lotion, lip balm, lipstick, mascara, moisturizer, mouthwash, nail varnish, perfume, sanitary products, shampoos, shaving products, skin-care products (creams, lubricants, preparations), soap, suncreams, toothpaste
- Photoallergenic contact dermatitis – perfume
- Inflammation – bath products, blusher, body lotion/oil, conditioner (hair), contraceptive creams, deodorant, depilatories, douches, eye creams, eye liner, eye shadow, face powder, foundation, hair-care products (dye, gel, spray, wax), hand cream/lotion, lip balm, lipstick, mascara, moisturizer, mouthwash, nail varnish, perfume, sanitary products, shampoos, shaving products, skin-care products (creams, lubricants, preparations), soap, suncreams, toothpaste
- Itching – bath products, blusher, body lotion/oil, conditioner (hair), contraceptive creams, deodorant, depilatories, douches, eye creams, eye liner, eye shadow, face powder, foundation,

hair-care products (dye, gel, spray, wax), hand cream/lotion, lip balm, lipstick, mascara, moisturizer, mouthwash, nail varnish, perfume, sanitary products, shampoos, shaving products, skin-care products (creams, lubricants, preparations), soap, suncreams, toothpaste

- Skin irritation – bath products, blusher, body lotion/oil, conditioner (hair), contraceptive creams, deodorant, depilatories, douches, eye creams, eye liner, eye shadow, face powder, foundation, hair-care products (dye, gel, spray, wax), hand cream/lotion, lip balm, lipstick, mascara, moisturizer, mouthwash, nail varnish, perfume, sanitary products, shampoos, shaving products, skin-care products (creams, lubricants, preparations), soap, suncreams, toothpaste
- Skin stinging – bath products, blusher, body lotion/oil, conditioner (hair), contraceptive creams, deodorant, depilatories, douches, eye creams, eye liner, eye shadow, face powder, foundation, hair-care products (dye, gel, spray, wax), hand cream/lotion, lip balm, lipstick, mascara, moisturizer, mouthwash, nail varnish, perfume, sanitary products, shampoos, shaving products, skin-care products (creams, lubricants, preparations), soap, suncreams, toothpaste

Other
- Cystitis (perfumed talc, bath products and douches, contraceptive creams, deodorant, sanitary products, soap)

Tests
- Skin test: patch test (bath products, blusher, body lotion/oil, conditioner (hair), contraceptive creams, deodorant, depilatories, douches, eye creams, eye liner, eye shadow, face powder, foundation, hair-care products (dye, gel, spray, wax), hand cream/ lotion, lip balm, lipstick, mascara, mouthwash, nail varnish, perfume, shampoos, shaving products, skin-care products (creams, lubricants, preparations), soap, suncreams, toothpaste)

Treatments
Avoidance:
- In occupational situations, use protective equipment such as gloves or masks
- Check labels for any ingredients to which you are sensitive

Prescription medication
- Conjunctivitis: antihistamines, cromoglycate, nedocromil sodium, steroids, sympathomimetics
- Rhinitis: antihistamines, decongestants, sodium cromoglycate, immunotherapy
- Asthma: anticholinergic drugs, antihistamines (exercise-induced), Beta2 (ß2) adrenoreceptor agonists, cromoglycate, nedocromil sodium, steroids, xanthine derivatives, zafirlukast
- Angioedema: adrenaline, antihistamines, steroids
- Blisters: antihistamines
- Inflammation: antihistamines, emollients, steroids
- Itching: antihistamines, emollients
- Contact dermatitis: steroids, antihistamines
- Photoallergenic contact dermatitis: *emo*llients, steroids
- Skin irritation: emollients
- Skin stinging: emollients
- Cystitis: antibiotics (for infection)

OTC remedies:
- Conjunctivitis: antihistamines
- Rhinitis: decongestants
- Angioedema: antihistamines
- Blisters: antihistamines
- Contact dermatitis: coal tar, emollients, steroids
- Inflammation: antihistamines, emollients
- Itching: antihistamines, emollients
- Skin irritation: emollients
- Cystitis: potassium citrate

Alternative remedies
- Conjunctivitis: herbalism, homeopathy
- Rhinitis: aromatherapy
- Asthma: acupuncture (mild asthma only), Buteyko method, homeopathy, relaxation techniques, yoga
- Blisters: aromatherapy
- Contact dermatitis: aromatherapy, Bach flower remedies, homeopathy
- Itching: aromatherapy, herbalism
- Cystitis: aromatherapy, herbalism, homeopathy

Self-help tips
- Choose cosmetics without perfume and with the minimum of pigments

- Don't use products after the expiry date
- Read all labels carefully
- Wash off all make-up thoroughly at night
- For symptom relief see *Conjunctivitis, Rhinitis, Cystitis, Asthma, Angioedema , Blisters, Contact Dermatitis, Photoallergenic contact dermatitis, Inflammation, Itching, Skin irritation* in the section on *Symptoms*

See also: *Balsam of Peru, Benzoyl peroxide, Bithionol, Castor oil, Cetyl alcohol, Chromium, Cinnamon bark, Cinammon oil, Cobalt, Colophony, Coriander oil, Dichlorophen, Digalloyl trioleate, Formaldehyde, Hexachlorophene, Isopropanol, Lavender oil, Nickel, Oils (cosmetic), Parabens, Patchouli oil, Peppermint oil, Perfume, Phenethyl alcohol, Phenol, Pphthalic acid, Paraphenylenediamine (ppda), Salicylanides, Solvents – alcohol solvents, Solvents – glycols, talc, Turpentine, Wool alcohol*

Co-trimoxazole
See *Drugs, Sulphonamides*

Cotton

The problem with cotton tends to be the finish (see *Formaldehyde*); dust from cotton is also an inhalant allergen that can cause occupational asthma.

Type of allergen: inhalant

Symptoms
Respiratory reactions: asthma

Tests
- CAP-RAST

Treatments
Avoidance: in occupational situations, use protective equipment such as masks; improved ventilation may also help.

Prescription medication: anticholinergic drugs, antihistamines (exercise-induced), Beta2 (ß2) adrenoreceptor agonists, cromo-glycate, nedocromil sodium, steroids, xanthine derivatives, zafirlukast

Alternative remedies: acupuncture (mild asthma only), Buteyko method, homeopathy, relaxation techniques, yoga

Self-help tips: for symptom relief see *Asthma* in the section on *Symptoms*

Cotton seed

Cotton seed is often found in animal feed and fertilizers.

Type of allergen: inhalant

Symptoms
Anaphylactic shock

Tests
* Skin prick test
* Blood test: CAP-RAST
* Symptom diary (including peak flow meter readings)

Treatments
Prescription medication
* Anaphylactic shock: adrenaline, antihistamines, steroids

Self-help tips: in occupational situations, use protective equipment such as masks.

Courgette

Courgette is a small marrow from the *Cucurbitaceae* family, also known as zucchini.

Type of allergen: consumed

Symptoms, tests, treatments and self-help tips, see *Vegetables*

You might also react to: others in the *Cucurbitaceae* family, such as cucumber, marrow, melon, pumpkin, squash, watermelon

Couscous
See *Wheat, grain*

Cow
See *Animal hair, Animal protein*

Crab
See *Shellfish*

Cranberry

Cranberry is the fruit of the shrub *Vaccinium oxycoccos*. It contains *salicylates*.

Type of allergen: consumed

Symptoms, tests, treatments and self-help tips, see *Fruit*

Crayfish
See *Shellfish*

Creosote
See *Phenol, volatile organic compounds*

Cress

Cress is a cruciferous leafy plant used in salads.

Type of allergen: consumed

Symptoms, tests, treatments and self-help tips, see *Vegetables*

Cucumbers

Cucumbers are the fruit of the plant *Cucumis sativus*. They contain *salicylates*, which have been linked to hyperactivity in children.

Type of allergen: consumed

Symptoms, tests, treatments and self-help tips, see *Vegetables*

You might also react to: others in the *Cucurbitaceae* family, such as courgette, marrow, melon, pumpkin, squash, watermelon; you might also react to banana and ragweed

Cumin

Cumin is the spice *Cuminum cyminum*. It contains *salicylates*, which have been linked to hyperactivity in children.

Type of allergen: inhalant, consumed, contact

Symptoms, treatments and self-help tips, see *Spices*

You might also react to: others in the *Umbelliferae* family, such as aniseed, caraway, carrot, celery, celeriac, coriander, dill, fennel, parsley, parsnip

Currants

Currants are the dried fruit of seedless grapes. They contain *salicylates*, which have been linked to hyperactivity in children. They may also contain sulphur dioxide, which causes problems with some asthmatics.

Type of allergen: consumed

Symptoms, tests, treatments and self-help tips, see *Fruit*

Curry powder

Curry powder contains *salicylates*, which have been linked to hyperactivity in children. The majority of reactions to curry powder are caused by the individual component spices caraway, cayenne, coriander and mustard.

Type of allergen: inhalant, contact, consumed

Symptoms, tests, treatments and self-help tips, see *Spices*

Cutlery

See *Chromium, metals*

Cutting oil

See *Cobalt*

Cyclohexane

See *Solvents – aliphatic hydrocarbons*

Cyclohexanone

See *Solvents – ketone solvents*

Dahlias

See *Plants*

Dairy produce

See *Cheese, Milk*

Damp treatment

See *Isocyanates*

Dates

Dates are the fruit of the date palm tree *Phoenix dactylifera*. They contain *salicylates*, which have been linked to hyperactivity in children.

Type of allergen: consumed

Symptoms, tests, treatments and self-help tips, see *Fruit*

You might also react to: coconut

Deer

See *Animal hair*

Degreasing solvents

See *Solvents – halogenated solvents*

Demeclocycline
See *Antibiotics, tetracycline, drugs*

Dental amalgam
See *Fillings, mercury*

Dental treatment
See *Fluoride*

Denture adhesives
See *Benzocaine*

Denture bases
See *Epoxy resin*

Deodorants
Perfumes and preservatives tend to cause most problems.

Type of allergen: contact, inhaled

Symptoms, tests, treatments and self-help tips, see *Cosmetics*
See also *Aluminium chloride, Ammonia*

Depilatories
Perfumes and preservatives tend to cause most problems.

Type of allergen: contact

Symptoms, tests, treatments and self-help tips, see *Cosmetics*

Detergent
Detergent is used in cleaning materials. Some of the problems are caused by enzymes and some by benzene, as detergent is also source of benzene.

Type of allergen: contact

Symptoms
Skin reactions: irritant contact dermatitis

Tests
- Blood test: ELISA (alkalase)
- Skin patch
- Symptom diary

Treatments
Avoidance: use protective equipment such as gloves to protect your skin

Prescription medication: steroids, antihistamines

OTC remedies: coal tar, emollients, steroids

Alternative remedies: aromatherapy, Bach flower remedies, homeopathy

Self-help tips: for symptom relief see *Contact dermatitis* in the section on *Symptoms*
See also *Alkalase, Alkalis, Benzene, Chromium (phosphate), Enzymes, Perfume*

Dichlorobenzene
See *Solvents – halogenated solvents*

Dichloromethane
See *Solvents – chlorinated hydrocarbons, Solvents – halogenated solvents*

Dichlorophen
Dichlorophen – also known as 2,2'-methylenebis(4-chloro-phenol) – is a non-toxic laxative vermicide. It is also used as a veterinary fungicide.

Type of allergen: contact

Likely sources of dichlorophen: antiseptic soaps, cosmetics

Symptoms
Gastrointestinal reactions: abdominal pain, nausea
Skin reactions: photoallergenic contact dermatitis

Tests
- Photopatch testing (the allergen is placed on two skin sites; one is exposed to sunlight after 48 hours, and then both areas are examined for a rash)
- Symptom diary

Treatments
Avoidance

Prescription medication
- Abdominal pain and swelling: antacids, anti-spasmodic drugs
- Nausea: antihistamines
- Photoallergenic contact dermatitis: emollients, steroids

OTC remedies
- Abdominal pain and swelling: antacids
- Nausea: antihistamines

Alternative remedies
- Abdominal pain and swelling: aromatherapy, herbalism, homeopathy
- Nausea: aromatherapy, herbalism, homeopathy

Self-help tips: for symptom relief see *Abdominal pain, Nausea, Photoallergenic contact dermatitis* in the section on *Symptoms*

Diethylbenzene
See *Solvents (aromatic hydrocarbons)*

Diethylene glycol
See *Solvents (glycols)*

Diethylene glycol monobutyl ether (DGMBE)
See *Solvents (glycol ether)*

Diethyl maleate

See *Solvents – esters*

Digalloyl trioleate

Digalloyl trioleateis a chemical used in antiseptic soaps and some cosmetics; it can cause skin rashes.

Type of allergen: contact

Likely sources of digalloyl trioleate: antiseptic soaps, cosmetics

Symptoms
Skin reactions: photoallergenic contact dermatitis

Tests
- Photopatch testing (the allergen is placed on two skin sites; one is exposed to sunlight after 48 hours, and then both areas are examined for a rash)
- Symptom diary

Treatments
Avoidance
- Use protective equipment, such as gloves

Prescription medication
- Photoallergenic contact dermatitis: emollients, steroids

Symptom relief, see *Photoallergenic contact dermatitis* in the section on *Symptoms*

Dill

Dill is the aromatic herb *Anethum graveolens*. It contains *salicylates*, which have been linked to hyperactivity in children.

Type of allergen: consumed

Symptoms, tests, treatments and self-help tips, see *Herbs*

You might also react to: others in the *Umbelliferae* family, such as aniseed, caraway, carrot, celery, celeriac, cumin, coriander, fennel, parsley, parsnip

Dimethyl ketone

See *Solvents – ketone solvents*

Dimethyl sulphoxide

Dimethyl sulphoxide is a colourless solid (chemical symbol $(CH_3)_2SO$).

Type of allergen: contact

Likely sources of dimethyl sulphoxide: solvents

Symptoms
Skin reactions: contact urticaria

Tests
• Skin patch
• Symptom diary

Treatments
Avoidance

Prescription medication: antihistamines, emollients, steroids

OTC remedies: calamine lotion, witch hazel

Alternative remedies: aromatherapy, herbalism, homeopathy

Self-help tips: for symptom relief see *Urticaria* in the section on *Symptoms*

Disinfectant

See *Ammonia, Chlorine, Formaldehyde, Mercury bichloride, Phenol*

Dodecyl gallate

See *Food additives – antioxidants*

Dogs
See *Pets*

Dopamine

Dopamine is a biogenic amine derived from the amino acid phenylalanine. It is a neurotransmitter in the brain and also produces *phenylethylamine*. The enzymes monoamine oxidase and catechol-O-methyl transferase break down dopamine in the body.

Type of allergen: consumed

Likely sources of dopamine: avocado, banana, grains, nuts, meat, fish, dairy products and beans

Symptoms
Skin reactions: flushing

Other reactions: weight gain
Tests
• Symptom diary

Treatments
Alternative remedies
• Flushing: herbalism

Douche preparations

Some people are sensitive to the ingredients in douche preparations, which can cause skin rashes.

Type of allergen: contact

Symptoms, tests, treatments and self-help tips, see *Cosmetics*

Doxycycline
See *Antibiotics, Tetracycline, Drugs*

Drugs

Not all reactions to medication are due to an allergy. Sometimes reactions are caused by:

- your body's inability to tolerate certain medication – for instance, some antibiotics such as erythromycin cause gastric upset
- your body's inability to break down a medication (for example, if you have liver or kidney damage)
- taking two types of medication at the same time which are broken down in the same way in the body – this may result in a higher level of one drug, and consequent side-effects (for example, if you take erythromycin and theophylline at the same time, the level of theophylline will increase, which could trigger a seizure)
- your body not having the enzyme responsible for metabolizing the drug (though this is rare)

Your GP or pharmacist will be able to advise on possible side-effects; if you are concerned by a reaction, talk to your GP immediately and he or she will be able to prescribe an alternative medication that won't have the same side-effects.

If you have reacted to medication in the past, always tell your GP or medical practitioner (e.g. dentist); he or she also needs to know if you have asthma or any other allergies.

The most likely causes of medication allergy are: ACE inhibitors, aspirin, antibiotics, anti-emetics, beta-blockers, sedatives.

Drugs can also cause occupational asthma for pharmaceutical workers and health care professionals (particularly cimetidine and piperazine). If symptoms start soon after beginning work and improve at weekends or on holidays, occupational asthma should be suspected.

See: *Ace inhibitors, Amoxycillin, Anaesthetic, Antibiotics, Anti-emetics, Antifungals, Antihistamines, Antimitotic compounds, Antiseptic, Arnica, Aspirin, Bacitracin, Benzocaine, Beta-blockers, Bithionol, Cephalosporins, Codeine, Dichlorophen, Digaylloyl trioleate, Erythromycin, Gentamycin, Hexachlorophene, Ibuprofen, Iodine, Insulin, Isphagula, Macrolides, Neomycin, Paracetamol, Penicillin, Phenoxymethilpenicillin, Sedatives, Streptomycin, Sulfamethoxazol, Sulphonamides, Tetracycline, Tobramycin*

Symptoms:

Anaphylactic shock: antibiotics, aspirin, insulin (rare), penicillin (rare), phenoxymethilpenicillin, sedatives, sulfamethoxazol, tetracycline – especially after sun exposure

Eye reactions: conjunctivitis (aspirin, sedatives)

Gastrointestinal reactions
• Diarrhoea (antibiotics, cephalosporin, tetracycline)
• Gastric upset/irritation (tetracycline)
• Heartburn (antibiotics, aspirin)
• Nausea (antibiotics)
• Vomiting (antibiotics)

Mouth, nasal and ear reactions
• Hay fever (isphagula)
• Itching mouth/palate (antibiotics)
• Rhinitis (aspirin, isphagula, sedatives)
• Nasal polyps (aspirin)
• Sinusitis (aspirin)
• Swollen mouth, lips and tongue (ACE inhibitors, amoxycillin, antibiotics, aspirin, cephalosporin, penicillin)

Respiratory reactions
• Asthma (occupational) (antibiotics, isphagula)
• Asthma (aspirin, beta-blockers, ibuprofen, paracetamol, tobramycin)
• Breathing problems (ACE inhibitors, amoxycillin, antibiotics, anti-emetics, aspirin, beta-blockers, cephalosporin, ibuprofen, insulin, penicillin)
• Cough (ACE inhibitors, aspirin)
• Wheezing (antibiotics, aspirin, beta-blockers, ibuprofen, insulin, phenoxymethilpenicillin)

Skin reactions
• Angioedema (aspirin, codeine, ibuprofen, iodine, paracetamol, penicillin, sulfamethoxazol)
• Atopic dermatitis (ACE inhibitors, amoxycillin, antibiotics, anti-emetics, antifungals, aspirin, cephalosporin, ibuprofen, insulin, iodine, macrolides, penicillin, phenoxymethil-penicillin, sedatives, sulphonamides, tetracycline)
• Blisters (sulphonamides)
• Contact dermatitis, including occupational (anaesthetics,

antibiotics, antifungals, *antihistamines*, antimitotic compounds, arnica, benzocaine, penicillin, sulfamethoxazol)
- Photoallergenic contact dermatitis (hexachlorophene, sulphonamides, sulfamethoxazol)
- Flushing (anti-emetics)
- Itching (amoxycillin, antibiotics, antifungals, aspirin, cephalosporin, gentamycin, tetracycline)
- Skin irritation (insulin)
- Urticaria (aspirin, bacitracin, benzocaine, gentamycin, insulin, neomycin, penicillin, streptomycin)

Other reactions
- Fever (ACE inhibitors, amoxycillin, antibiotics, cephalosporin, macrolides, penicillin, sulphonamides)
- Chest pain (ACE inhibitors, anti-emetics)
- Joint pain (antifungals, cephalosporin, penicillin)
- Rapid pulse (insulin)
- Sweating (insulin)

Tests
- Blood test: CAP-RAST (antibiotics (ampicilloyl, cefaclor, penicilloyl), cephalosporin, insulin (bovine, human, porcine), isphagula, penicillin, tetracycline)
- Blood test: ELISA (amoxycillin, erythromycin, insulin (bovine, human, porcine), penicillin, phenacetin, sulfamethoxazol, tetracycline)
- Skin test: patch test (anaesthetics, antifungals, *antihistamines*, antimitotic compounds, bacitracin, benzocaine, cephalosporin, neomycin, penicillin, tetracycline)
- Skin test: photopatch testing – the allergen is placed on two skin sites; one is exposed to sunlight after 48 hours, and then both areas are examined for a rash (hexachlorophene, sulphonamides)
- Symptom diary

Treatments
Avoidance
- In occupational situations, use protective equipment such as gloves or masks; improved ventilation may also help.
- Check labels of medication carefully and mention any sensitivities to a pharmacist before buying over the counter medication

Prescription medication
- Anaphylactic shock: adrenaline, antihistamines, steroids
- Diarrhoea: antidiarrhoeal drugs
- Gastric upset/irritation: painkillers (use paracetamol rather than aspirin)
- Heartburn: antacids, alginates
- Nausea: antihistamines
- Vomiting: anti-emetics
- Hay fever: antihistamines, cromoglycate, decongestants, nedocromil sodium, steroids, sympathomimetics
- Rhinitis: antihistamines, decongestants, sodium cromoglycate, immunotherapy
- Asthma: anticholinergic drugs, antihistamines (exercise-induced), Beta2 (ß2) adrenoreceptor agonists, cromoglycate, nedocromil sodium, steroids, xanthine derivatives, zafirlukast
- Breathing problems: bronchodilators, corticosteroids
- Cough: antihistamines, bronchodilators, corticosteroids
- Wheezing: bronchodilator
- Angioedema: adrenaline, antihistamines, steroids
- Itching: antihistamines, emollients
- Dermatitis: steroids, antihistamines
- Photoallergenic contact dermatitis: emollients, steroids
- Skin irritation: emollients
- Urticaria: antihistamines, emollients, steroids

OTC remedies:
- Conjunctivitis: antihistamines
- Diarrhoea: kaolin and morphine, calcium carbonate, pectin
- Gastric upset/irritation: as prescription medication
- Heartburn: as prescription medication
- Nausea: antihistamines
- Vomiting: oral rehydration solution
- Hay fever: antihistamines, decongestants
- Rhinitis: decongestants
- Cough: demulcents, antitussives, expectorants
- Dermatitis: coal tar, emollients, steroids
- Urticaria: calamine lotion, witch hazel

Alternative remedies
- Conjunctivitis: herbalism, homeopathy
- Diarrhoea: aromatherapy, herbalism, homeopathy
- Gastric upset/irritation: aromatherapy, herbalism

- Heartburn: aromatherapy, homeopathy, herbalism
- Nausea: aromatherapy, herbalism, homeopathy
- Vomiting: herbalism
- Hay fever: aromatherapy, herbalism, homeopathy
- Rhinitis: aromatherapy
- Asthma: acupuncture (mild asthma only), Buteyko method, homeopathy, relaxation techniques, yoga
- Cough: aromatherapy, homeopathy
- Angioedema: antihistamines
- Contact dermatitis: aromatherapy, Bach flower remedies, homeopathy
- Flushing: herbalism
- Itching: aromatherapy, herbalism
- Urticaria: aromatherapy, herbalism, homeopathy
- Desensitization: aspirin, cephalosporin, penicillin

Self-help tips: for symptom relief see *Diarrhoea, Gastric upset/ irritation, Heartburn, Gausea, Vomiting, Hay fever, Itching mouth/ palate, Rhinitis, Fever, Joint pain, Asthma, Breathing problems, Cough, Wheezing, Contact dermatitis, Photoallergenic contact dermatitis, Flushing, Itching, Skin irritation, Urticaria* in the section on *Symptoms*
See also *Balsam of Peru, Castor oil*

Dry-cleaning fluid
See *Benzene, isocyanates, Solvents – aliphatic hydrocarbons, Solvents – glycol ether, Solvents – halogenated solvents*

Duck
See *Meat and poultry*

Dust mites
Dust mites (*Dermatophagoides pteronnysimus*) are microscopic creatures (about fifty times smaller than the width of a human hair) that eat dust in our homes; they do not bite, sting or transmit diseases. When they eat bits of fabric, insect parts, skin scales and other components of house dust, they secrete enzymes which they then excrete; the two main allergens in mite droppings are contained in the proteins coating the droppings, called Der p1

and Der p2. The droppings are very small, so they become airborne and are inhaled.

Over 80 per cent of people with allergies show a positive skin reaction to dust mites. Dust mites increase during damp weather, when allergy to dust mites and moulds often seem to be worse.

Dust mites like warm and humid environments (25°C, 70-80 per cent humidity) because they absorb water from the air rather than drinking it; below 50 per cent humidity, they dry out and die. They have powerful suckers on their legs so they stick to fabric, particularly carpets, soft furnishings and curtains. Up to 2 million mites may live in just one mattress and a teaspoon of dust can contain more than 250,000 mite droppings! Mites are killed by sunlight, washing at high temperatures and humidity of less than 55 per cent.

Type of allergen: inhalant

Likely sources of dust mites: bedding, carpets, soft furnishings

Symptoms
Headaches

Mouth, nasal and ear reactions: blocked ears, rhinitis, sinusitis, sneezing

Respiratory reactions: asthma, breathing difficulty, cough, wheezing

Skin reactions: angioedema, eczema

Other reactions: joint pain, muscular aches

Tests
- Skin prick test
- CAP-RAST – dust mite (dermatophagoides farinae, dermatophagoides microceras, dermatophagoides pteronyssinus, euroglyphus maynei), storage mite (acarus siro, glycyphagus domesticus, lepidoglyphus destructor, tyrophagus putrescentiae)
- Blood test: ELISA (dust mite (dermatophagoides farinae, dermatophagoides microceras, dermatophagoides pteronys-

sinus, euroglyphus maynci), storage mite (acarus siro, lepido-
glyphus destructor), glycyphagus domesticus, tyrophagus
putrescentiae)
- Intradermal
- Inhalation challenge
- Nasal challenge
- Symptom diary (including peak flow meter readings)

Treatments
Prescription medication
- Headache: painkillers, non-steroidal anti-inflammatories
- Ear problems: sympathomimetics
- Rhinitis: antihistamines, decongestants, sodium cromoglycate, immunotherapy
- Sneezing: antihistamines, decongestants, sodium cromogylcate
- Asthma: anticholinergic drugs, antihistamines (exercise-induced), Beta2 (ß2) adrenoreceptor agonists, cromoglycate, nedocromil sodium, steroids, xanthine derivatives, zafirlukast
- Breathing problems: bronchodilators, corticosteroids
- Cough: antihistamines, bronchodilators, corticosteroids
- Wheezing: bronchodilator
- Angioedema: adrenaline, antihistamines, steroids
- Eczema: emollients, immune suppressants, steroids, UVA/UVB light treatment, wet wrapping, antihistamines
- Joint pain and swelling: anti-inflammatory drugs, painkillers, steroids
- Muscle pain: painkillers

OTC remedies
- Headache: as prescription medication
- Ear problems: painkillers
- Rhinitis: decongestants
- Cough: demulcents, antitussives, expectorants
- Angioedema: antihistamines
- Eczema: emollients, hydrocortisone cream
- Joint pain and swelling: aspirin, paracetamol
- Muscle pain: painkillers

Alternative remedies
- Headache: acupuncture, aromatherapy, herbalism, homeo-pathy
- Ear problems: aromatherapy, herbalism, homeopathy
- Rhinitis: aromatherapy

- Sneezing: acupuncture
- Joint pain and swelling: acupuncture, aromatherapy, herbalism, homeopathy
- Muscle pain: homeopathy
- Asthma: acupuncture (mild asthma only), Buteyko method, homeopathy, relaxation techniques, yoga
- Cough: aromatherapy, homeopathy
- Eczema: aromatherapy, evening primrose oil, relaxation, herbalism, homeopathy, Chinese herbal medicine, Bach flower remedies

Self-help tips: see the section on *Asthma* in the chapter *Allergic illnesses*. for symptom relief, see *Headache, Ear problems, Rhinitis, Sneezing, Fever, Joint pain, Muscular aches, Asthma, Breathing problems, Cough, Wheezing, Angioedema, Eczema* in the section on *Symptoms*

You might also react to: mites in food; mites in hay, grain and flour

Dyes

Dyes can cause occupational asthma for textile workers and dye manufacturers. If symptoms start soon after beginning work and improve at weekends or on holidays, occupational asthma should be suspected.

Some dyes can also cause contact dermatitis, particularly coal tar dyes; these include alizarin (derived from anthracene or madder plant root). Dyes such as gentian violet can also cause occupational contact dermatitis in pharmaceutical workers.

Henna is a natural vegetable dye which can cause sneezing, asthma and rhinitis.

For further information about the dyes themselves and cross-reactivity see *Acridine, Alizarin, Eosin, Fluorescein, Henna, Gentian violet, Methylene blue, Rose bengal*

Type of allergen: contact, inhaled

Symptoms:

Gastrointestinal reactions: nausea (methylene blue), vomiting (methylene blue)

Mouth/nasal/ear reactions: rhinitis (henna), Sneezing (henna)

Respiratory reactions: asthma (including occupational) (henna)

Skin reactions: contact dermatitis (including occupational) (alizarin, gentian violet), photoallergenic contact dermatitis (acridine, eosin, fluorescein, methylene blue, rose Bengal)

Tests
- Skin patch
- Skin tests – photopatch testing (acridine, eosin, fluorescein, rose Bengal)
- Symptom diary (including peak flow meter readings)

Treatments
Avoidance
- In an occupational situation, use protective equipment such as masks and gloves. Improved ventilation may help.

Prescription medication
- Nausea: antihistamines
- Vomiting: anti-emetics
- Rhinitis: antihistamines, decongestants, sodium cromoglycate, immunotherapy
- Sneezing: antihistamines, decongestants, sodium cromogylcate
- Asthma: anticholinergic drugs, antihistamines (exercise-induced), Beta2 (ß2) adrenoreceptor agonists, cromoglycate, nedocromil sodium, steroids, xanthine derivatives, zafirlukast
- Contact dermatitis: steroids, antihistamines
- Photoallergenic contact dermatitis: emollients, steroids (acridine)

OTC remedies
- Nausea: antihistamines
- Vomiting: oral rehydration solution
- Rhinitis: decongestants
- Contact dermatitis: coal tar, emollients, steroids

Alternative remedies
- Nausea: aromatherapy, herbalism, homeopathy
- Vomiting: herbalism
- Rhinitis: aromatherapy
- Sneezing: acupuncture
- Asthma: acupuncture (mild asthma only), Buteyko method, homeopathy, relaxation techniques, yoga

• Contact dermatitis: aromatherapy, Bach flower remedies, homeopathy

Self-help tips: for symptom relief see *Nausea, Vomiting, Rhinitis, Sneezing, Asthma, Contact dermatitis, Photoallergenic Contact dermatitis* in the section on *Symptoms*
See also: *Acridine, Ammonium dichromate, Chromium, Copper sulphate, Cobalt, Eosin, Copper sulphate, Fluorescein, Formaldehyde, Methyl alcohol, Methylene blue, Nickel, phenol, Phthalic anhydride, Paraphenylenediamine (PPDA), Rose Bengal, silver nitrate, Solvents – alcohol solvents*

E numbers
See *Food additives*

Eel
See *Fish*

Eggs

Eggs are one of the most common causes of food allergy in young children, though many outgrow it by the age of five. It tends to be intolerance rather than allergy in adults. The major effect is from eating the egg, although it can also be a contact allergen.

Most people are allergic to the proteins in the white of the egg rather than the yolk. Ovalbumin is the major allergen and makes up roughly half of the egg white; the other three main allergens in egg white are ovomucoid, ovotransferrin (or conalbumin), and lysozyme. Cooking reduces the allergenicity of eggs, though the allergen ovomucoid is resistant to heat.

Eggs also contain the vasoactive amine tyramine, which causes the blood vessels to widen and may trigger migraines.

Type of allergen: consumed, contact

Likely sources of eggs: advocaat, batter, brioche and rich breads cakes, egg noodles, ice cream, marzipan, mayonnaise, meringues, pastries, quiches, salad dressings, soufflés, waffles, Yorkshire pudding.

They may also be found in shampoo and photographic film; the MMR (mumps, measles and rubella) vaccine is cultured in hen egg.

Symptoms
Anaphylactic shock

Eye reactions: conjunctivitis

Gastrointestinal reactions: abdominal pain and swelling, diarrhoea, nausea, vomiting

Headache: headache, migraine

Mouth, nasal and ear reactions: ears blocked, rhinitis

Respiratory reactions: asthma, breathing problems, wheezing

Skin reactions: angioedema, contact dermatitis, eczema, flushing, urticaria, allergic contact urticaria (raw egg)

Tests
- Skin prick test – white, whole or yolk
- Blood test: ELISA – white, yolk, ovalbumin, ovomucoid
- Intradermal – whole, white and yolk; plus budgerigar, chicken, duck, goose
- CAP-RAST test – white, yolk
- Elimination diet
- Food challenge
- Symptom diary (including peak flow meter readings)

Treatments
Avoidance
- Check with a dietitian to ensure that your diet is still nutritionally sound. Check the ingredients on food package labels and ask about the ingredients in foods prepared in restaurants when you eat out. Avoid anything on the following list: albumin, egg, globulin, lecithin, livetin, lysozymne, ova-, ovo-, silici albuminate, simplesse, vitellin, white, yolk.

  In severe hen egg allergy, children should be skin tested with dilute (1:10) MMR vaccine before it is administered.

  Check the labels of cosmetics – some are egg-based.

Prescription medication
- Anaphylactic shock: adrenaline, antihistamines, steroids
- Conjunctivitis: antihistamines, cromoglycate, nedocromil sodium, steroids, sympathomimetics

- Abdominal pain and swelling: antacids, anti-spasmodic drugs
- Diarrhoea: antidiarrhoeal drugs
- Nausea: antihistamines
- Vomiting: anti-emetics
- Headache: painkillers, non-steroidal anti-inflammatories
- Migraine: painkillers, anti-sickness drugs, ergotamine, 5-HT agonists, beta-blockers, sodium valproate, sumatryptan
- Ear problems: sympathomimetics
- Rhinitis: antihistamines, decongestants, sodium cromoglycate, immunotherapy
- Asthma: anticholinergic drugs, antihistamines (exercise-induced), Beta2 (ß2) adrenoreceptor agonists, cromoglycate, nedocromil sodium, steroids, xanthine derivatives, zafirlukast
- Breathing problems: bronchodilators, corticosteroids
- Wheezing: bronchodilator
- Angioedema: adrenaline, antihistamines, steroids
- Contact dermatitis: steroids, antihistamines
- Eczema: emollients, immune suppressants, steroids, UVA/UVB light treatment, wet wrapping, antihistamines
- Urticaria: antihistamines, emollients, steroids

OTC remedies
- Conjunctivitis: antihistamines
- Abdominal pain and swelling: antacids
- Diarrhoea: kaolin and morphine, calcium carbonate, pectin
- Nausea: antihistamines
- Vomiting: oral rehydration solution
- Headache: as prescription medication
- Migraine: aspirin, ibuprofen, paracetamol
- Ear problems: painkillers
- Rhinitis: decongestants
- Angioedema: antihistamines
- Contact dermatitis: coal tar, emollients, steroids
- Eczema: emollients, hydrocortisone cream, calamine lotion, witch hazel

Alternative remedies
- Conjunctivitis: herbalism, homeopathy
- Abdominal pain and swelling: aromatherapy, herbalism, homeopathy
- Diarrhoea: aromatherapy, herbalism, homeopathy
- Nausea: aromatherapy, herbalism, homeopathy

- Vomiting: herbalism
- Headache: acupuncture, aromatherapy, herbalism, homeopathy
- Migraine: acupuncture, Alexander technique, aromatherapy, chiropractic, herbalism, homeopathy, hypnosis, osteopathy, reflexology
- Ear problems: aromatherapy, herbalism, homeopathy
- Rhinitis: aromatherapy
- Asthma: acupuncture (mild asthma only), Buteyko method, homeopathy, relaxation techniques, yoga
- Contact dermatitis: aromatherapy, Bach flower remedies, homeopathy
- Eczema: aromatherapy, evening primrose oil, relaxation, herbalism, homeopathy, Chinese herbal medicine, Bach flower remedies
- Flushing: herbalism
- Urticaria: aromatherapy, herbalism, homeopathy

Self-help tips: for symptom relief see *Conjunctivitis, Abdominal pain, Diarrhoea, Nausea, Vomiting, Headache, Migraine, Ear problems, Rhinitis, Asthma, Breathing problems, Wheezing, Angioedema, Contact dermatitis, Eczema, Flushing, Urticaria* in the section on *Symptoms*

You might also react to: bird feathers. If you're allergic to the proteins in egg yolk (apovitellenins I, apovitellenins VI, and phosvitin), it's known as "bird-egg syndrome" and you'll react to the inhaled antigens. If you react to the livetin protein in egg yolk, you may also react to chicken meat. If your allergy is seasonal, you may react to the pollen of oak trees, ragweed and goosefoot weeds. You might also react to apples.

Elastic
See *Paraphenylenediamine (ppda)*

Electrical cleaning solvents
See *solvents – halogenated solvents*

Embalming fluid
See *Glutaraldehyde*

Emollients
See *Linseed oil*

Endive

Endive is the salad vegetable *Cichorium endivia*.

Type of allergen: contact

Symptoms, tests, treatments and self-help tips, see *Vegetables*

You might also react to: artichoke chicory, dandelion, lettuce, sunflower seeds, tarragon

Engine cleaners

See *Solvents (aromatic hydrocarbons)*

Envelopes (self-adhesive)

See *Latex*

Environmental pollutants

For further information about the environmental pollutants themselves and cross-reactivity see *Ozone, Sulphur dioxide*.

Nitrogen dioxode (NO_2) is formed when fuel is burned at high temperatures; it is also released from gas pilot lights.

Sulphur dioxide (SO_2) is formed when fuel containing sulphur (usually coal or oil) is burned, and during industrial processes such as metal smelting.

Ozone (O_3) is formed during fuel combustion.

Type of allergen: inhalant

Symptoms
Anaphylactic shock (sulphur dioxide)

Gastrointestinal reactions: irritable bowel syndrome (sulphur dioxide)

Headache

Faintness: (sulphur dioxide), neurological problems (Sulphur dioxide)

Respiratory reactions: asthma (ozone, sulphur dioxide), breathing difficulties (ozone, nitrogen dioxide, sulphur dioxide), cough (nitrogen dioxide, sulphur dioxide), wheezing (ozone, nitrogen dioxide, sulphur dioxide)

Tests
• Symptom diary (including peak flow meter readings)

Treatments
Avoidance

Prescription medication
• Anaphylactic shock: adrenaline, antihistamines, steroids
• Gastric upset/irritation: painkillers (use paracetamol rather than aspirin)
• Faintness: adrenaline (as part of anaphylaxis)
• Asthma: anticholinergic drugs, antihistamines (exercise-induced), Beta2 (ß2) adrenoreceptor agonists, cromoglycate, nedocromil sodium, steroids, xanthine derivatives, zafirlukast
• Breathing problems: bronchodilators, corticosteroids
• Cough: antihistamines, bronchodilators, corticosteroids
• Wheezing: bronchodilator

OTC remedies
• Gastric upset/irritation: as prescription medication
• Cough: demulcents, antitussives, expectorants

Alternative remedies
• Gastric upset/irritation: aromatherapy, herbalism
• Faintness: aromatherapy, Bach flower remedies
• Asthma: acupuncture (mild asthma only), Buteyko method, homeopathy, relaxation techniques, yoga
• Cough: aromatherapy, homeopathy

Self-help tips
• Avoid smoking in the house
• Avoid walking or cycling on busy roads – ozone is concentrated at ground level and nitrogen oxides from car fumes can also make asthma worse
• Keep car windows closed if you pull up behind a lorry or a bus, as more particles will be emitted from the vehicle as it sets off
• Breathe through your nose if you're in polluted air
• For symptom relief see *Gastric upset/irritation, Faintness,*

Asthma, Breathing problems, Cough, Wheezing in the section on *Symptoms*

Enzymes

An enzyme is a protein molecule produced by a living organism. It catalyzes the chemical reactions of other substances (i.e. makes them possible or speeds them up) without being destroyed or altered. It is either a protein-splitting enzyme or biological, and can cause occupational asthma for detergent workers, pharmaceutical workers, bakers and food technology workers. If symptoms start soon after beginning work and improve at weekends or on holidays, occupational asthma should be suspected.

Enzymes are classified according to the type of reaction they catalyze:

- Oxidoreductases – these catalyze oxidation-reduction reactions; they are involved in the transfer of hydrogen or electrons between molecules
- Transferases – these catalyze the transfer of a group of atoms between molecules
- Hydrolases – these catalyze the addition or removal of water from molecules; they are important in the breakdown of materials such as starch and include enzymes such as alpha-amylase
- Lyases – these catalyze double bonds between molecules
- Isomerases – these catalyze the rearrangement of atoms within a molecule
- Ligases – these catalyze the formation of covalent bonds (where atoms share one or more pairs of electrons in a molecule); they are important in the synthesis and repair of molecules, including DNA, and are used in genetic engineering

For further information about the enzymes themselves and cross-reactivity see *Alpha-amylase, Benzophenones, Chymopapain, Papain*

Symptoms

Anaphylactic shock (chymopapain, papain)

Respiratory reactions: occupational asthma

Skin reactions: contact dermatitis (benzophenones); urticaria (benzophenones)

Tests
- CAP-RAST (alpha amylase, chymopapain)
- Blood test: ELISA (alpha amylase, papain)
- Patch test (benzophenones, papain)
- Symptom diary (including peak flow meter readings)

Treatments
Avoidance
- Use protective equipment such as masks and gloves. Improved ventilation may also help.

Prescription medication
- Anaphylactic shock: adrenaline, antihistamines, steroids
- Asthma: anticholinergic drugs, antihistamines (exercise-induced), Beta2 (ß2) adrenoreceptor agonists, cromoglycate, nedocromil sodium, steroids, xanthine derivatives, zafirlukast
- Contact dermatitis: steroids, antihistamines
- Urticaria: antihistamines, emollients, steroids

OTC remedies:
- Contact dermatitis: coal tar, emollients, steroids
- Urticaria: calamine lotion, witch hazel

- **Alternative remedies**
- Asthma: acupuncture (mild asthma only), Buteyko method, homeopathy, relaxation techniques, yoga
- Dermatitis: aromatherapy, Bach flower remedies, homeopathy
- Urticaria: aromatherapy, herbalism, homeopathy

Self-help tips: for symptom relief see *Asthma, Contact Dermatitis, Urticaria* in the section on *Symptoms*

Eosin

Eosin is a red dye used in toner and cosmetics. The potassium or sodium salts of eosin are used in pharmaceuticals.

Type of allergen: contact

Likely sources of eosin: chemical dyes, lipsticks

Symptoms, tests, treatments and self-help tips, see *Dyes*

Epoxy resin

Epoxy resin is a synthetic plastic material produced by the polymerizing of epoxide compounds and phenols (i.e. amines or amides). It is resistant to chemical attack and is very tough; it is also used as an adhesive and in some vinyl and plastic.

Epoxy coatings contain strong solvents such as *ketones, esters* and *aromatic hydrocarbons*. Resin and hardener, the two components of epoxy glue, are generally allergenic only in their unmixed states.

It can cause occupational asthma; if symptoms start soon after beginning work and improve at weekends or on holidays, occupational asthma should be suspected.

Type of allergen: inhalant, contact

Likely sources of epoxy resin: adhesives and adhesive tapes; denture bases; flame retardants; floorings (particularly seamless); industrial coatings; inks; vinyl, plastic and polyvinylchloride products (e.g. spectacle frames, vinyl gloves); wall panel coatings; wires in transformers and motor windings

Symptoms
Mouth/nasal/ear reactions: hay fever

Respiratory reactions: asthma (including occupational)

Skin reactions: contact dermatitis, itching, skin irritation

Other reactions: fever, muscle pain

Tests
• Skin patch test
• Symptom diary (including peak flow meter readings)

Treatments
Avoidance
• In an occupational situation, use protective equipment such as gloves and masks. Improved ventilation can also help.

Prescription medication
• Hay fever: antihistamines, cromoglycate, decongestants, nedocromil sodium, steroids, sympathomimetics

- Asthma: anticholinergic drugs, antihistamines (exercise-induced), Beta2 (ß2) adrenoreceptor agonists, cromoglycate, nedocromil sodium, steroids, xanthine derivatives, zafirlukast
- Contact dermatitis: steroids, antihistamines
- Itching: antihistamines, emollients
- Skin irritation: emollients
- Fever: aspirin, ibuprofen, paracetamol
- Muscle pain: painkillers

OTC remedies
- Hay fever: antihistamines, decongestants
- Fever: aspirin, ibuprofen, paracetamol
- Muscle pain: painkillers
- Contact dermatitis: coal tar, emollients, steroids
- Itching: antihistamines, emollients
- Skin irritation: emollients

Alternative remedies
- Hay fever: aromatherapy, herbalism, homeopathy
- Fever: herbalism, homeopathy
- Muscle pain: homeopathy
- Asthma: acupuncture (mild asthma only), Buteyko method, homeopathy, relaxation techniques, yoga
- Contact dermatitis: aromatherapy, Bach flower remedies, homeopathy
- Itching: aromatherapy, herbalism

Self-help tips: epoxy resin can penetrate rubber gloves, so use heavy duty vinyl gloves if you use it at work.

Check product listings and avoid those listing: 4,4'-Isopropylidenediphenol-epichlorohydrin; diglycidyl ether; bisphenol A [2,2-bis (4-hydroxyphenyl)propane] (diphenylpropane); epichlorohydrin (1-chloro-2,3-epoxypropane) (8-chloropropylene oxide)

For symptom relief, see *Hay fever, Fever, Muscle pain, Asthma, Contact dermatitis, Itching, Skin irritation* in the section on *Symptoms*

Alternative products that won't cause a reaction:
Epoxy-free bonding agents
See also *Anhydrides, Phenol*

Epoxythane
See *Ethylene oxide*

Erasers
See *Latex*

Erythromycin
Erythromycin is a macrolide antibiotic.

Type of allergen: consumed

Symptoms, tests, treatments and self-help tips, see *Drugs*

Erythrosine
Erythrosine is a disodium salt which is used in dentistry as a colouring agent to disclose plaque. It is also used as a dye in foods. See *Food additives – colourings*

Ethyl acetate
See *Solvents – esters*

Ethyl acrylate
See *Solvents – esters*

Ethyl alcohol
Ethyl alcohol is a grain alcohol also known as ethanol (chemical symbol C_2H_5OH). It is made by fermenting sugar, starch and other carbohydrates. It is used as a solvent.

Type of allergen: contact

Likely sources of ethyl acetate: solvents

Symptoms
Skin reactions: contact urticaria

Tests
• Symptom diary

Treatments

Avoidance: use protective equipment such as gloves

Prescription medication: antihistamines, emollients, steroids

OTC remedies: calamine lotion, witch hazel

Alternative remedies: aromatherapy, herbalism, homeopathy

Self-help tips: for symptom relief see *Urticaria* in the section on *Symptoms*

Ethylbenzene

See *Solvents – aromatic hydrocarbons*

Ethylene diamine

Ethylene diamine tetraacetic acid (EDTA) is a compound used as a chelating agent in chemical reactions; it is used to bind iron, magnesium and other metallic ions.

Type of allergen: contact

Likely sources of ethylene diamine: Preservatives in creams and paints

Symptoms

Skin reactions: contact dermatitis, skin irritation

Tests

- Skin patch test
- Symptom diary

Treatments

Avoidance
- Check labels

Prescription medication
- Contact dermatitis: steroids, antihistamines
- Skin irritation: emollients

OTC remedies
• Contact dermatitis: coal tar, emollients, steroids
• Skin irritation: emollients

Alternative remedies
• Contact dermatitis: aromatherapy, Bach flower remedies, homeopathy

Self-help tips: for symptom relief see *Contact dermatitis, Skin irritation* in the section on *Symptoms*

Ethylene dichloride
See *Solvents (chlorinated hydrocarbons),*
Solvents (halogenated solvents)

Ethylene glycol
See *Solvents (glycols)*

Ethylene glycol monobutyl ether (EGMBE) and Ethylene glycol monoethyl ether (EGMEE)
See *Solvents (glycol ether)*

Ethylene oxide
Ethylene oxide – also known as epoxyethane – is a colourless flammable gas, chemical symbol C_2H_4O. It is used to sterilize heat-sensitive medical equipment.

Type of allergen: inhalant

Symptoms, tests, treatments and self-help tips, see *Chemicals*

Ethyl 4-Hydroxy-Benzoate, Ethyl 4-Hydroxy-Benzoate sodium salt
See *Food additives – preservatives*

Ethyl silicate
See *Solvents (esters)*

Eugenol
Eugenol is a colourless aromatic hydrocarbon, chemical symbol $C_{10}H_{12}O_2$, found in the oil of pimento and cloves.

Type of allergen: contact, inhaled

Likely sources of eugenol: perfumes

Symptoms, test, treatments and self-help tips: See *Perfumes, Cosmetics*

Explosives
See *Phenol*

Eye creams
Perfumes and preservatives tend to cause most problems.

Type of allergen: contact

Symptoms, tests, treatments and self-help tips, see *Cosmetics*
See also Bitter almond oil

Eye liner
Perfumes and preservatives tend to cause most problems.

Type of allergen: contact

Symptoms, tests, treatments and self-help tips, see *Cosmetics*

Eye shadow
Perfumes and preservatives tend to cause most problems.

Type of allergen: contact

Symptoms, tests, treatments and self-help tips, see *Cosmetics*

Fabric/textiles

Curtain and furniture fabrics can contain volatile chemicals such as hydrocarbons from treatments, preservatives and some free monomers from the synthetic fibres or the treatments such as stain resistant coatings. The fibres can absorb volatile chemicals and release them slowly, causing a continued exposure of low concentration.

Vinyl fabrics are generally made from vinyl chloride organosols adhered to woven cotton backings. The vinyl chloride polymer is blended with a plastisizer to give it flexibility and softness. The residual free monomer from the polymer and the plastisizer give the finished product its particular odour, which is most noticeable in new car upholstery.

Alternative products that may not cause a reaction: untreated, natural fibre fabrics such as cotton, wool, silk and linen
See also *Chlorine, Chlorocresol (preservative), Chromium, Formaldehyde, Mould, Plastic, PVC, Wool alcohol*

Fabric conditioner
See *Formaldehyde*

Face powder

Perfumes and preservatives tend to cause most problems.

Type of allergen: contact.

Symptoms, tests, treatments and self-help tips, see *Cosmetics*

Fastenings, metal
See *Nickel*

Feathers

If symptoms start soon after beginning work and improve at weekends or on holidays, occupational asthma should be suspected.

Type of allergen: inhalant

Likely sources of feathers: birds (pet or occupational); soft furnishings – cushions, pillows

Symptoms
Mouth, nasal and ear reactions: rhinitis, sneezing

Respiratory reactions: asthma (including occupational), breathing problems

Tests
- CAP-RAST test – budgerigar, canary chicken, duck, goose, finch, parrot, pigeon, turkey)
- Blood test: ELISA – budgerigar, chicken, canary, duck, duck down, finch, goose, goose down, lovebird, parrot, pigeon, turkey
- Skin prick test – budgerigar, duck, goose, poultry
- Intradermal – budgerigar, chicken, duck, goose
- Symptom diary (including peak flow meter readings)

Treatments
Avoidance
- In an occupational situation, use protective equipment such as masks.

Prescription medication
- Rhinitis: antihistamines, decongestants, sodium cromoglycate, immunotherapy
- Sneezing: antihistamines, decongestants, sodium cromogylcate
- Asthma: anticholinergic drugs, antihistamines (exercise-induced), Beta2 (ß2) adrenoreceptor agonists, cromoglycate, nedocromil sodium, steroids, xanthine derivatives, zafirlukast
- Breathing problems: bronchodilators, corticosteroids

OTC remedies
- Rhinitis: decongestants

Alternative remedies
- Rhinitis: aromatherapy
- Sneezing: acupuncture
- Asthma: acupuncture (mild asthma only), Buteyko method, homeopathy, relaxation techniques, yoga

Self-help tips: use pillows and cushions stuffed with hypo-allergenic material or encase them in plastic.

For symptom relief, see *Rhinitis, Sneezing, Asthma, Breathing problems* in the section on *Symptoms*

You might also react to: egg

Fennel

Fennel is the herb *Foeniculum vulgare*; the root is often used as a vegetable and the leaves as flavouring. The main constituent is anethole, which can cause food intolerance in some people.

Type of allergen: consumed

Symptoms, tests, treatments and self-help tips, see *Herbs*

You might also react to: others in the *Umbelliferae* family, such as aniseed, caraway, carrot, celery, celeriac, cumin, coriander, dill, parsley, parsnip; you might also react to birch pollen

Fenugreek

Fenugreek is the spice *Trigonella foenum-graecum*.

For those who work with foodstuffs, if symptoms start soon after beginning work and improve at weekends or on holidays, occupational asthma should be suspected.

Type of allergen: inhalant, consumed

Symptoms, treatments and self-help tips, see *Spices*

Fermented food

Fermented food contains the vasoactive *amine tyramine*, which causes the blood vessels to widen and may trigger migraines.

Type of allergen: consumed

Symptoms
Headache/psychological problems: migraine

Skin reactions: flushing, urticaria

Tests
- Elimination diet
- Food challenge
- Symptom diary

Treatments
Avoidance
- Check labels carefully and check with a dietitian to ensure that your diet is still nutritionally sound

Prescription medication
- Migraine: painkillers, anti-sickness drugs, ergotamine, 5-HT agonists, beta-blockers, sodium valproate, sumatryptan
- Urticaria: antihistamines, emollients, steroids

OTC remedies
- Migraine: aspirin, ibuprofen, paracetamol
- Urticaria: calamine lotion, witch hazel

Alternative remedies
- Migraine: acupuncture, Alexander technique, aromatherapy, chiropractic, herbalism, homeopathy, hypnosis, osteopathy, reflexology
- Flushing: herbalism
- Urticaria: aromatherapy, herbalism, homeopathy

Self-help tips: for symptom relief see *Migraine, Flushing, Urticaria* in the section on *Symptoms*

Ferret
See *Animal hair*

Fibreglass resin
See *Benzoyl peroxide*

Figs

Figs are the fruit of the tree *Ficus carica*. They contain the vasoactive *amine tyramine*, which causes the blood vessels to widen and may trigger migraines.

Type of allergen: consumed

Symptoms, tests, treatments and self-help tips, see *Fruit*

You might also react to: latex – which has a similar protein to that in figs

Fillings, mercury

Dental amalgam fillings are 50 per cent mercury; mercury can leak from the fillings, but it is not known whether the amount released is enough to affect patients. Symptoms tend to develop gradually, so they are difficult to notice. The British Dental Association, World Health Organisation and American Dental Association support continued use of amalgam fillings, and the Swedish Medical Research Council found no link between health problems and the use of amalgam.

Type of allergen: inhalant, consumed

Symptoms
Gastrointestinal reactions: diarrhoea, gastric upset/irritation, nausea, vomiting

Mouth, nasal and ear reactions: gingivitis and spongy gums

Psychological problems: depression, mood swings, memory loss, inability to concentrate

Respiratory reactions: breathing problems, cough

Skin reactions: itching, rash

Other reactions: tremor

Tests
- Mercury blood test – this must be done within a day or so of exposure, as mercury remains in the bloodstream for only a couple of days
- Symptom diary – check this against your dental records; if there is a correlation between fillings and your symptoms, you may suspect mercury-related illness
- Provocation – keep a note of your symptoms for a month, then have the filling replaced with a non-amalgam filling and note your symptoms for the next month; although your symptoms may seem worse out of expectation, if they do not get worse then mercury can be crossed off your list of suspects

Treatments
Avoidance

Prescription medication:
- Diarrhoea: antidiarrhoeal drugs
- Gastric upset/irritation: painkillers (use paracetamol rather than aspirin)
- Nausea: antihistamines
- Vomiting: anti-emetics
- Depression: antidepressants
- Breathing problems: bronchodilators, corticosteroids
- Cough: antihistamines, bronchodilators, corticosteroids
- Contact dermatitis: steroids, antihistamines
- Itching: antihistamines, emollients

OTC remedies:
- Diarrhoea: kaolin and morphine, calcium carbonate, pectin
- Gastric upset/irritation – as prescription medication
- Nausea: antihistamines
- Vomiting: oral rehydration solution
- Cough: demulcents, antitussives, expectorants
- Contact dermatitis: coal tar, emollients, steroids
- Itching: antihistamines, emollients

Alternative remedies:
- Diarrhoea: aromatherapy, herbalism, homeopathy
- Gastric upset/irritation: aromatherapy, herbalism
- Nausea: aromatherapy, herbalism, homeopathy
- Vomiting: herbalism
- Depression: aromatherapy, Bach flower remedies, herbalism

- Cough: aromatherapy, homeopathy
- Contact dermatitis: aromatherapy, Bach flower remedies, homeopathy
- Itching: aromatherapy, herbalism

Self-help tips: for symptom relief, see *Diarrhoea*, *Gastric upset*, *Nausea*, *Vomiting*, *Depression*, *Breathing problems*, *Cough*, *Itching*, *Rash* in the section on *Symptoms*

Alternative products that won't cause a reaction: Composite, glass ionomer cement, ceramic, gold

Fireworks
See *Colophony*

Fish

Fish and shellfish are the third most common cause of food allergy, after eggs and milk. Allergy to fish is more common in areas where fish consumption is high.

Histamine – produced by bacteria – can be found in fish, particularly mackerel.

Fish can cause occupational asthma in fish and shellfish workers, particularly if automatic gutting machines are used. If symptoms start soon after beginning work and improve at weekends or on holidays, occupational asthma should be suspected.

The fish that are most likely to cause problems include cod, salmon, trout, herring, sardine, bass, swordfish and tuna; the allergen is thought to be a parvalbumin in the protein muscle of fish (particularly cod). If you are allergic to fresh salmon or tuna, you may be able to tolerate tinned fish; the length of cooking time may deactivate the allergenic components. If you are very sensitive, you may have problems from inhaling the steam from cooking fish.

There is no connection between allergy to fish and iodine.

Some pickled fish contains the vasoactive amines tyramine and *phenylethylamine*, which widens the blood vessels and may trigger migraine

Type of allergen: consumed, contact, inhalant

Symptoms
Anaphylactic shock

Eye reactions: itching

Gastrointestinal reactions: abdominal pain and swelling, diarrhoea, gastric upset/irritation, heartburn, nausea, wind

Headache: migraine

Mouth, nasal and ear reactions: rhinitis

Respiratory reactions: asthma (including occupational), wheezing

Skin reactions: angioedema, contact dermatitis (including occupational), eczema, flushing, itching, urticaria, allergic contact urticaria (raw fish)

Tests
- CAP-RAST tests (anchovy, blue mussel, chub mackerel, clam, cod, crayfish, eel, hake, herring, jack mackerel, mackerel, megrim, octopus, oyster, pilchard, plaice, salmon, sardine, snail, sole, squid, swordfish, trout, tuna)
- Blood test: ELISA (anchovy, carp, caviar, cod, crayfish, eel, haddock, halibut, herring, mackerel, perch, pike, plaice, salmon, sardine, squid, sole, trout, tuna)
- Skin prick tests (carp, cod, eel, halibut, herring, lobster, mackerel, mussels, plaice, salmon, sole, trout, tuna)
- Patch test (raw fish)
- Intradermal – cod, carp, eel, halibut, lobster, salmon, sole, trout, tuna
- Elimination diet
- Food challenge
- Symptom diary (including peak flow meter readings)

Treatments
Avoidance
- Avoid eating fish and any dish that may contain fish (or has been cooked in the same pan as fish, if your reaction is severe) – check labels and check with a dietitian to ensure that your diet is still nutritionally sound

- In an occupational situation, use protective equipment such as gloves and masks.

Prescription medication
- Anaphylactic shock: adrenaline, antihistamines, steroids
- Conjunctivitis: antihistamines, cromoglycate, nedocromil sodium, steroids, sympathomimetics
- Abdominal pain and swelling: antacids, anti-spasmodic drugs
- Diarrhoea: antidiarrhoeal drugs
- Gastric upset/irritation: painkillers (use paracetamol rather than aspirin)
- Heartburn: antacids, alginates
- Nausea: antihistamines
- Wind: antacids
- Migraine: painkillers, anti-sickness drugs, ergotamine, 5-HT agonists, beta-blockers, sodium valproate, sumatryptan
- Rhinitis: antihistamines, decongestants, sodium cromoglycate, immunotherapy
- Asthma: anticholinergic drugs, antihistamines (exercise-induced), Beta2 (ß2) adrenoreceptor agonists, cromoglycate, nedocromil sodium, steroids, xanthine derivatives, zafirlukast
- Angioedema: adrenaline, antihistamines, steroids
- Contact dermatitis: steroids, antihistamines
- Eczema: emollients, immune suppressants, steroids, UVA/UVB light treatment, wet wrapping, antihistamines
- Itching: antihistamines, emollients
- Urticaria: antihistamines, emollients, steroids

OTC remedies
- Conjunctivitis: antihistamines
- Abdominal pain and swelling: antacids
- Diarrhoea: kaolin and morphine, calcium carbonate, pectin
- Gastric upset/irritation: as prescription medication
- Heartburn: as prescription medication
- Nausea: antihistamines
- Wind: antacids
- Migraine: aspirin, ibuprofen, paracetamol
- Rhinitis: decongestants
- Angioedema: antihistamines
- Contact dermatitis: coal tar, emollients, steroids
- Eczema: emollients, hydrocortisone cream

- Itching: antihistamines, emollients
- Urticaria: calamine lotion, witch hazel

Alternative remedies
- Conjunctivitis: herbalism, homeopathy
- Abdominal pain and swelling: aromatherapy, herbalism, homeopathy
- Diarrhoea: aromatherapy, herbalism, homeopathy
- Gastric upset/irritation: aromatherapy, herbalism
- Heartburn: aromatherapy, homeopathy, herbalism
- Nausea: aromatherapy, herbalism, homeopathy
- Wind: aromatherapy, herbalism, homeopathy
- Migraine: acupuncture, Alexander technique, aromatherapy, chiropractic, herbalism, homeopathy, hypnosis, osteopathy, reflexology
- Rhinitis: aromatherapy
- Asthma: acupuncture (mild asthma only), Buteyko method, homeopathy, relaxation techniques, yoga
- Contact dermatitis: aromatherapy, Bach flower remedies, homeopathy
- Eczema: aromatherapy, evening primrose oil, relaxation, herbalism, homeopathy, Chinese herbal medicine, Bach flower remedies
- Flushing: herbalism
- Itching: aromatherapy, herbalism
- Urticaria: aromatherapy, herbalism, homeopathy

Self-help tips: Check the ingredients on food package labels and ask about the ingredients in foods prepared in restaurants when you eat out – avoid any specific fish or shellfish name, imitation crab or lobster (surimi). Avoid glues and fertilizers made with fish extracts.

For symptom relief, see *Conjunctivitis, Abdominal pain and Swelling, Diarrhoea, Gastric upset/irritation, Heartburn, Nausea, Wind, Migraine, Rhinitis, Asthma, Wheezing, Angioedema, Contact dermatitis, Eczema, Flushing, Itching, Urticaria* in the section on *Symptoms*
See also *Shellfish*

Fish, pickled
See *Fish*

Flame retardants
See *Epoxy resin*

Flax seed

Flax is the plant *Linum usitatissimum*. Its seed can cause occupational asthma, and is also used to produce *linseed oil*.

Type of allergen: inhalant

Tests
• Blood test: ELISA
• Symptom diary (including peak flow meter readings)

Treatments
Avoidance: in occupational situations, use protective equipment such as masks; improved ventilation may also help.

Prescription medication: *a*nticholinergic drugs, antihistamines (exercise-induced), Beta2 (ß2) adrenoreceptor agonists, cromo-glycate, nedocromil sodium, steroids, xanthine derivatives, zafirlukast

Alternative remedies: acupuncture (mild asthma only), Buteyko method, homeopathy, relaxation techniques, yoga

Self-help tips: for symptom relief see *Asthma* in the section on *Symptoms*

Fleas
The saliva from flea bites causes the reaction.

Type of allergen: injectant

Symptoms
Skin reactions: itching, skin irritation

Tests
• Skin patch
• Symptom diary

Treatments
Avoidance

Prescription medication
- Itching: antihistamines, emollients
- Skin irritation: emollients

OTC remedies
As Prescription medication

Alternative remedies
- Itching: aromatherapy, herbalism

Self-help tips: for symptom relief see *Itching, Skin irritation* in the section on *Symptoms*

Flooring
See *Adhesives, epoxy resin, PVC*

Flour
Flour can cause occupational asthma; as well as being an airborne irritant, it contains other allergens such as fungal mites, spores and finely chopped wheat hairs. Twenty per cent of bakers exposed to it will develop asthma, and caterers may also be affected. If symptoms start soon after beginning work and improve at weekends or on holidays, occupational asthma should be suspected. Flour can also cause eczema and rhinitis in those allergic to wheat.

Type of allergen: inhalant, contact, consumed

Symptoms
Nasal reactions: rhinitis

Respiratory reactions: occupational asthma

Skin reactions: eczema, irritant contact dermatitis

Tests
- Skin prick tests (oat, rye, wheat)
- Elimination diet

- Food challenge
- Symptom diary (including peak flow meter readings)

Treatments
Immunotherapy (for inhaled allergen only – not if it's caused when eaten)

Avoidance
- Check labels carefully and check with a dietitian to ensure that your diet is still nutritionally sound
- In an occupational situation, use protective equipment such as masks and gloves. Improved ventilation may help.

Prescription medication
- Rhinitis: antihistamines, decongestants, sodium cromoglycate, immunotherapy
- Asthma: anticholinergic drugs, antihistamines (exercise-induced), Beta2 (ß2) adrenoreceptor agonists, cromoglycate, nedocromil sodium, steroids, xanthine derivatives, zafirlukast
- Contact dermatitis: steroids, antihistamines
- Eczema: emollients, immune suppressants, steroids, UVA/UVB light treatment, wet wrapping, antihistamines

OTC remedies
- Rhinitis: decongestants
- Contact dermatitis: coal tar, emollients, steroids
- Eczema: emollients, hydrocortisone cream

Alternative remedies
- Rhinitis: aromatherapy
- Asthma: acupuncture (mild asthma only), Buteyko method, homeopathy, relaxation techniques, yoga
- Contact dermatitis: aromatherapy, Bach flower remedies, homeopathy
- Eczema: aromatherapy, evening primrose oil, relaxation, herbalism, homeopathy, Chinese herbal medicine, Bach flower remedies

Self-help tips: for symptom relief see *Rhinitis, Asthma, Eczema, Contact dermatitis* in the section on *Symptoms*

You might also react to: wheat
See also *Grain*

Flucanozole
See *Antifungal drugs*
Symptoms, tests, treatments and self-help tips, see
Drugs

Fluorescein

Fluorescein is a yellowish-red dye that produces green flurores-cence. It is used in tracing water flow and in microscopy.

Type of allergen: contact

Likely sources of fluorescein: chemical dyes, lipsticks

Symptoms, tests, treatments and self-help tips, see
Dyes

Fluorescent dye solvent
See *Solvents – aromatic hydrocarbons*

Fluoride

Fluoride is an ion which is added to drinking water to help decrease dental caries. It is also a byproduct of industrial processes including the production of fertilizer, glass, cement and aluminium, and has been linked with occupational asthma. If symptoms start soon after beginning work and improve at weekends or on holidays, occupational asthma should be suspected.

Type of allergen: inhalant, consumed

Likely sources of fluoride: dental treatments, drinking water, toothpaste, steelworks

Tests
• Symptom diary (including peak flow meter readings)

Treatments

Avoidance: in an occupational situation, use protective equipment such as masks. Improved ventilation may also help.

Prescription medication: anticholinergic drugs, antihistamines (exercise-induced), Beta2 (ß2) adrenoreceptor agonists, cromoglycate, nedocromil sodium, steroids, xanthine derivatives, zafirlukast

Alternative remedies: acupuncture (mild asthma only), Buteyko method, homeopathy, relaxation techniques, yoga

Self-help tips: for symptom relief see *Asthma* in the section on *Symptoms*

Fluxes

Flux is a substance used in soldering metals to avoid oxidization, and in smelting metals to remove impurities. It can cause occupational asthma for electronic workers. If symptoms start soon after beginning work and improve at weekends or on holidays, occupational asthma should be suspected.

Type of allergen: inhalant

Symptoms

Respiratory reactions: asthma (occupational)

Tests

• Symptom diary (including peak flow meter readings)

Treatments

Avoidance

• In an occupational situation, use protective equipment such as masks and gloves. Improved ventilation may help.

Prescription medication

• Asthma: anticholinergic drugs, antihistamines (exercise-induced), Beta2 (ß2) adrenoreceptor agonists, cromoglycate, nedocromil sodium, steroids, xanthine derivatives, zafirlukast

Alternative remedies
• Asthma: acupuncture (mild asthma only), Buteyko method, homeopathy, relaxation techniques, yoga

Self-help tips for symptom relief see *Asthma* in the section on *Symptoms*

Foam

There are two basic types of foam: closed cell and open cell. Closed cell types are used for impact resistance in products such as athletic protective equipment, flotation devices and shoe soles. Open cell types (which are more common) are generally softer and more pliable; they can contain residual styrene, vinyl acetate, isocyanate and hydrocarbon agents which are released slowly as the cells are broken down by use. Synthetic stuffing for pillows, mattresses, quilts and furniture can contain preservatives, free monomers (from the stuffing or from absorbed from packaging materials), stain and fire proofing treatments.
See *Isocyanates, Solvents, Vinyl acetate*

Foam rubber

See *Formaldehyde, Isocyanates, Polyurethane*

Food additives – anti-caking agents (E500-579)

These stop powdered foods clumping together.

Type of allergen: consumed

Symptoms
Gastrointestinal reactions
• Gastric upset – 500 (Sodium carbonates)
• Nausea – 508 (Potassium chloride)
• Vomiting – 508 (Potassium chloride)

Mouth/nasal/ear reactions
• Irritation of mucous membranes – 503 Ammonium carbonates

Tests
- Elimination diet
- Food challenge
- Symptom diary

Treatments
Avoidance
- Check labels carefully and check with a dietitian to ensure that your diet is still nutritionally sound

Prescription medication
- Irritation of mucous membranes: painkillers
- Gastric upset/irritation: painkillers (use paracetamol rather than aspirin)
- Nausea: antihistamines
- Vomiting: anti-emetics

OTC remedies
- Irritation of mucous membranes: painkillers
- Gastric upset/irritation: as prescription medication
- Nausea: antihistamines
- Vomiting: oral rehydration solution

Alternative remedies
- Irritation of mucous membranes: herbalism
- Gastric upset/irritation: aromatherapy, herbalism
- Nausea: aromatherapy, herbalism, homeopathy
- Vomiting: herbalism

Food additives – antioxidants (E300-321)

These stop food going rancid, particularly oils and fats, and prevent undesirable colour changes in foods that are high in carbohydrates (i.e. when the food reacts with oxygen in the air). BHA and BHT (E320 and E321) are the most likely culprits.

Type of allergen: contact, consumed

Symptoms
Gastrointestinal reactions
- Gastric irritation – E310 (Propyl gallate); E311 (Octyl gallate);

E312 (Dodecyl gallate)
- Nausea – E319 (tert-Butylhydroquinone)
- Vomiting – E319 tert-Butylhydroquinone

Respiratory reactions
- Asthma – E310 (Propyl gallate); E311 (Octyl gallate); E312 (Dodecyl gallate)

Skin reactions
- Skin irritation – E310 (Propyl gallate); E311 (Octyl gallate); E312 (Dodecyl gallate)
- Skin rashes – E320 Butulated hydroxyanisole (BHA); E321 Butylated hydroxytoluene (BHT)

Tests
- Skin patch test
- Elimination diet
- Food challenge
- Symptom diary (including peak flow meter readings)

Treatments
Avoidance
- Check labels carefully and check with a dietitian to ensure that your diet is still nutritionally sound

Prescription medication
- Gastric upset/irritation: painkillers (use paracetamol rather than aspirin)
- Nausea: antihistamines
- Vomiting: anti-emetics
- Asthma: anticholinergic drugs, antihistamines (exercise-induced), Beta2 (ß2) adrenoreceptor agonists, cromoglycate, nedocromil sodium, steroids, xanthine derivatives, zafirlukast
- Contact dermatitis: steroids, antihistamines
- Skin irritation: emollients

OTC remedies
- Gastric upset/irritation: as prescription medication
- Nausea: antihistamines
- Vomiting: oral rehydration solution
- Contact dermatitis: coal tar, emollients, steroids
- Skin irritation: emollients

Alternative remedies
- Gastric upset/irritation: aromatherapy, herbalism
- Nausea: aromatherapy, herbalism, homeopathy
- Vomiting: herbalism
- Asthma: acupuncture (mild asthma only), Buteyko method, homeopathy, relaxation techniques, yoga
- Contact dermatitis: aromatherapy, Bach flower remedies, homeopathy

Self-help tips for symptom relief see *Gastric upset/irritation, Nausea, Vomiting, Asthma, Contact dermatitis, Skin irritation* in the section on *Symptoms*

You might also react to: aspirin if you are sensitive to the gallates (E310-12) or BHT (E321)

Food additives – colours
(E100-180)

The food colour additives most likely to affect you are the azo dyes and "coal tar" dyes; these are dyes that were originally derived from coal tar, but are now produced synthetically. See *Appendix 4* for a list of E numbers with likely sources of food and possible symptoms.

Type of allergen: contact, consumed

Symptoms
Gastrointestinal reactions
- Diarrhoea – E110 (Sunset yellow FCF)
- Nausea – E131 (Patent blue); E132 (Indigo Carmine);
- Vomiting – E110 (Sunset yellow FCF); E131 (Patent blue); E132 (Indigo Carmine)

Headache
- Migraine – E102 (Tartrazine)

Mouth/nasal/ear reactions
- Rhinitis – E110 (Sunset yellow FCF); E122 (Carmoisine); E129 (Allura red AC)

Psychological problems
- Hyperactivity – E102 (Tartrazine); E104 (Quinoline Yellow);

E110 (Sunset yellow FCF); E120 (Cochineal or carminic acid); 128 (Red 2G; E131 (Patent blue); E132 (Indigo Carmine); E133 (Brilliant blue FCF); E151 (Brilliant black BN); E160b (Annatto)

Respiratory reactions:
- Asthma – E102 (Tartrazine); E104 (Quinoline Yellow); 107 (Yellow 2G); E120 (Cochineal or carminic acid); E122 (Carmoisine); E123 (Amaranth); E124 (Brilliant scarlet 4R or Ponceau); E129 (Allura red AC); E132 (Indigo Carmine); E133 (Brilliant blue FCF); E154 (Brown FK); E155 (Chocolate brown HT)

Breathing problems
- Wheezing – E102 (Tartrazine); E131 (Patent blue); E132 (Indigo Carmine)

Skin reactions
- Angioedema – E110 (Sunset yellow FCF); E122 (Carmoisine); E123 (Amaranth); E160b (Annatto)
- Contact dermatitis – E104 (Quinoline Yellow)
- Itching – E102 (Tartrazine); E131 (Patent blue); E132 (Indigo Carmine)
- Skin rashes/urticaria – E102 (Tartrazine); E110 (Sunset yellow FCF); E122 (Carmoisine); E123 (Amaranth); E129 (Allura red AC); E131 (Patent blue); E132 (Indigo Carmine); E154 (Brown FK); E155 (Chocolate brown HT); E160b (Annatto)

Other reactions
- Sensitivity to light – E127 (Erythrosine)

Tests
- Blood tests: CAP-RAST
- Skin patch test
- Elimination diet
- Food challenge
- Symptom diary (including peak flow meter readings)

Treatments
Avoidance
- Check labels carefully and check with a dietitian to ensure that your diet is still nutritionally sound

Prescription medication
- Diarrhoea: antidiarrhoeal drugs
- Nausea: antihistamines
- Vomiting: anti-emetics
- Migraine: painkillers, anti-sickness drugs, ergotamine, 5-HT agonists, beta-blockers, sodium valproate, sumatryptan
- Rhinitis: antihistamines, decongestants, sodium cromoglycate, immunotherapy
- Hyperactivity: stimulant drugs
- Asthma: anticholinergic drugs, antihistamines (exercise-induced), Beta2 (ß2) adrenoreceptor agonists, cromoglycate, nedocromil sodium, steroids, xanthine derivatives, zafirlukast
- Breathing problems: bronchodilators, corticosteroids
- Angioedema: adrenaline, antihistamines, steroids
- Contact dermatitis: steroids, antihistamines
- Itching: antihistamines, emollients
- Urticaria: antihistamines, emollients, steroids

OTC remedies
- Diarrhoea: kaolin and morphine, calcium carbonate, pectin
- Nausea: antihistamines
- Vomiting: oral rehydration solution
- Migraine: aspirin, ibuprofen, paracetamol
- Rhinitis: decongestants
- Angioedema: antihistamines
- Contact dermatitis: coal tar, emollients, steroids
- Itching: antihistamines, emollients
- Urticaria: calamine lotion, witch hazel

Alternative remedies
- Diarrhoea: aromatherapy, herbalism, homeopathy
- Nausea: aromatherapy, herbalism, homeopathy
- Vomiting: herbalism
- Migraine: acupuncture, Alexander technique, aromatherapy, chiropractic, herbalism, homeopathy, hypnosis, osteopathy, reflexology
- Rhinitis: aromatherapy
- Hyperactivity: herbalism
- Asthma: acupuncture (mild asthma only), Buteyko method, homeopathy, relaxation techniques, yoga
- Contact dermatitis: aromatherapy, Bach flower remedies, homeopathy

- Itching: aromatherapy, herbalism
- Urticaria: aromatherapy, herbalism, homeopathy

Self-help tips: for symptom relief see *Diarrhoea, Nausea, Vomiting, Migraine, Rhinitis, Hyperactivity, Asthma, Breathing problems, Angioedema, Contact dermatitis, Itching, Urticaria* in the section on *Symptoms*

You might also react to: preservatives (Benzoates – E210-219) and aspirin if you are sensitive to Tartrazine (E102)

Food additives – emulsifiers, stabilizers and thickeners (E322-495)

These improve texture.

Type of allergen: contact, consumed

Symptoms
Gastrointestinal reactions
- Abdominal cramps – E385 (Calcium disodium); E412 (Guar gum)
- Colitis – E407 (Carrageenan); 430 (Polyoxyetheylene (8) Stearate)
- Diarrhoea – E385 (Calcium disodium); E421 (Mannitol); E422 (Glycerin)
- Gastric upset – E327 (Calcium lactate); E407 (Carrageenan); E420 (Sorbitol); 430 (Polyoxyetheylene (8) Stearate); E450 (Sodium pyrophosphate); E451 (Potassium polyphosphates)
- Nausea – E412 (Guar gum); E421 (Mannitol); E422 (Glycerin)
- Vomiting – E385 (Calcium disodium); E421 (Mannitol); E422 (Glycerin)
- Wind – E412 (Guar gum)

Headache
- Headaches – E422 (Glycerin)

Mouth/nasal/ear reactions
- Irritation of mucous membranes – E414 Acacia (Gum Arabic)
- Rhinitis – E416 Karaya gum

Respiratory reactions
- Asthma – E416 Karaya gum

Skin reactions
- Dermatitis – E416 Karaya gum
- Skin irritation – E413 (Tragacanth)
- Urticaria – E416 Karaya gum

Tests
- Skin patch test
- Elimination diet
- Food challenge
- Symptom diary (including peak flow meter readings)

Treatments
Avoidance
- Check labels carefully and check with a dietitian to ensure that your diet is still nutritionally sound

Prescription medication
- Abdominal pain and swelling: antacids, anti-spasmodic drugs
- Colitis: aminosalicylates, immunosuppressants, steroids, sulphasalazine
- Diarrhoea: antidiarrhoeal drugs
- Gastric upset/irritation: painkillers (use paracetamol rather than aspirin)
- Nausea: antihistamines
- Vomiting: anti-emetics
- Wind: antacids
- Headache: painkillers, non-steroidal anti-inflammatories
- Irritation of mucous membranes: painkillers
- Rhinitis: antihistamines, decongestants, sodium cromoglycate, immunotherapy
- Asthma: anticholinergic drugs, antihistamines (exercise-induced), Beta2 (ß2) adrenoreceptor agonists, cromoglycate, nedocromil sodium, steroids, xanthine derivatives, zafirlukast
- Contact dermatitis: steroids, antihistamines
- Skin irritation: emollients
- Urticaria: antihistamines, emollients, steroids

OTC remedies
- Abdominal pain and swelling: antacids

- Diarrhoea: kaolin and morphine, calcium carbonate, pectin
- Gastric upset/irritation: as prescription medication
- Nausea: antihistamines
- Vomiting: oral rehydration solution
- Wind: antacids
- Headache: as prescription medication
- Irritation of mucous membranes: painkillers
- Rhinitis: decongestants
- Contact dermatitis: coal tar, emollients, steroids
- Skin irritation: emollients
- Urticaria: calamine lotion, witch hazel

Alternative remedies
- Abdominal pain and swelling: aromatherapy, herbalism, homeopathy
- Colitis: herbalism
- Diarrhoea: aromatherapy, herbalism, homeopathy
- Gastric upset/irritation: aromatherapy, herbalism
- Nausea: aromatherapy, herbalism, homeopathy
- Vomiting: herbalism
- Wind: aromatherapy, herbalism, homeopathy
- Headache: acupuncture, aromatherapy, herbalism, homeopathy
- Irritation of mucous membranes: herbalism
- Rhinitis: aromatherapy
- Asthma: acupuncture (mild asthma only), Buteyko method, homeopathy, relaxation techniques, yoga
- Contact dermatitis: aromatherapy, Bach flower remedies, homeopathy
- Urticaria: aromatherapy, herbalism, homeopathy

Self-help tips: for symptom relief see *Abdominal pain and swelling, Colitis, Diarrhoea, Gastric upset/irritation, Nausea, Vomiting, Wind, Headaches, Irritation of mucous membranes, Rhinitis, Asthma, Contact dermatitis, Skin irritation, Urticaria* in the section on *Symptoms*

Self-help tips: for symptom relief see *Irritation of mucous membranes, Gastric upset/irritation, Nausea, Vomiting* in the section on *Symptoms*

Food additives – flavour enhancers (E620-635)

These are used to improve the "taste" of foods. Most of the problems are caused by monosodium glutamate (MSG), which can give you "Chinese restaurant syndrome" (so-called because MSG is heavily used in the preparation of Chinese food) and is thought to be intolerance rather than an allergic reaction.

MSG, when consumed in large amounts, can cause flushing, sensations of warmth, headache, facial pressure, chest pain, or feelings of detachment in some people.

Type of allergen: consumed

Symptoms
Gastrointestinal reactions
- Abdominal cramps – 622 (Monopotassium glutamate)
- Nausea – 622 (Monopotassium glutamate)
- Vomiting – 622 (Monopotassium glutamate

Headache
- Headaches – 621 (Monosodium glutamate); 622 (Mono-potassium glutamate)

Respiratory reactions
- Asthma – 621 (Monosodium glutamate); 622 (Monopotassium glutamate); E623 (Calcium glutamate); E627 (Sodium guanylate); 631 (Sodium 5'-inosinate); 634 (Sodium 5'-ribonucleotide)

Skin reactions:
- Flushing – 621 (Monosodium glutamate)

Other reactions
- Palpitations – 621 (Monosodium glutamate)

Tests
- Elimination diet
- Food challenge
- Symptom diary (including peak flow meter readings)

Treatments
Avoidance
- Check labels carefully and check with a dietitian to ensure that your diet is still nutritionally sound

Prescription medication
- Abdominal pain and swelling: antacids, anti-spasmodic drugs
- Nausea: antihistamines
- Vomiting: anti-emetics
- Headache: painkillers, non-steroidal anti-inflammatories
- Asthma: anticholinergic drugs, antihistamines (exercise-induced), Beta2 (ß2) adrenoreceptor agonists, cromoglycate, nedocromil sodium, steroids, xanthine derivatives, zafirlukast
- Palpitations: beta-blockers, calcium channel blockers, digitalis drugs

OTC remedies
- Abdominal pain and swelling: antacids
- Nausea: antihistamines
- Vomiting: oral rehydration solution
- Headache: as prescription medication

Alternative remedies
- Abdominal pain and swelling: aromatherapy, herbalism, homeopathy
- Nausea: aromatherapy, herbalism, homeopathy
- Vomiting: herbalism
- Headache: acupuncture, aromatherapy, herbalism, homeopathy
- Asthma: acupuncture (mild asthma only), Buteyko method, homeopathy, relaxation techniques, yoga
- Flushing: herbalism
- Palpitations: aromatherapy, herbalism, homeopathy

Self-help tips: for symptom relief see *Abdominal pain/swelling, Nausea, Vomiting, headaches, Palpitations, Asthma, Flushing* in the section on *Symptoms*

You might also react to: aspirin, if you are sensitive to 621 (MSG), 622 (Monopotassium glutamate), E623 (Calcium glutamate); E627 (Sodium Guanylate); 631 (Sodium 5'-inosinate); 634 (Sodium 5'-ribonucleotide).

Food additives – preservatives
(E200-297)

These prevent the growth of bacteria and fungi which spoil food. Sulphites inhibit the enzyme reaction that causes food to turn brown (e.g. apples) and also browning caused by non-enzyme reactions in dried fruits, wine and vinegar.

Type of allergen: contact, consumed.

Symptoms
Gastrointestinal reactions
- Abdominal pain – E252 Potassium nitrate
- Diarrhoea – E221 (Sodium sulphite); E235 (Natamycin)
- Gastric upset/irritation – E210 (Benzoic acid); E220 (Sulphur dioxide); E221 (Sodium sulphite); E222 (Sodium bisulsulphite); E223 (Sodium metabisulphite); E224 (Potassium metabisulphite); E226 (Calcium sulphite); E227 (Calcium hydrogen sulphite); E239 (Hexamine); E252 (Potassium nitrate)
- Nausea – E221 (Sodium sulphite); E235 (Natamycin); E249 (Potassium nitrite); E250 (Sodium nitrite); E251 (Sodium nitrate); E252 (Potassium nitrate); E264 (Ammonium acetate)
- Vomiting – E235 (Natamycin); E264 (Ammonium acetate)

Headache
- Headaches – E249 (Potassium nitrite); E250 (Sodium nitrite); E251 (Sodium nitrate); E281 (Sodium propionate); E282 (Calcium propionate); E283 (Potassium propionate)
- Migraine – E281 (Sodium propionate); E282 (Calcium propionate); E283 (Potassium propionate)
- Neurological problems – E210 (Benzoic acid)

Mouth/nasal/ear reactions
- Mouth ulcers – E218 (Methyl paraben)

Psychological problems
- Hyperactivity – E210 (Benzoic acid); E211 (Sodium benzoate); E212 (Potassium benzoate); E213 (Calcium benzoate); E214 (Ethyl 4-Hydroxy-Benzoate)

Respiratory reactions
- Asthma – E210 (Benzoic acid); E211 (Sodium benzoate); E212 (Potassium benzoate); E213 (Calcium benzoate); E214 (Ethyl

4-Hydroxy-Benzoate); E216 (Propyl4-hydroxybenzoate); E217 (Propyl4-hydroxybenzoate sodium salt); E218 (Methyl paraben); E219 (Methyl 4-hydroxybenzoate); E220 (Sulphur dioxide); E221 (Sodium sulphite); E222 (Sodium bisulsulphite); E223 (Sodium metabisulphite); E224 (Potassium metabisulphite); E226 (Calcium sulphite); E227 (Calcium hydrogen sulphite); E249 (Potassium nitrite); E250 (Sodium nitrite); E251 (Sodium nitrate)

- Breathing problems – E249 (Potassium nitrite); E250 (Sodium nitrite); E251 (Sodium nitrate)

Skin reactions
- Angioedema – E221 (Sodium sulphite)
- Contact dermatitis – E214 (Ethyl 4-Hydroxy-Benzoate); E215 (Ethyl 4-Hydroxy-Benzoate sodium salt); E216 (Propyl4-hydroxybenzoate); E218 (Methyl paraben); E219 (Methyl 4-hydroxybenzoate); E282 (Calcium propionate)
- Skin rashes/urticaria – E200 (Sorbic acid); E210 (Benzoic acid); E211 (Sodium benzoate); E212 (Potassium benzoate); E213 (Calcium benzoate); E214 (Ethyl 4-Hydroxy-Benzoate); E217 (Propyl4-hydroxybenzoate sodium salt); E218 (Methyl paraben); E221 (Sodium sulphite); E222 (Sodium bisulsulphite); E223 (Sodium metabisulphite); E224 (Potassium metabisulphite); E226 (Calcium sulphite); E227 (Calcium hydrogen sulphite); E235 (Natamycin); E235 (Natamycin); E239 (Hexamine)
- Skin sensitivity – E217 (Propyl4-hydroxybenzoate sodium salt)

Tests
- Skin patch test
- Elimination diet
- Food challenge
- Symptom diary (including peak flow meter readings)

Treatments
See under *Food additives – colours* above, plus:

Prescription medication
- Abdominal pain and swelling: antacids, anti-spasmodic drugs
- Gastric upset/irritation: painkillers (use paracetamol rather than aspirin)
- Headache: painkillers, non-steroidal anti-inflammatories
- Mouth ulcers: antiseptic mouthwash, folic acid, hydrocortisone pellets

OTC remedies
- Abdominal pain and swelling: antacids
- Gastric upset/irritation: as prescription medication
- Headache: as prescription medication
- Mouth ulcers: as prescription medication

Alternative remedies
- Abdominal pain and swelling: aromatherapy, herbalism, homeopathy
- Gastric upset/irritation: aromatherapy, herbalism
- Headache: acupuncture, aromatherapy, herbalism, homeopathy
- Mouth ulcers: aromatherapy, herbalism, homeopathy

Self-help tips: for symptom relief see *Abdominal pain and swelling, Diarrhoea, Gastric upset/irritation, Nausea, Vomiting, Headaches, Migraine, Mouth ulcers, Hyperactivity, Asthma, Breathing problems, Angioedema, Contact dermatitis, Itching, Urticaria* in the section on *Symptoms*

You might also react to: Tartrazine (E102) if you react to benzoates

Formaldehyde

Formaldehyde – also known as methanal – is a colourless gas, chemical symbol HCHO. It is an *aldehyde* commonly used as a solution in water (formalin) as a disinfectant and preservative.

Formaldehyde gas can be also generated by the burning of organic fuels such as wood, oil, gas, coal, tobacco, diesel and gasoline or from the burning of formaldehyde-based plastics such as urea formaldehyde, phenol formaldehyde and polyacetal resins.

It can cause occupational asthma for hospital staff and embalmers; if symptoms start soon after beginning work and improve at weekends or on holidays, occupational asthma should be suspected.

Type of allergen: inhalant, contact

Likely sources of formaldehyde:
- Cosmetics and body care products: antiperspirants, cosmetics,

deodorants, hair treatments, nail varnish, shampoos, toothpaste
- Home care materials: adhesives, disinfectant, fabric conditioner, fungicides, insecticides, moth-proofing, paper towels, polishes, waxes
- Fabrics (used to protect against stains, grease, water, fading dye and creasing): dyes, leather goods, permanent-press clothing, wrinkle-resistant clothes, shoes, textiles
- Paper, ink and paint: duplicating paper, ink, newsprint, paints, paint stripper, photographic chemicals and paper
- Home construction: blockboard, carpeting, cavity wall or foam insulation, chipboard, foam rubber, fibreglass insulation, melamine, plaster, plywood, resin adhesive, synthetic resin, wallpaper, wood varnish,
- Other: burning of gas, wood or oil; cigarette smoke, preservatives in pharmaceuticals, spray aerosols

Symptoms
Eye reactions: allergic conjunctivitis

Gastrointestinal reactions: nausea

Headache: drowsiness, headache

Mouth, nasal and ear reactions: irritation of mucous membranes

Respiratory reactions: asthma (occupational), breathing problems, cough, wheezing

Skin reactions: contact dermatitis, inflammation, itching, photoallergenic contact dermatitis, skin irritation, urticaria

Tests
- Skin patch test
- Blood test: CAP-RAST
- Blood test: ELISA
- Inhalation challenge
- Symptom diary (including peak flow meter readings)

Treatments
Avoidance
- In an occupational situation, use protective equipment such as gloves and masks.

Prescription medication

- Conjunctivitis: antihistamines, cromoglycate, nedocromil sodium, steroids, sympathomimetics
- Nausea: antihistamines
- Headache: painkillers, non-steroidal anti-inflammatories
- Irritation of mucous membranes: painkillers
- Asthma: anticholinergic drugs, antihistamines (exercise-induced), Beta2 (ß2) adrenoreceptor agonists, cromoglycate, nedocromil sodium, steroids, xanthine derivatives, zafirlukast
- Breathing problems: bronchodilators, corticosteroids
- Cough: antihistamines, bronchodilators, corticosteroids
- Wheezing: bronchodilator
- Contact dermatitis: steroids, antihistamines
- Inflammation: antihistamines, emollients, steroids
- Itching: antihistamines, emollients
- Photoallergenic contact dermatitis: emollients, steroids
- Skin irritation: emollients
- Urticaria: antihistamines, emollients, steroids

OTC remedies

- Conjunctivitis: antihistamines
- Nausea: antihistamines
- Headache: as prescription medication
- Irritation of mucous membranes: painkillers
- Cough: demulcents, antitussives, expectorants
- Angioedema: antihistamines
- Contact dermatitis: coal tar, emollients, steroids
- Inflammation: antihistamines, emollients
- Itching: antihistamines, emollients
- Urticaria: calamine lotion, witch hazel

Alternative remedies

- Conjunctivitis: herbalism, homeopathy
- Nausea: aromatherapy, herbalism, homeopathy
- Headache: acupuncture, aromatherapy, herbalism, homeopathy
- Irritation of mucous membranes: herbalism
- Asthma: acupuncture (mild asthma only), Buteyko method, homeopathy, relaxation techniques, yoga
- Cough: aromatherapy, homeopathy
- Contact dermatitis: aromatherapy, Bach flower remedies, homeopathy

- Itching: aromatherapy, herbalism
- Urticaria: aromatherapy, herbalism, homeopathy

Self-help tips: check labels and avoid anything listing: Paratertiary butylphenol formaldehyde resin, PTBP formaldehyde, Butylphen, 4(1,1-dimethylethyl)phenol, Oxymethylene, Methanal, Formalin.

For symptom relief, see *Conjunctivitis, Nausea, Headaches, Irritation of mucous membranes, Asthma, Breathing problems, Cough, Wheezing, Contact dermatitis, Inflammation, Itching, Photoallergenic contact dermatitis, Skin irritation, Urticaria* in the section on *Symptoms*

Formaldehyde releasers (cosmetics)
See *Formaldehyde*

Self-help tips: check labels and avoid anything listing: imidazolidinyl urea, diazolidinyl urea, DMDM (dimethylolmethyl) hydantoin, 2-bromo-2-nitropropane-1,3-diol, tris (hydroxymethyl) nitromethane

Foundation
Perfumes and preservatives tend to cause most problems.

Type of allergen: contact

Symptoms, tests, treatments and self-help tips, see *Cosmetics*

Fox
See *Animal hair*

Fragrance
See *Perfume*

Fruit
For further information about the fruits themselves and cross-reactivity see *Apple, Apricot, Avocado, Banana, Blackberries, Blackcurrants, Blueberries, Carambola, Cherries, Citrus fruit,*

Cranberry, Currants, Dates, Figs, Gooseberries, Grape, Grapefruit, Guava, Jack fruit, Kiwi fruit, Lemon, Lime, Mandarin, Mango, Melon, Nectarine, Olive, Orange, Papaya, Passion Fruit, Peach, Pear, Pineapple, Plum, Prune, Raisin, Raspberry, Redcurrant, Rhubarb, Strawberry

Symptoms:
Anaphylactic shock
- Apple, avocado, banana (rare), cherries, citrus fruit, grapes (especially red), kiwi fruit, mango, melon (rare), orange, papaya, peach, pear, persimmon, pineapple, plum

Anaphylactic shock
- Exercise-induced – apple

Eye reactions
- Conjunctivitis – avocado, kiwi fruit, mango

Gastrointestinal reactions
- Abdominal pain and swelling – avocado, banana, blackberries, gooseberries, kiwi fruit, mango, orange, peach, pineapple, redcurrants, rhubarb, strawberries
- Colitis – papaya, strawberries
- Diarrhoea – apple, banana, blackberries, blackcurrant, cranberry, gooseberries, kiwi fruit, melon, orange, passion fruit, peach, pineapple, redcurrants, rhubarb, strawberries
- Gastric upset/irritation – blackcurrant, cranberry, kiwi fruit, orange, passion fruit, peach
- Heartburn –citrus fruit, grapefruit, orange
- Nausea – orange, peach, strawberries
- Vomiting – apple, banana, blackberries, cherries, gooseberries, kiwi fruit, melon, orange, peach, pineapple, redcurrants, rhubarb, strawberries

Headaches:
- Headache – avocado, banana, citrus fruit, figs, grapefruit, pineapple, plum, prune
- Migraine – avocado, banana, citrus fruit, figs, grapefruit, plum, prune, strawberries

Mouth, nasal and ear reactions:
- Ears blocked – citrus fruit, grapefruit

- Hay fever – grapes (occupational, to pollen)
- Irritation of mucous membranes – apple, grapes, kiwi fruit, mango, strawberries
- Itching mouth/palate – apple, banana, cherries, grapes, guava, jack fruit, kiwi fruit, mango, orange, peach, pear, plum, strawberries
- Rhinitis – apple, avocado, banana, blackcurrant, cranberry, grapes, guava, mandarin, melon, orange, passion fruit, peach
- sneezing – banana, grapes

Psychological problems:
- Hyperactivity – apple, apricots, banana, blackberries, blackcurrant, blueberries, cherries, citrus fruit, cranberry, currants, dates, gooseberries, grapefruit, grapes, melon, nectarines, orange, passion fruit, peach, pineapple, plum, prune, raisins, raspberry, strawberries
- Sleep problems – carambola

Respiratory reactions:
- Asthma (occupational) – mandarin
- Asthma – apple, avocado, blackcurrant, cranberry, currants, melon, passion fruit, strawberries
- Breathing problems – orange
- Cough – grapes
- Wheezing – apple, apricots, banana, blackberries, blackcurrant, blueberries, cherries, citrus fruit, cranberry, currants, dates, gooseberries, grapes, mango, melon, nectarines, orange, passion fruit, peach, pineapple, plum, prune, raisins, raspberry, strawberries)

Skin reactions:
- Angioedema – apple, apricots, banana, blackberries, blackcurrant, blueberries, cherries, citrus fruit, cranberry, currants, dates, gooseberries, grapes, kiwi fruit, mango, melon, nectarines, orange, passion fruit, pear, pineapple, plum, prune, raisins, raspberry, strawberries
- Atopic dermatitis – melon, strawberries
- Contact dermatitis, including occupational – citrus fruit peel (including grapefruit, lemon, lime, orange), grapes, kiwi fruit, olive, orange (oil), pear, plum, strawberries
- Photoallergenic contact dermatitis – lemon, lime
- Eczema – avocado, grapes, plum, strawberries
- Flushing – avocado, banana, citrus fruit, figs, grapefruit,

grapes, mango, plum, prune, strawberries)
- Itching – apple, blackcurrant, cranberry, kiwi fruit, mango, melon, orange, passion fruit, pear, pineapple
- Skin irritation – mango)
- Urticaria (this has been dismissed by some experts – it's more likely to be the stone than the fruit in stone fruit) – apple, apricots, avocado, banana, blackberries, blackcurrant, blueberries, cherries, citrus fruit, cranberry, currants, dates, figs, gooseberries, grapefruit, grapes, kiwi fruit, mango, melon, nectarines, orange, papaya, passion fruit, peach (exercise-induced), pineapple, plum, prune, raisins, raspberry, strawberries

Tests

- Blood test: CAP-RAST (apple, apricots, avocado, banana, blackberries, blueberries, carambola, cherries, citrus fruit, cranberry, dates, figs, grapefruit, grapes, guava, jack fruit, kiwi fruit, lemon, lime, mandarin, mango, melon, orange, papaya, passion fruit, peach, pear, persimmon, pineapple, redcurrants, strawberries)
- Blood test: ELISA (apple, apricots, avocado, banana, blackberries, blackcurrants, blueberries, cranberry, dates, figs, gooseberries, grapefruit, grapes, guava, kiwi fruit, lemon, mandarin, mango, melon (including canteloupe and watermelon), nectarines, olive, orange, papaya, peach, pear, pineapple, raisins, raspberry, redcurrants, rhubarb, strawberries)
- Skin test: skin prick (apple, avocado, banana, cherries, grapefruit, grapes, kiwi fruit, lemon, lime, mango, orange, peach, pear, pineapple, strawberries)
- Skin test: Intradermal (banana, grapefruit, grapes, orange, peach, pear, pineapple, strawberries)
- Hydrogen breath test: if your body can't absorb fructose, your breath will have a higher concentration of hydrogen (apple)
- Elimination diet (apple, apricots, avocado, banana, blackberries, blueberries, carambola, cherries, citrus fruit, cranberry, dates, figs, gooseberries, grapefruit, grapes, guava, jack fruit, kiwi fruit, lemon, lime, mango, melon, nectarines, orange, papaya, passion fruit, peach, pear, persimmon, pineapple, prune, raisins, raspberry, redcurrants, rhubarb, strawberries)
- Food challenge (apple, apricots, avocado, banana, blackberries, blueberries, carambola, cherries, citrus fruit, cranberry, dates,

figs, gooseberries, grapefruit, grapes, guava, jack fruit, kiwi fruit, lemon, lime, mango, melon, nectarines, orange, papaya, passion fruit, peach, pear, persimmon, pineapple, prune, raisins, raspberry, redcurrants, rhubarb, strawberries)
- Symptom diary (including peak flow meter readings)
- Exercise challenge

Treatments
Avoidance
- In occupational situations, use protective equipment such as gloves or masks; improved ventilation may also help.
- Check labels carefully and check with a dietitian to ensure that your diet is still nutritionally sound

Prescription medication
- Anaphylactic shock: adrenaline, antihistamines, steroids
- Abdominal pain and swelling: antacids, anti-spasmodic drugs
- Colitis: aminosalicylates, immunosuppressants, steroids, sulphasalazine
- Diarrhoea: antidiarrhoeal drugs
- Gastric upset/irritation: painkillers (use paracetamol rather than aspirin)
- Heartburn: antacids, alginates
- Nausea: antihistamines
- Vomiting: anti-emetics
- Headache: painkillers, non-steroidal anti-inflammatories
- Migraine: painkillers, anti-sickness drugs, ergotamine, 5-HT agonists, beta-blockers, sodium valproate, sumatryptan
- Ear problems: sympathomimetics
- Hay fever: antihistamines, cromoglycate, decongestants, nedocromil sodium, steroids, sympathomimetics
- Irritation of mucous membranes: painkillers
- Itching/burning mouth/palate: painkillers
- Rhinitis: antihistamines, decongestants, sodium cromoglycate, immunotherapy
- Hyperactivity: stimulant drugs
- Sleep problems: benzodiazepenes
- Asthma: anticholinergic drugs, antihistamines (exercise-induced), Beta2 (ß2) adrenoreceptor agonists, cromoglycate, nedocromil sodium, steroids, xanthine derivatives, zafirlukast
- Breathing problems: bronchodilators, corticosteroids
- Cough: antihistamines, bronchodilators, corticosteroids
- Wheezing: bronchodilators

- Angioedema: adrenaline, antihistamines, steroids
- Itching: antihistamines, emollients
- Dermatitis: steroids, antihistamines
- Photoallergenic contact dermatitis: emollients, steroids
- Eczema: emollients, immune suppressants, steroids, UVA/UVB light treatment, wet wrapping, antihistamines
- Skin irritation: emollients
- Urticaria: antihistamines, emollients, steroids

OTC remedies
- Conjunctivitis: antihistamines
- Abdominal pain and swelling: antacids
- Diarrhoea: kaolin and morphine, calcium carbonate, pectin
- Gastric upset/irritation: as prescription medication
- Heartburn: as prescription medication
- Nausea: antihistamines
- Vomiting: oral rehydration solution
- Headache: as prescription medication
- Migraine: aspirin, ibuprofen, paracetamol
- Hay fever: antihistamines, decongestants
- Irritation of mucous membranes: painkillers
- Itching/burning mouth/palate: painkillers
- Rhinitis: decongestants
- Sleep problems: various remedies (most of them include antihistamines)
- Cough: demulcents, antitussives, expectorants
- Dermatitis: coal tar, emollients, steroids
- Eczema: emollients, hydrocortisone cream
- Urticaria: calamine lotion, witch hazel

Alternative remedies
- Conjunctivitis: herbalism, homeopathy
- Abdominal pain and swelling: aromatherapy, herbalism, homeopathy
- Colitis: herbalism
- Diarrhoea: aromatherapy, herbalism, homeopathy
- Gastric upset/irritation: aromatherapy, herbalism
- Heartburn: aromatherapy, homeopathy, herbalism
- Nausea: aromatherapy, herbalism, homeopathy
- Vomiting: herbalism
- Headache: acupuncture, aromatherapy, herbalism, homeopathy
- Migraine: acupuncture, Alexander technique, aromatherapy,

chiropractic, herbalism, homeopathy, hypnosis, osteopathy, reflexology
- Ear problems: aromatherapy, herbalism, homeopathy
- Hay fever: aromatherapy, herbalism, homeopathy
- Irritation of mucous membranes: herbalism
- Rhinitis: aromatherapy
- Hyperactivity: herbalism
- Sleep problems: aromatherapy, Bach flower remedies, herbalism, homeopathy, relaxation exercises, meditation
- Asthma: acupuncture (mild asthma only), Buteyko method, homeopathy, relaxation techniques, yoga
- Cough: aromatherapy, homeopathy
- Angioedema: antihistamines
- Contact dermatitis: aromatherapy, Bach flower remedies, homeopathy
- Eczema: aromatherapy, evening primrose oil, relaxation, herbalism, homeopathy, Chinese herbal medicine, Bach flower remedies
- Flushing: herbalism
- Itching: aromatherapy, herbalism
- Urticaria: aromatherapy, herbalism, homeopathy

Self-help tips: for symptom relief see *Conjunctivitis, Abdominal pain and swelling, Colitis, Diarrhoea, Gastric upset/irritation, Heartburn, Nausea, Vomiting, Headaches, Migraine, Ear problems, Hay fever, Itching mouth/palate, Irritation of mucous membranes, Rhinitis, Sneezing, Hyperactivity, Asthma, Breathing problems, Cough, Wheezing, Angioedema, Contact dermatitis, Photoallergenic contact dermatitis, Eczema, Flushing, Itching, Skin irritation, Urticaria* in the section on *Symptoms*
See also Yeast

Fruit juice
Type of allergen: consumed

Symptoms
Other: cystitis

Tests
- Elimination diet
- Food challenge
- Symptom diary

Treatments
Avoidance: Check labels carefully and check with a dietitian to ensure that your diet is still nutritionally sound

Prescription medication: antibiotics (for infection)

OTC remedies: potassium citrate

Alternative remedies: aromatherapy, herbalism, homeopathy

Self-help tips: for symptom relief see *Cystitis* in the section on *Symptoms*

Frusemide
Frusemide (or Furosemide) is a diuretic.

Type of allergen: consumed

Symptoms
Gastrointestinal reactions: nausea, vomiting

Respiratory reactions: breathing problems

Skin reactions: angioedema, rash, itching, urticaria

Tests
• Blood test: ELISA

Treatments
Avoidance

Prescription medication
• Nausea: antihistamines
• Vomiting: anti-emetics
• Breathing problems: bronchodilators, corticosteroids
• Angioedema: adrenaline, antihistamines, steroids
• Contact dermatitis: steroids, antihistamines
• Itching: antihistamines, emollients
• Urticaria: antihistamines, emollients, steroids

OTC remedies
- Nausea: antihistamines
- Vomiting: oral rehydration solution
- Angioedema: antihistamines
- Contact dermatitis: coal tar, emollients, steroids
- Itching: antihistamines, emollients
- Urticaria: calamine lotion, witch hazel

Alternative remedies
- Nausea: aromatherapy, herbalism, homeopathy
- Vomiting: herbalism
- Contact dermatitis: aromatherapy, Bach flower remedies, homeopathy
- Itching: aromatherapy, herbalism
- Urticaria: aromatherapy, herbalism, homeopathy

Self-help tips: for symptom relief see *Nausea, Vomiting, Breathing problems, Angioedema, Rash, Itching, Urticaria* in the section on *Symptoms*

Fuel additives
See *Methyl alcohol, Solvents (alcohol solvents)*

Fungicides
See *Chlorine, Chlorsalicylamide, Formaldehyde*

Furniture made from particle board
See *Solvents (aromatic hydrocarbons), Solvents (ketone solvents)*

Furniture oils
See *Volatile organic compounds*

Furniture stuffing
See *Volatile organic compounds*

Game
Hung game (such as pheasant, grouse or venison) contains the vasoactive amine tyramine, which causes the blood vessels to widen and may trigger migraines.

Type of allergen: consumed

Symptoms
Headache: headache, migraine

Skin reactions: flushing, urticaria

Tests
- Elimination diet
- Food challenge
- Symptom diary

Treatments
Avoidance
- Check labels carefully

Prescription medication
- Headache: painkillers, non-steroidal anti-inflammatories
- Migraine: painkillers, anti-sickness drugs, ergotamine, 5-HT agonists, beta-blockers, sodium valproate, sumatryptan
- Urticaria: antihistamines, emollients, steroids

OTC remedies
- Headache: as prescription medication
- Migraine: aspirin, ibuprofen, paracetamol
- Urticaria: calamine lotion, witch hazel

Alternative remedies
- Headache: acupuncture, aromatherapy, herbalism, homeopathy
- Migraine: acupuncture, Alexander technique, aromatherapy, chiropractic, herbalism, homeopathy, hypnosis, osteopathy, reflexology
- Flushing: herbalism
- Urticaria: aromatherapy, herbalism, homeopathy

Self-help tips: for symptom relief see *Headache, Migraine, Flushing, Urticaria* in the section on *Symptoms*

Garlic
Garlic is a herb from the *lilacea* family, botanical name *Allium sativum*. The allergens in garlic are diallyldisulphide, allylpropyldisulphide, allylmercaptan and allicin.

Type of allergen: contact, consumed

Symptoms, tests, treatments and self-help tips, see *Herbs*

You might also react to: asparagus, chives, leek, onion, shallot

Gentamycin

Gentamycin is an aminoglycoside antibiotic used for treatment of serious or complicated infections such as lung infections, septicaemia and meningitis. It is also used as drops for ear and eye infections, and as ointment for infected burns or ulcers.

Type of allergen: consumed, contact

Symptoms, tests, treatments and self-help tips, see *Drugs*

You might also react to: neomycin, netilmycin, streptomycin and tobramycin

Gentian violet

Gentian violet is a dye used in pharmaceuticals which can cause occupational contact dermatitis.

Type of allergen: contact

Symptoms, tests, treatments and self-help tips, see *Dyes*

Geraniol
See *Perfumes*

Geraniol 10-hydroxylase
See *Enzymes*

Geranium oil
Geranium oil is derived from the plant *Pelargonium*.

Type of allergen: contact, inhalant

Likely sources of geranium oil: Perfumes, toiletries

Symptoms, tests, treatments and self-help tips, see *Oils, cosmetic*

Gerbils
See *Pets*

Ginger
Ginger is the spice *Zingiber officinale*.

Type of allergen: contact, consumed

Symptoms, treatments and self-help tips, see *Spices*

You might also react to: cardamom, turmeric

Ginger beer
See *Yeast*

Glass
See *Cobalt*

Glass cleaner
See *Methyl alcohol, solvents – alcohol solvents*

Gloves
See *Latex, Mercaptobenzothiazole*

Glues
See *Adhesives, Isocyanates, Solvents – aliphatic hydrocarbons*

Glutaraldehyde
Glutaraldehyde is a dialdehyde used as a fixative. It is also used in solutions used to sterilize instruments. It goes through latex and vinyl gloves, so medical workers may suffer from dermatitis. It can also cause occupational asthma for medical staff; if symptoms

start soon after beginning work and improve at weekends or on holidays, occupational asthma should be suspected.

Type of allergen: inhalant, contact

Likely sources of glutaraldehyde: Embalming fluid, sterilizing fluid, waterless hand cleaners

Symptoms
Respiratory reactions: occupational asthma

Skin reactions: contact dermatitis

Tests
• Skin patch
• Symptom diary (including peak flow meter readings)

Treatments
Avoidance: in occupational situations, use protective equipment.

Prescription medication
• Asthma: anticholinergic drugs, antihistamines (exercise-induced), Beta2 (ß2) adrenoreceptor agonists, cromoglycate, nedocromil sodium, steroids, xanthine derivatives, zafirlukast
• Contact dermatitis: steroids, antihistamines

OTC remedies
• Contact dermatitis: coal tar, emollients, steroids

Alternative remedies
• Asthma: acupuncture (mild asthma only), Buteyko method, homeopathy, relaxation techniques, yoga
• Contact dermatitis: aromatherapy, Bach flower remedies, homeopathy

Self-help tips: for symptom relief see *Asthma, Contact dermatitis* in the section on *Symptoms*

Gluten

The soluble grain proteins in gluten cause an IgE reaction; in coeliac disease, gliadin-specific IgA and IgG is developed.

Type of allergen: contact, consumed

Likely sources of gluten: breads, flour, cakes, biscuits, pancakes, semolina, pastry, sauces, gravy, pasta, cereals, muesli, couscous, bulgar wheat

Symptoms
Gastrointestinal reactions: abdominal pain and swelling, diarrhoea, nausea, vomiting, wind

Skin reactions: angioedema, contact dermatitis, eczema, itching, urticaria

Tests
- CAP-RAST test
- Blood test: ELISA
- Skin prick tests
- Elimination diet
- Food challenge
- Symptom diary

Treatments
Avoidance
- Check labels carefully and check with a dietitian to ensure that your diet is still nutritionally sound

Prescription medication
- Abdominal pain and swelling: antacids, anti-spasmodic drugs
- Diarrhoea: antidiarrhoeal drugs
- Nausea: antihistamines
- Vomiting: anti-emetics
- Wind: antacids
- Angioedema: adrenaline, antihistamines, steroids
- Contact dermatitis: steroids, antihistamines
- Eczema: emollients, immune suppressants, steroids, UVA/UVB light treatment, wet wrapping, antihistamines
- Itching: antihistamines, emollients
- Urticaria: antihistamines, emollients, steroids

OTC remedies
- Abdominal pain and swelling: antacids
- Diarrhoea: kaolin and morphine, calcium carbonate, pectin

- Nausea: antihistamines
- Vomiting: oral rehydration solution
- Wind: antacids
- Angioedema: antihistamines
- Contact dermatitis: coal tar, emollients, steroids
- Eczema: emollients, hydrocortisone cream
- Itching: antihistamines, emollients
- Urticaria: calamine lotion, witch hazel

Alternative remedies
- Abdominal pain and swelling: aromatherapy, herbalism, homeopathy
- Diarrhoea: aromatherapy, herbalism, homeopathy
- Nausea: aromatherapy, herbalism, homeopathy
- Vomiting: herbalism
- Wind: aromatherapy, herbalism, homeopathy
- Contact dermatitis: aromatherapy, Bach flower remedies, homeopathy
- Eczema: aromatherapy, evening primrose oil, relaxation, herbalism, homeopathy, Chinese herbal medicine, Bach flower remedies
- Itching: aromatherapy, herbalism
- Urticaria: aromatherapy, herbalism, homeopathy

Self-help tips: for symptom relief see *Abdominal pain and swelling, Diarrhoea, Nausea, Vomiting, Wind, Angioedema, Contact dermatitis, Eczema, Itching, Urticaria* in the section on *Symptoms*

Alternative products that won't cause a reaction: rice, maize and gluten-free products

You might also react to: barley, rye, wheat and possibly oats – see *Grain*

Glycerine
See *Food additives – emulsifiers, stabilizers and thickeners*

Glycerol
See *Solvents – glycols*

Goats
See *Animal hair*

Gold
Gold is the metal, chemical symbol Au.

Type of allergen: contact

Symptoms, tests, treatments and self-help tips, see *Metals*

Goose
See *Meat and poultry*

Gooseberries
Gooseberries are the fruit of the plant *Ribes grossularia*. They contain *salicylates*, which have been linked to hyperactivity in children. They also contain oxalates, a derivative of oxalic acid.

Type of allergen: consumed

Symptoms, tests, treatments and self-help tips, see *Fruit*

Grain
Grain can cause occupational asthma in farmers, dock workers, bakers and millers. If symptoms start soon after beginning work and improve at weekends or on holidays, occupational asthma should be suspected.

Some grains can also cause anaphylactic shock, including barley (found in breakfast cereals and beer).

For further information about the grains themselves and cross-reactivity see *Barley, Buckwheat, Corn, Millet, Oats, Rye, Spelt, Wheat*

Symptoms:
Anaphylactic shock
- Barley, millet, wheat
- Exercise-induced – corn, barley, buckwheat, oats, rye, wheat

Eye reactions
- Conjunctivitis – buckwheat, wheat

Gastrointestinal reactions
- Abdominal pain and swelling – corn, oats, rye, spelt, wheat
- Diarrhoea – rye, spelt, wheat
- Gastric upset/irritation – corn, barley, buckwheat, oats, rye
- Nausea – corn, oats, rye, spelt, wheat
- Vomiting – corn, oats, rye, spelt, wheat
- Wind – wheat

Mouth, nasal and ear reactions:
- Ears blocked – wheat
- Itching mouth/palate/throat – buckwheat
- Rhinitis – corn, barley, buckwheat, oats, rye, spelt, wheat
- Sneezing – corn, barley, buckwheat, rye, spelt, wheat

Other:
- Fever – oats
- Weight loss – wheat

Respiratory reactions:
- Asthma (occupational) – corn, barley, buckwheat, oats, rye, spelt, wheat
- Breathing problems – corn, barley, oats, spelt, wheat
- Cough – corn, barley, oats, wheat
- Wheezing (corn, barley, buckwheat, oats, rye, wheat

Skin reactions:
- Angioedema – corn, barley, millet, oats, rye, spelt, wheat
- Contact dermatitis, including occupational – corn, barley, buckwheat, millet, oats, rye, spelt, wheat
- Eczema – barley, spelt, wheat
- Itching – barley, buckwheat, oats, rye, spelt, wheat
- Urticaria – corn, barley, buckwheat, oats, spelt, wheat

Tests
- Blood test: CAP-RAST (barley, buckwheat, corn, millet (common, foxtail, Japanese), oats, rye, wheat)
- Blood test: ELISA (barley, buckwheat, corn, millet, oats, rye, spelt, wheat and wheat bran)
- Skin test: skin prick (barley, barley bran and barley flour, buckwheat, corn bran and corn flour, oat and oat flour, rye bran and rye flour, wheat, wheat bran and wheat flour)
- Skin test: Intradermal (corn bran and corn flour, oat and oat flour, rye bran and rye flour, wheat, wheat bran and wheat flour)

- Nasal challenge (barley bran and barley flour, corn bran and corn flour, oat and oat flour, rye bran and rye flour, wheat, wheat bran and wheat flour)
- Inhalation challenge (barley bran and barley flour, corn bran and corn flour, oat and oat flour, rye bran and rye flour, wheat, wheat bran and wheat flour)
- Elimination diet (barley, buckwheat, corn, millet, oats, rye, wheat)
- Food challenge (barley, buckwheat, corn, millet, oats, rye, wheat)
- Symptom diary (including peak flow meter readings)
- Exercise challenge

Treatments
Avoidance
- In occupational situations, use protective equipment such as gloves or masks; improved ventilation may also help.
- Check labels carefully and check with a dietitian to ensure that your diet is still nutritionally sound

Prescription medication
- Anaphylactic shock: adrenaline, antihistamines, steroids
- Abdominal pain and swelling: antacids, anti-spasmodic drugs
- Diarrhoea: antidiarrhoeal drugs
- Gastric upset/irritation: painkillers (use paracetamol rather than aspirin)
- Nausea: antihistamines
- Vomiting: anti-emetics
- Wind: antacids
- Ear problems: sympathomimetics
- Fever: aspirin, ibuprofen, paracetamol
- Itching/burning mouth/palate: painkillers
- Rhinitis: antihistamines, decongestants, sodium cromoglycate, immunotherapy
- Asthma: anticholinergic drugs, antihistamines (exercise-induced), Beta2 (ß2) adrenoreceptor agonists, cromoglycate, nedocromil sodium, steroids, xanthine derivatives, zafirlukast
- Breathing problems: bronchodilators, corticosteroids
- Cough: antihistamines, bronchodilators, corticosteroids
- Wheezing: bronchodilators
- Angioedema: adrenaline, antihistamines, steroids
- Itching: antihistamines, emollients
- Dermatitis: steroids, antihistamines

- Eczema: emollients, immune suppressants, steroids, UVA/UVB light treatment, wet wrapping, antihistamines
- Urticaria: antihistamines, emollients, steroids

OTC remedies:
- Abdominal pain and swelling: antacids
- Diarrhoea: kaolin and morphine, calcium carbonate, pectin
- Gastric upset/irritation: as prescription medication
- Nausea: antihistamines
- Vomiting: oral rehydration solution
- Wind: antacids
- Itching/burning mouth/palate: painkillers
- Rhinitis: decongestants
- Fever: aspirin, ibuprofen, paracetamol
- Cough: demulcents, antitussives, expectorants
- Angioedema: antihistamines
- Dermatitis: coal tar, emollients, steroids
- Eczema: emollients, hydrocortisone cream
- Itching: antihistamines, emollients
- Urticaria: calamine lotion, witch hazel

Alternative remedies
- Abdominal pain and swelling: aromatherapy, herbalism, homeopathy
- Diarrhoea: aromatherapy, herbalism, homeopathy
- Gastric upset/irritation: aromatherapy, herbalism
- Nausea: aromatherapy, herbalism, homeopathy
- Vomiting: herbalism
- Wind: aromatherapy, herbalism, homeopathy
- Ear problems: aromatherapy, herbalism, homeopathy
- Rhinitis: aromatherapy
- Fever: herbalism, homeopathy
- Asthma: acupuncture (mild asthma only), Buteyko method, homeopathy, relaxation techniques, yoga
- Cough: aromatherapy, homeopathy
- Angioedema: antihistamines
- Contact dermatitis: aromatherapy, Bach flower remedies, homeopathy
- Eczema: aromatherapy, evening primrose oil, relaxation, herbalism, homeopathy, Chinese herbal medicine, Bach flower remedies
- Itching: aromatherapy, herbalism
- Urticaria: aromatherapy, herbalism, homeopathy

Self-help tips: for symptom relief see *Abdominal pain and swelling, Diarrhoea, Gastric upset/irritation, Nausea, Vomiting, Wind, Ear problems, Itching mouth/palate, Rhinitis, Sneezing, Fever, Weight loss, Asthma, Breathing problems, Cough, Wheezing, Angioedema, Contact dermatitis, Eczema, Itching, Urticaria* in the section on *Symptoms*

See also *Flour*

Grain mite

The grain mite, found in grain with a high water content, can cause occupational asthma in farmers and dock workers. If symptoms start soon after beginning work and improve at weekends or on holidays, occupational asthma should be suspected.

Type of allergen: inhalant, contact

Symptoms
Respiratory reactions: asthma (occupational)

Skin reactions: eczema ("grain itch")

Tests
- Skin prick tests
- Intradermal
- Inhalation challenge
- Symptom diary (including peak flow meter readings)

Treatments
Avoidance
- In occupational situations, use protective equipment such as gloves and masks. Improved ventilation may help.

Prescription medication
- Asthma: anticholinergic drugs, antihistamines (exercise-induced), Beta2 (ß2) adrenoreceptor agonists, cromoglycate, nedocromil sodium, steroids, xanthine derivatives, zafirlukast
- Eczema: emollients, immune suppressants, steroids, UVA/UVB light treatment, wet wrapping, antihistamines

OTC remedies
- Eczema: emollients, hydrocortisone cream

Alternative remedies
- Asthma: acupuncture (mild asthma only), Buteyko method, homeopathy, relaxation techniques, yoga
- Eczema: aromatherapy, evening primrose oil, relaxation, herbalism, homeopathy, Chinese herbal medicine, Bach flower remedies

Self-help tips: for symptom relief see *Asthma, Eczema*, in the section on *Symptoms*

Grapefruit

Grapefruit is the fruit *Citrus paradisi*.

Type of allergen: contact, consumed

Symptoms, tests, treatments and self-help tips, see *Fruit*
See also *Citrus fruits*

Grapes

Grapes are the fruit of the vine, *Vitis vinifera*. They contain *salicylates*, which have been linked to hyperactivity in children. They also contain *histamine*.

Type of allergen: contact, consumed

Symptoms, tests, treatments and self-help tips, see *Fruit*

Gravy
See *Wheat*

Grease remover
See *Colophony*

Grease solvent
See *Solvents – chlorinated hydrocarbons*

Guar gum
See *Food additives – emulsifiers, stabilizers and thickeners*

Guava
Guava is the fruit *Psidium guajava*.

Type of allergen: consumed

Symptoms, tests, treatments and self-help tips, see *Fruit*

Guinea pigs
See *Pets, animal hair*

Gum acacia
Gum acacia is used in colour printing to separate printed sheets and prevent smearing; it can cause occupational asthma for printers. If symptoms start soon after beginning work and improve at weekends or on holidays, occupational asthma should be suspected.

Type of allergen: inhalant, contact

Symptoms
Respiratory reactions: asthma (occupational)

Skin reactions: rashes

Tests
• Skin patch test
• Symptom diary (including peak flow meter readings)

Treatments

Avoidance
- In occupational situations, use protective equipment such as masks and gloves. Improved ventilation may also help.

Prescription medication
- Asthma: anticholinergic drugs, antihistamines (exercise-induced), Beta2 (ß2) adrenoreceptor agonists, cromoglycate, nedocromil sodium, steroids, xanthine derivatives, zafirlukast
- Contact dermatitis: steroids, antihistamines

OTC remedies
- Contact dermatitis: coal tar, emollients, steroids

Alternative remedies
- Asthma: acupuncture (mild asthma only), Buteyko method, homeopathy, relaxation techniques, yoga
- Contact dermatitis: aromatherapy, Bach flower remedies, homeopathy

Self-help tips: for symptom relief see *Asthma, Contact dermatitis* in the section on *Symptoms*

Gum Arabic
See *Food additives – emulsifiers, stabilizers and thickeners*

Gums
Gums include tragacanth, gum acacia and gum Arabic. They can cause occupational asthma for carpet makers, pharmaceutical workers and printers; if symptoms start soon after beginning work and improve at weekends or on holidays, occupational asthma should be suspected.

Type of allergen: inhalant, contact

Symptoms
Respiratory reactions: occupational asthma

Skin reactions: rashes

Tests
- CAP-RAST test
- Skin patch test
- Symptom diary (including peak flow meter readings)

Treatments
Avoidance
- In occupational situations, use protective equipment such as masks and gloves. Improved ventilation may also help.

Prescription medication
- Asthma: anticholinergic drugs, antihistamines (exercise-induced), Beta2 (ß2) adrenoreceptor agonists, cromoglycate, nedocromil sodium, steroids, xanthine derivatives, zafirlukast
- Contact dermatitis: steroids, antihistamines

OTC remedies
- Contact dermatitis: coal tar, emollients, steroids

Alternative remedies
- Asthma: acupuncture (mild asthma only), Buteyko method, homeopathy, relaxation techniques, yoga
- Contact dermatitis: aromatherapy, Bach flower remedies, homeopathy

Self-help tips: for symptom relief see *Asthma, Contact dermatitis* in the section on *Symptoms*
See also *Chlorocresol (preservative), Colophony*

Haddock
See *Fish*

Hair dye
See *Cobalt, Cosmetics, Paraphenylenediamine (ppda)*

Hair spray
See *Benzophenones, Cosmetics, Hair care products*

Hair treatments
See *Cosmetics, Formaldehyde, Persulphate, Quinine*

Hake, Halibut
See *Fish*

Hamsters
See *Animal hair, Pets*

Hand cleaners
See *Glutaraldehyde*

Hand cream/lotion
Perfumes and preservatives tend to cause most problems.

Type of allergen: contact

Symptoms, tests, treatments and self-help tips, see *Cosmetics*

Hare
See *Animal hair*

Hay
Hay can cause occupational asthma in farmers, due to mould spores in the hay. If symptoms start soon after beginning work and improve at weekends or on holidays, occupational asthma should be suspected.

Type of allergen: inhalant

Symptoms
Respiratory reactions:
• Asthma (occupational), hypersensitivity pneumonitis

Tests
• Blood test: ELISA
• Symptom diary (including peak flow meter readings)

Treatments
Avoidance: in occupational situations, use protective equipment such as gloves and masks.

Prescription medication: anticholinergic drugs, antihistamines (exercise-induced), Beta2 (ß2) adrenoreceptor agonists, cromoglycate, nedocromil sodium, steroids, xanthine derivatives, zafirlukast

Alternative remedies: acupuncture (mild asthma only), Buteyko method, homeopathy, relaxation techniques, yoga

Self-help tips
- Keep harvested crops dry
- Ventilate storage area
- Avoid colds and viral infections
- Humidify the air
- Maintain your recommended weight
- For symptom relief, see *Asthma* in the section on *Symptoms*

Hazelnut

Hazelnut is the fruit of the tree *Corylus avellana*.

Type of allergen: consumed

Symptoms, tests, treatments and self-help tips, see *Nuts*

Heat

See *Temperature*

Henna

Henna is a natural vegetable dye which can cause sneezing, asthma and rhinitis.

Type of allergen: inhalant

Symptoms, tests, treatments and self-help tips, see *Dyes*

Herbs

For further information about the herbs themselves and cross-reactivity, see *Angelica, Basil, Bay leaf, Camomile, Chives, Coriander, Dill, Fennel, Garlic, Marjoram, Mint, Oregano, Parsley, Peppermint, Rosemary, Sage, Tarragon, Thyme*

Symptoms:

Anaphylactic shock
* Coriander, oregano (rare), parsley
* Exercise-induced – fennel, garlic

Eye reactions
* Conjunctivitis – fennel, parsley

Gastrointestinal reactions
* Abdominal pain and swelling – coriander
* Diarrhoea – chives, garlic
* Gastric upset/irritation – coriander
* Heartburn – peppermint
* Nausea – garlic
* Headaches: migraine – parsley

Mouth, nasal and ear reactions:
* Hay fever – camomile, peppermint
* Irritation of mucous membranes – garlic
* Itching mouth/palate – fennel, parsley
* Rhinitis – coriander, garlic
* Sneezing – garlic

Psychological problems
* Hyperactivity – dill, oregano, rosemary, tarragon, thyme

Respiratory reactions:
* Asthma (occupational) – bay leaf, garlic, rosemary
* Asthma – coriander, fennel, mint, oregano, rosemary, tarragon
* Wheezing – coriander, dill, garlic, oregano, parsley, rosemary, tarragon, thyme

Skin reactions:
* Angioedema – coriander, dill, fennel, oregano, parsley, rosemary, tarragon, thyme
* Atopic dermatitis – coriander
* Contact dermatitis, including occupational – angelica, garlic,

marjoram, oregano, parsley, peppermint, rosemary, sage
- Photoallergenic contact dermatitis – angelica, coriander, dill, parsley oil
- Eczema – coriander, garlic
- Flushing – garlic, parsley
- Skin irritation – basil, oregano, rosemary, tarragon
- Urticaria (this has been dismissed by some experts) – dill, fennel (exercise-induced), oregano, parsley, rosemary, tarragon, thyme

Tests
- Blood test: CAP-RAST (basil, bay leaf, coriander, dill, fennel (fresh and seed), garlic, lovage, marjoram, mint, oregano, parsley, tarragon, thyme)
- Blood test: ELISA (basil, bay leaf, dill, fennel, garlic, lovage, marjoram, mint, oregano, parsley, rosemary, sage, tarragon, thyme)
- Skin test: skin prick (camomile, coriander, fennel, garlic, parsley)
- Skin test: intradermal (parsley)
- Skin test: patch test (basil, coriander, oregano)
- Skin test: photopatch test (angelica)
- Elimination diet (coriander, dill, fennel, garlic, lovage, mint, parsley, rosemary, tarragon, thyme)
- Food challenge (coriander, dill, fennel, garlic, lovage, mint, parsley, rosemary, tarragon, thyme)
- Symptom diary (including peak flow meter readings)
- Exercise challenge

Treatments
Avoidance
- In occupational situations, use protective equipment such as gloves or masks; improved ventilation may also help.
- Check labels carefully and check with a dietitian to ensure that your diet is still nutritionally sound

Prescription medication
- Anaphylactic shock: adrenaline, antihistamines, steroids
- Abdominal pain and swelling: antacids, anti-spasmodic drugs
- Diarrhoea: antidiarrhoeal drugs
- Gastric upset/irritation: painkillers (use paracetamol rather than aspirin)

- Heartburn: antacids, alginates
- Nausea: antihistamines
- Migraine: painkillers, anti-sickness drugs, ergotamine, 5-HT agonists, beta-blockers, sodium valproate, sumatryptan
- Hay fever: antihistamines, cromoglycate, decongestants, nedocromil sodium, steroids, sympathomimetics
- Irritation of mucous membranes: painkillers
- Itching/burning mouth/palate: painkillers
- Rhinitis: antihistamines, decongestants, sodium cromoglycate, immunotherapy
- Hyperactivity: stimulant drugs
- Asthma: anticholinergic drugs, antihistamines (exercise-induced), Beta2 (ß2) adrenoreceptor agonists, cromoglycate, nedocromil sodium, steroids, xanthine derivatives, zafirlukast
- Wheezing: bronchodilator
- Angioedema: adrenaline, antihistamines, steroids
- Dermatitis: steroids, antihistamines
- Photoallergenic contact dermatitis: emollients, steroids
- Eczema: emollients, immune suppressants, steroids, UVA/UVB light treatment, wet wrapping, antihistamines
- Skin irritation: emollients
- Urticaria: antihistamines, emollients, steroids

OTC remedies:
- Conjunctivitis: antihistamines
- Abdominal pain and swelling: antacids
- Diarrhoea: kaolin and morphine, calcium carbonate, pectin
- Gastric upset/irritation: as prescription medication
- Heartburn: as prescription medication
- Nausea: antihistamines
- Migraine: aspirin, ibuprofen, paracetamol
- Hay fever: antihistamines, decongestants
- Irritation of mucous membranes: painkillers
- Itching/burning mouth/palate: painkillers
- Rhinitis: decongestants
- Dermatitis: coal tar, emollients, steroids
- Eczema: emollients, hydrocortisone cream
- Urticaria: calamine lotion, witch hazel

Alternative remedies
- Conjunctivitis: herbalism, homeopathy
- Abdominal pain and swelling: aromatherapy, herbalism, homeopathy

379

- Diarrhoea: aromatherapy, herbalism, homeopathy
- Gastric upset/irritation: aromatherapy, herbalism
- Heartburn: aromatherapy, homeopathy, herbalism
- Nausea: aromatherapy, herbalism, homeopathy
- Migraine: acupuncture, Alexander technique, aromatherapy, chiropractic, herbalism, homeopathy, hypnosis, osteopathy, reflexology
- Hay fever: aromatherapy, herbalism, homeopathy
- Irritation of mucous membranes: herbalism
- Rhinitis: aromatherapy
- Angioedema: antihistamines
- Contact dermatitis: aromatherapy, Bach flower remedies, homeopathy
- Eczema: aromatherapy, evening primrose oil, relaxation, herbalism, homeopathy, Chinese herbal medicine, Bach flower remedies
- Flushing: herbalism
- Urticaria: aromatherapy, herbalism, homeopathy

Self-help tips: for symptom relief see *Conjunctivitis, Abdominal pain and swelling, Diarrhoea, Gastric upset/irritation, Heartburn, nausea, Migraine, Hay fever, Irritation of mucous membranes, Itching mouth/palate, Rhinitis, Sneezing, Hyperactivity, asthma, Wheezing, Angioedema, Contact dermatitis, Photoallergenic contact dermatitis, Eczema, Flushing, Skin irritation, Urticaria* in the section on *Symptoms*

Herring
See *Fish*

Hexachlorophene

Hexachlorophene is a skin antiseptic or germicide which kills or prevents the growth of bacteria and other micro-organisms.

Type of allergen: contact

Likely sources of hexachlorophene: antiseptic soaps, creams and cosmetics

Symptoms, tests, treatments and self-help tips, see *Drugs*

Hexamethylene diisocyanate
See *Isocyanates*

Hexamine
See *Food additives – preservatives*

Hexylene glycol
See *Solvents – glycols*

Histamine

Histamine is an amine derived from the amino acid histidine, which is found in eggs, herbs, cheese, potatoes, nuts and fish. It is formed when bacteria break down the amino acid and remove the acid group. It is stored in mast cells in the body and released when the immune system recognizes an allergen.

Histamine poisoning is also known as "scombroid poisoning", named after the *Scomberesocidae* family of fish (which includes mackerel and tuna) which are the most likely sources of the problem. It can start any time between ten minutes and twelve hours after the food in question has been eaten, and is usually caused if the fish has been left unrefrigerated.

Type of allergen: consumed

Likely sources of histamine: cheese (particularly blue), eggs, fish, herbs, nuts, potatoes, sauerkraut, salami, sausages, spinach, tomatoes, red wine, yeast products

Symptoms
Gastrointestinal reactions: abdominal pain and swelling, diarrhoea, nausea, vomiting

Headache: headache, migraine

Mouth, nasal and ear reactions: burning sensation in mouth

Skin reactions: angioedema (particularly facial), flushing, rash, sweating

Tests
- Elimination diet
- Food challenge
- Symptom diary

Treatments
Avoidance
- Check labels carefully and check with a dietitian to ensure that your diet is still nutritionally sound

Prescription medication
- Abdominal pain and swelling: antacids, anti-spasmodic drugs
- Diarrhoea: antidiarrhoeal drugs
- Nausea: antihistamines
- Vomiting: anti-emetics
- Headache: painkillers, non-steroidal anti-inflammatories
- Migraine: painkillers, anti-sickness drugs, ergotamine, 5-HT agonists, beta-blockers, sodium valproate, sumatryptan
- Angioedema: adrenaline, antihistamines, steroids
- Dermatitis: steroids, antihistamines

OTC remedies
- Abdominal pain and swelling: antacids
- Diarrhoea: kaolin and morphine, calcium carbonate, pectin
- Nausea: antihistamines
- Vomiting: oral rehydration solution
- Headache: as prescription medication
- Migraine: aspirin, ibuprofen, paracetamol
- Dermatitis: coal tar, emollients, steroids

Alternative remedies
- Abdominal pain and swelling: aromatherapy, herbalism, homeopathy
- Diarrhoea: aromatherapy, herbalism, homeopathy
- Nausea: aromatherapy, herbalism, homeopathy
- Vomiting: herbalism
- Headache: acupuncture, aromatherapy, herbalism, homeopathy
- Migraine: acupuncture, Alexander technique, aromatherapy, chiropractic, herbalism, homeopathy, hypnosis, osteopathy, reflexology
- Dermatitis: aromatherapy, Bach flower remedies, homeopathy
- Flushing: herbalism

Self-help tips: for symptom relief see *Abdominal pain and swelling, Diarrhoea, Nausea, Vomiting, Headache, Migraine, Angio-edema, Contact dermatitis, Flushing* in the section on *Symptoms*

Honey

The problem can be with the honey itself, or pollen, venom or bee allergens contained within the honey.

Type of allergen: consumed

Symptoms

Gastrointestinal reactions: diarrhoea, vomiting

Mouth, nasal and ear reactions: rhinitis

Skin reactions: urticaria

Tests
- Blood test: CAP-RAST
- Blood test: ELISA
- Symptom diary
- Elimination diet
- Food challenge

Treatments
Avoidance
- Check labels carefully and check with a dietitian to ensure that your diet is still nutritionally sound

Prescription medication
- Diarrhoea: antidiarrhoeal drugs
- Vomiting: anti-emetics
- Rhinitis: antihistamines, decongestants, sodium cromoglycate, immunotherapy
- Urticaria: antihistamines, emollients, steroids

OTC remedies
- Diarrhoea: kaolin and morphine, calcium carbonate, pectin
- Vomiting: oral rehydration solution
- Rhinitis: decongestants
- Urticaria: calamine lotion, witch hazel

Alternative remedies
- Diarrhoea: aromatherapy, herbalism, homeopathy
- Vomiting: herbalism
- Rhinitis: aromatherapy
- Urticaria: aromatherapy, herbalism, homeopathy

Self-help tips: for symptom relief see *Diarrhoea, Vomiting, Rhinitis, Urticaria* in the section on *Symptoms*

You might also react to: birch pollen, ragweed pollen

Hops

Hops are from the plant *Humulus lupulus*.

Type of allergen: inhalant, consumed

Likely sources of hops: brewing

Symptoms
Respiratory reactions: asthma

Skin reactions: angioedema, urticaria

Tests
- Blood test: CAP-RAST
- Blood test: ELISA
- Skin prick tests
- Symptom diary (including peak flow meter readings)

Treatments
Avoidance

Prescription medication
- Asthma: anticholinergic drugs, antihistamines (exercise-induced), Beta2 (ß2) adrenoreceptor agonists, cromoglycate, nedocromil sodium, steroids, xanthine derivatives, zafirlukast
- Angioedema: adrenaline, antihistamines, steroids
- Urticaria: antihistamines, emollients, steroids

OTC remedies
- Angioedema: antihistamines
- Urticaria: calamine lotion, witch hazel

Alternative remedies
- Asthma: acupuncture (mild asthma only), Buteyko method, homeopathy, relaxation techniques, yoga
- Urticaria: aromatherapy, herbalism, homeopathy

Self-help tips: for symptom relief see *Asthma, Angioedema, Urticaria* in the section on *Symptoms*

Horse
See *Animal hair, Meat*

Horseradish
Horseradish is the condiment *Armoracia rusticana*.

Type of allergen: contact, consumed

Symptoms, tests, treatments and self-help tips, see *Spices*

You might also react to: cabbage, broccoli, Brussels sprouts, cauliflower, mustard, radish, swede, turnip, watercress

Hot water bottles
See *Latex*

House dust mite
See *Dust mite*

Hydraulic brake fluids
See *Solvents – glycol ether*

Hydraulic fluids
See *Solvents – glycol ether*

Hydrocarbon propellants
See *Volatile organic compounds*

Hydroxycitronellal
See *Perfumes*

Ibuprofen

Ibuprofen is a non-steroidal anti-inflammatory drug (NSAID); it is used as a painkiller and in the treatment of rheumatism and arthritis to relieve inflammation and stiffness. One in 20 asthma sufferers has a severe attack after taking ibuprofen.

Type of allergen: consumed

Symptoms, tests, treatments and self-help tips, see *Drugs*

You might also react to: aspirin

Indigo Carmine

See *Food additives – colourings*

Industrial coatings

See *Epoxy resin*

Inks

See *Chlorocresol (preservative), Chromium, Cobalt, Epoxy resin, Formaldehyde, Isocyanates, Methyl alcohol, Phenol, Solvents – alcohol solvents, Solvents – glycol ether, Solvents – halogenated solvents, Wool alcohol*

Insects and parasites

See *Bee and wasp stings*

Insect bites

See *Bee and wasp stings, Fleas*

Insecticide

Alternative products that might not cause a reaction: Use eucalyptus oil to deter moths, silverfish and ants; use lavender or eucalyptus sachets among clothes.
See *Benzene, Copper sulphate, Formaldehyde, Solvents – glycol ether*

Insect repellent
See *Camphor oil, Cedarwood oil, Citronella oil,*
Volatile organic compounds

Insulation materials
See *Formaldehyde*

Instruments
See *Cobalt*

Insulin

Insulin is a hormone produced by the pancreas in response to high blood sugar levels; diabetics are deficient in insulin, and may need to inject it into their system. If you are an insulin-dependent diabetic, you may react to the insulin (which may be derived from beef or pork). Your reaction may be local (i.e. it will appear as a red and itchy area of skin around the place where you have injected the insulin) or it may be systemic (where the whole body is affected, including breathing difficulty, heartbeat changes and urticaria). You may need to change the type of insulin used.

Type of allergen: injected, consumed

Symptoms, tests, treatments and self-help tips, see *Drugs*

Iodine

Iodine is a non-metallic element, chemical symbol I. It is soluble in ethanol and other organic solvents, but not in water. It is used as a mild antiseptic; it is also contained in some prescription medication for thyroid problems and coughs. Iodine and its salts may cause allergic reactions.

Some foods contain iodine (such as seafood, bread, dairy products and iodized table salt), but there is no connection between allergy to iodine and allergy to fish.

Type of allergen: contact, consumed

Symptoms, tests, treatments and self-help tips, see *Drugs*

Iron

Iron is a metallic element, chemical symbol Fe. It is used in metal-working and smelting.

Type of allergen: contact

Symptoms, tests, treatments and self-help tips, see *Metals*

Isobutyl acetate

See *solvents – esters*

Isocyanates

Isocyanates are the salts and esters of cyanic acid; they are aromatic and aliphatic compounds (see *Solvents*). The most common forms are:
- toluene diisocyanate (TDI)
- methylene bisphenyl isocyanate (MDI)
- hexamethylene diisocyanate (HDI)

They are used in manufacture of polyurethane foams, paints, wire and electrical components. Problems tend to be occupational, through inhaling the vapour or skin contact while handling the liquid forms. They can cause occupational asthma for spray painters, insulation installers, plastics, foam and rubber industry workers; approximately 10 per cent of people exposed to isocyanates suffer from asthma. If symptoms start soon after beginning work and improve at weekends or on holidays, occupational asthma should be suspected.

Type of allergen: inhaled, contact

Likely sources of isocyanates: cleaning products, damp treatment, dry-cleaning fluid, glues, ink (printers) nail varnish, paint stripper, paint thinners, pens and markers, polyurethane, stain removers

Symptoms
Eye reactions: conjunctivitis

Gastrointestinal reactions: gastric upset/irritation

Headache: dizziness, headache

Other: fever, muscle pain, weight loss

Psychological problems: fatigue

Respiratory reactions: asthma (occupational), hypersensitivity pneumonitis, breathing problems, chest tightness, cough, wheezing

Skin reactions: contact dermatitis, inflammation

Tests
- Blood test: CAP-RAST (HDI, MDI, TDI)
- Blood test: ELISA (HDI, MDI, TDI)
- Symptom diary (including peak flow meter readings)

Treatments
Avoidance
- In occupational situations, use protective equipment such as gloves and masks. Improved ventilation may also help.

Prescription medication
- Conjunctivitis: antihistamines, cromoglycate, nedocromil sodium, steroids, sympathomimetics
- Gastric upset/irritation: painkillers (use paracetamol rather than aspirin)
- Headache: painkillers, non-steroidal anti-inflammatories
- Fever: aspirin, ibuprofen, paracetamol
- Muscle pain: painkillers
- Asthma: anticholinergic drugs, antihistamines (exercise-induced), Beta2 (ß2) adrenoreceptor agonists, cromoglycate, nedocromil sodium, steroids, xanthine derivatives, zafirlukast
- Breathing problems: bronchodilators, corticosteroids
- Cough: antihistamines, bronchodilators, corticosteroids
- Wheezing: bronchodilator
- Contact dermatitis: steroids, antihistamines
- Inflammation: antihistamines, emollients, steroids

OTC remedies
- Conjunctivitis: antihistamines
- Gastric upset/irritation: as prescription medication
- Headache: as prescription medication
- Fever: aspirin, ibuprofen, paracetamol
- Muscle pain: painkillers
- Cough: demulcents, antitussives, expectorants
- Contact dermatitis: coal tar, emollients, steroids
- Inflammation: antihistamines, emollients

Alternative remedies
- Conjunctivitis: herbalism, homeopathy
- Gastric upset/irritation: aromatherapy, herbalism
- Faintness: aromatherapy, Bach flower remedies
- Headache: acupuncture, aromatherapy, herbalism, homeopathy
- Fever: herbalism, homeopathy
- Muscle pain: homeopathy
- Asthma: acupuncture (mild asthma only), Buteyko method, homeopathy, relaxation techniques, yoga
- Cough: aromatherapy, homeopathy
- Contact dermatitis: aromatherapy, Bach flower remedies, homeopathy

Self-help tips: for symptom relief, see *Conjunctivitis, Gastric upset/irritation, Headache, Fever, Muscle pain, Weight loss, Fatigue, Asthma, Breathing problems, Cough, Wheezing, Contact dermatitis, Inflammation* in the section on *Symptoms*

Isoeugenol
See *Perfumes*

Isophorone
See *Solvents – ketone solvents*

Isopropanol
Isopropanol – also known as rubbing alcohol – is a *solvent*.

Type of allergen: inhalant

Likely sources of isopropanol: cosmetics, perfumes, some types of coatings, cleaners, liniments, antiseptic solutions, liquid soaps and medications

Symptoms
Eye reactions: conjunctivitis

Respiratory reactions: breathing problems

Test: Symptom diary

Treatments
Avoidance
* In occupational situations, use protective equipment such as goggles and masks. Improved ventilation may also help

Prescription medication
* Conjunctivitis: antihistamines, cromoglycate, nedocromil sodium, steroids, sympathomimetics
* Breathing problems: bronchodilators, corticosteroids

OTC remedies
* Conjunctivitis: antihistamines

Alternative remedies
* Conjunctivitis: herbalism, homeopathy

Self-help tips: for symptom relief see *Conjunctivitis, Breathing problems* in the section on *Symptoms*
See also *Solvents – alcohol solvents*

Isphagula
Isphagula is a bulk-forming agent used in the treatment of diarrhoea and constipation by absorbing water from the large intestine.

Type of allergen: inhalant, consumed

Symptoms, tests, treatments and self-help tips, see *Drugs*

Jack fruit

Jack fruit is the fruit *Artocarpus heterophyllus*.

Type of allergen: consumed

Symptoms, tests, treatments and self-help tips, see *Fruit*

You might also react to: plantain

Jack mackerel

See *Fish*

Jewellery

See *Cobalt, Nickel, Palladium, Metals*

Jujube

Jujube is the fruit *Ziziphus jujuba*, also known as the Chinese date − see *Date*

Juniper berry

Juniper berries − used as flavourings in gin − are the berries of the evergreen shrub of the genus *Juniperus*, particularly *J. communis*

Type of allergen: contact, consumed

Symptoms, tests, treatments and self-help tips, see *Spices*

Karaya gum

See *Food additives − emulsifiers, stabilizers and thickeners*

Keys

See *Nickel, Metals*

Kitchen utensils

See *Cobalt, Metals*

Kiwi fruit

Kiwi fruit is the fruit *Actinidia chinensis*. It is also known as Chinese gooseberry.

Actinidin is the major allergen in kiwi fruit; it has similar chemical properties to papain.

Type of allergen: contact, consumed

Symptoms, tests, treatments and self-help tips, see *Fruit*

You might also react to: latex

Knives
See *Chromium, Nickel, Metals*

Kohlrabi

Kohlrabi is a variety of cabbage.

Type of allergen: consumed

Symptoms, tests, treatments and self-help tips, see *Vegetables*

Lacquer
See *Solvents (ketone solvents)*

Lacquer coatings
See *Solvents (esters)*

Lacquer solvents
See *Methyl alcohol, Solvents (alcohol solvents), Solvents (esters)*

Lacquer thinners
See *Amyl alcohol, Solvents (alcohol solvents),
Solvents (aromatic hydrocarbons)*

Lactose

Lactose is the major sugar in human and bovine milk.

Intolerance to lactose isn't due to allergy but to insufficient quantities in the body of the enzyme lactase (which breaks down lactose); undigested lactose molecules are not absorbed by the body and are fermented in the bowel, with the result of diarrhoea, abdominal pain, bloating and wind. It is hard to distinguish between lactose intolerance and milk protein allergy; however, milk allergy often has symptoms not seen in lactose intolerance such as rhinitis, ear pain, eczema and urticaria.

Products containing casein, lactalbumin, lactate or lactic acid do not contain lactose and should pose no problems. Fermented milk products such as yoghurt and buttermilk may be tolerated, as the level of lactose is reduced by the action of bacterial enzymes.

If you have coeliac disease, you may be lactose-intolerant until the coeliac disease has been treated.

Type of allergen: consumed

Likely sources of lactose: butter, cheese, cheese flavour, chocolate, cream, curd, fermented milk products, margarine (containing milk solids), milk, milk solids, milk powder, yoghurt, whey

Symptoms
Gastrointestinal reactions: abdominal pain and swelling, diarrhoea, wind

Tests
- Blood test: CAP-RAST (not particularly reliable for children)
- Skin prick test (not particularly reliable for children)
- Lactose tolerance test – you fast for 24 hours; a blood sample is taken and the glucose level tested. Then you're given a drink of lactose and blood samples are taken for the next 2-3 hours to see how much glucose is in your blood and if lactase is present in your digestive system
- Hydrogen breath test – if lactose is undigested, hydrogen is produced and can be measured in the breath. The test can be affected by undigested sucrose, maltose or starch, the presence of sugar diabetes and smoking
- Acid stool test – if lactose is undigested, it ferments in the lower bowel and creates lactic acid, which can be measured in faeces. This test is used for children.
- Endoscopy – a small piece from the lining of the small intestine is removed and examined by the doctor
- Symptom diary

Treatments
Avoidance
• Check labels carefully and check with a dietitian to ensure that your diet is still nutritionally sound

Prescription medication
• Abdominal pain and swelling: antacids, anti-spasmodic drugs
• Diarrhoea: antidiarrhoeal drugs
• Wind: antacids

OTC remedies
• Abdominal pain and swelling: antacids
• Diarrhoea: kaolin and morphine, calcium carbonate, pectin
• Wind: antacids

Alternative remedies
• Abdominal pain and swelling: aromatherapy, herbalism, homeopathy
• Diarrhoea: aromatherapy, herbalism, homeopathy
• Wind: aromatherapy, herbalism, homeopathy

Self-help tips: add lactase to milk before drinking it – this breaks down lactose into glucose and galactose, which the body will be able to tolerate.

For symptom relief, see *Abdominal pain and swelling, Diarrhoea, Wind* in the section on *Symptoms*

Lamb
Type of allergen: contact, consumed

Symptoms, tests, treatments and self-help tips, see *Meat and poultry*

You might also react to: beef

Laminates
See *Adhesives*

Langoustines
See *Shellfish*

Lanolin

Lanolin is an emulsion of purified wool fat in water. It contains cholesterol, terpene alcohols and esters. See *Wool alcohol*

Latex

Latex is derived from the rubber tree, *Hevea brasiliensis*.

Latex allergy tends to start with an allergic rash on the hands after using gloves; don't turn them inside out, as the powder will be released into the air and the resultant sensitization will lead to asthma (particularly for health care professionals). It has been estimated that up to 6 per cent of the general population is sensitized to latex and up to 12 per cent of health care workers who are regularly exposed to it. If your symptoms start soon after beginning work and improve at weekends or on holidays, occupational asthma should be suspected.

Type of allergen: contact, inhalant

Likely sources of latex: adhesives and self-adhesive envelopes, baby bottle teats, balloons, condoms, dummies, gloves, goggles, hot water bottles, mattresses and pillows, medical equipment, pencil erasers, rubber-soled shoes, rubber bands, rubber toys, sports equipment handles, tyres

Symptoms
Anaphylactic shock (rare)

Eye reactions: conjunctivitis – caused by sensitivity to the natural proteins in latex, which become airborne when they adhere to powder (e.g. in gloves)

Mouth/nasal/ear reactions: irritation of mucous membranes – caused by sensitivity to the natural proteins in latex, which become airborne when they adhere to powder (e.g. in gloves)

Respiratory reactions: asthma (occupational)

Skin reactions: angioedema, contact dermatitis (reddening, itching and swelling of the skin 1-2 days after contact), urticaria

Tests
- Skin prick test
- Patch test
- Blood test: CAP-RAST
- Blood test: ELISA
- Symptom diary (including peak flow meter readings)

Treatments
Avoidance
- In occupational situations, use protective equipment such as masks; improved ventilation may help

Prescription medication
- Anaphylactic shock: adrenaline, antihistamines, steroids
- Conjunctivitis: antihistamines, cromoglycate, nedocromil sodium, steroids, sympathomimetics
- Irritation of mucous membranes: painkillers
- Asthma: anticholinergic drugs, antihistamines (exercise-induced), Beta2 (ß2) adrenoreceptor agonists, cromoglycate, nedocromil sodium, steroids, xanthine derivatives, zafirlukast
- Angioedema: adrenaline, antihistamines, steroids
- Contact dermatitis: steroids, antihistamines
- Urticaria: antihistamines, emollients, steroids

OTC remedies
- Conjunctivitis: antihistamines
- Irritation of mucous membranes: painkillers
- Angioedema: antihistamines
- Contact dermatitis: coal tar, emollients, steroids
- Urticaria: calamine lotion, witch hazel

Alternative remedies
- Conjunctivitis: herbalism, homeopathy
- Irritation of mucous membranes: herbalism
- Asthma: acupuncture (mild asthma only), Buteyko method, homeopathy, relaxation techniques, yoga
- Contact dermatitis: aromatherapy, Bach flower remedies, homeopathy
- Urticaria: aromatherapy, herbalism, homeopathy

Self-help tips: use non-powdered gloves
For symptom relief, see *Conjunctivitis, Irritation of mucous*

membranes, Asthma, Angioedema, Contact dermatitis, Urticaria in the section on *Symptoms*

Alternative products that won't cause a reaction
• Leather shoes
• Plastic erasers and toys
• Non-latex condoms
• Synthetic rubber (though you may be allergic to some of the additives)

You might also react to: avocado, bananas, chestnuts, figs, kiwi fruit (all contain proteins found in *latex*); also almonds, apple, carrot, celery, cherry, hazelnut, melons, papaya, peaches, pear, plum, potato (raw), tomato; and possibly apricots, cherries, figs, grapes, hazel nuts, passion fruit, peaches, pears, pineapple, rye, strawberries, walnuts
See also *Talc, Thuriams*

Latex emulsion polymers
See *Solvents – esters*

Lavender oil
Lavender oil is derived from the plant *Lavendula officinalis*.

Type of allergen: contact, inhaled

Likely sources of lavender oil: aromatherapy oil, cosmetics, toiletries

Symptoms, tests, treatments and self-help tips, see *Oils, cosmetic*

Lead
Lead is a metallic element, chemical symbol Pb. It is used in building construction work.

Type of allergen: contact

Likely sources of lead: alloys, bullets, shot, lead-plate accumulators, pewter, solder

Symptoms, tests, treatments and self-help tips, see *Metals*

Leather goods

Type of allergen: contact

Symptoms
Skin reactions: contact dermatitis

Tests
• Skin patch test
• Symptom diary

Treatments
Avoidance

Prescription medication: steroids, antihistamines

OTC remedies: coal tar, emollients, steroids

Alternative remedies: aromatherapy, Bach flower remedies, homeopathy

Self-help tips: for symptom relief see *Contact dermatitis* in the section on *Symptoms*

Alternative products that might not cause a reaction: PVC goods, natural fabrics such as cotton

See *Chlorocresol (preservative), Chromate, Chromium, Formaldehyde, Potassium dichromate, Wool alcohol*

Leek

Leek is the vegetable *Allium porrum*. It contains oxalates, a derivative of oxalic acid.

Type of allergen: consumed

Symptoms, tests, treatments and self-help tips, see *Vegetables*

You might also react to: asparagus, chives, garlic, onion, shallot

Legumes

For further information about the legumes themselves and cross-reactivity see *Chick peas, Lentil*

Symptoms
Anaphylactic shock
• Chick peas, lentil

Eye reactions
• Conjunctivitis (chick peas, lentil)

Gastrointestinal reactions
• Abdominal pain and swelling (chick peas)
• Gastric upset/irritation (chick peas)
• Vomiting (lentil)

Mouth, nasal and ear reactions
• Rhinitis (chick peas, lentil)

Respiratory reactions
• Asthma (chick peas, lentil)
• Cough (chick peas, lentil)
• wheezing (chick peas)

Skin reactions
• Angioedema (chick peas, lentil)
• urticaria (chick peas, lentil)

Tests
• Blood test: CAP-RAST (chick peas, lentil)
• Blood test: ELISA (lentil)
• Elimination diet (chick peas, lentil)
• Food challenge (chick peas, lentil)
• Symptom diary (including peak flow meter readings)

Treatments
Avoidance
• Check labels carefully and check with a dietitian to ensure that your diet is still nutritionally sound

Prescription medication
- Anaphylactic shock: adrenaline, antihistamines, steroids
- Conjunctivitis: antihistamines, cromoglycate, nedocromil sodium, steroids, sympathomimetics
- Abdominal pain and swelling: antacids, anti-spasmodic drugs
- Gastric upset/irritation: painkillers (use paracetamol rather than aspirin)
- Vomiting: anti-emetics
- Rhinitis: antihistamines, decongestants, sodium cromoglycate, immunotherapy
- Asthma: anticholinergic drugs, antihistamines (exercise-induced), Beta2 (ß2) adrenoreceptor agonists, cromoglycate, nedocromil sodium, steroids, xanthine derivatives, zafirlukast
- Cough: antihistamines, bronchodilators, corticosteroids
- Wheezing: bronchodilator
- Angioedema: adrenaline, antihistamines, steroids
- Urticaria: antihistamines, emollients, steroids

OTC remedies
- Conjunctivitis: antihistamines
- Abdominal pain and swelling: antacids
- Gastric upset/irritation: as prescription medication
- Vomiting: oral rehydration solution
- Rhinitis: decongestants
- Cough: demulcents, antitussives, expectorants
- Angioedema: antihistamines
- Urticaria: calamine lotion, witch hazel

Alternative remedies
- Conjunctivitis: herbalism, homeopathy
- Abdominal pain and swelling: aromatherapy, herbalism, homeopathy
- Gastric upset/irritation: aromatherapy, herbalism
- Vomiting: herbalism
- Rhinitis: aromatherapy
- Asthma: acupuncture (mild asthma only), Buteyko method, homeopathy, relaxation techniques, yoga
- Cough: aromatherapy, homeopathy
- Urticaria: aromatherapy, herbalism, homeopathy

Self-help tips: for symptom relief see *Conjunctivitis, Abdominal pain and swelling, Gastric upset/irritation, Vomiting, Asthma, Cough, Wheezing, Angioedema, Urticaria* in *Symptoms*

Lemon

Lemon is the fruit of the tree *Citrus limon*. The reaction may be to acid present in the lemon (e.g. chlorogenic acid).

Type of allergen: contact, consumed

Symptoms, tests, treatments and self-help tips, see *Fruit, Citrus fruit*

Lentil

Lentils are the leguminous plant *Ervum lens*.

Type of allergen: consumed

Symptoms, tests, treatments and self-help tips, see *Legumes*

You might also react to: beans, chick peas, liquorice, pea, peanut, senna, soy

Lettuce

Lettuce is the salad vegetable *Lactuca sativa*. The problem is in the milky sap.

Type of allergen: contact, consumed

Symptoms, tests, treatments and self-help tips, see *Vegetables*

You might also react to: ragweed pollen; artichoke, chicory, dandelion, endive, sunflower seeds, tarragon

Lime

Lime is the fruit of the tree *Citrus aurantifolia*. The reaction may be to acid present in the lime (e.g. chlorogenic acid).

Type of allergen: contact, consumed

Symptoms, tests, treatments and self-help tips, see *Fruit*
See also *Citrus fruit*

Liniments
See *Isopropanol, Solvents — alcohol solvents*

Linoleum
See *Colophony, Linseed oil*
Linoleum is made from linseed oil and ground cork.

Linseed oil
Linseed oil is derived from the flax plant genus *Linum*. Is used in the manufacture of paint, varnish and linoleum.

Type of allergen: contact, inhalant

Likely sources of linseed oil: emollients, medicinal soaps, shaving cream, depilatories, patent leather, insulating materials, cloth, cough remedies

Symptoms
Skin reactions: angioedema, urticaria

Tests
• Blood test: CAP-RAST
• Symptom diary

Treatments
Avoidance
• Check labels; in occupational situations, use protective equipment such as gloves and masks. Improved ventilation may also help.

Prescription medication
• Angioedema: adrenaline, antihistamines, steroids
• Urticaria: antihistamines, emollients, steroids

OTC remedies
- Angioedema: antihistamines
- Urticaria: calamine lotion, witch hazel

Alternative remedies
- Urticaria: aromatherapy, herbalism, homeopathy

Self-help tips: for symptom relief see *Angioedema, Urticaria* in the section on *Symptoms*

Lip balm
Perfumes and preservatives tend to cause most problems.

Type of allergen: contact

Symptoms, tests, treatments and self-help tips, see *Cosmetics*

Lipstick
Perfumes and preservatives tend to cause most problems.

Type of allergen: contact

Symptoms, tests, treatments and self-help tips, see *Cosmetics*

Liquorice
Liquorice contains *salicylates*, which have been linked to hyperactivity in children.

Type of allergen: consumed

Symptoms
Psychological problems: hyperactivity

Respiratory reactions: wheezing

Skin reactions: angioedema, urticaria (this has been dismissed by some experts)

Tests
- Blood test: ELISA
- Elimination diet
- Food challenge
- Symptom diary (including peak flow meter readings)

Treatments
Avoidance
- Check labels carefully and check with a dietitian to ensure that your diet is still nutritionally sound

Prescription medication
- Hyperactivity: stimulant drugs
- Wheezing: bronchodilator
- Angioedema: adrenaline, antihistamines, steroids
- Urticaria: antihistamines, emollients, steroids

OTC remedies
- Angioedema: antihistamines
- Urticaria: calamine lotion, witch hazel

Alternative remedies
- Hyperactivity: herbalism
- Urticaria: aromatherapy, herbalism, homeopathy

Self-help tips: for symptom relief see *Hyperactivity, Wheezing, Angioedema, Urticaria* in the section on *Symptoms*

You might also react to: beans, chick peas, lentil, pea, peanut, senna, soy

Liver
See *Phenylethylamine*

Llama
See *Animal hair*

Lobster
See *Shellfish*

Lubricants
See *Solvents – glycols, Wool alcohol*

Lubricating oils
See *Cobalt*

Lymecycline
See *Antibiotics, Tetracycline, Drugs*

Lysozyme
See *Egg*

Macadamia nuts

Macadamia nuts are the fruit of the tree *Macadamia spp.* It is not a common allergen.

Type of allergen: contact, consumed

Symptoms, tests, treatments and self-help tips, see *Nuts*

Mace

Mace is a spice *Myristica fragrans*. It contains *salicylates*, which have been linked to hyperactivity in children.

Type of allergen: inhalant, contact, consumed

For symptoms, tests, treatments and self-help tips, see *Spices*

Mackerel
See *Fish*

Macrolides

Macrolides are broad-spectrum *antibiotics* used to treat respiratory tract infections, middle ear infections, pelvic infections and wound infections. They inhibit the production of protein in bacteria and stop them multiplying. They are often prescribed as an alternative to penicillin. Macrolides include: azithromycin, clarithromycin, erythromycin.

Type of allergen: consumed

Symptoms, tests, treatments and self-help tips, see *Drugs*

Make-up, eye
See *Cosmetics*

Maize
See *Corn*

Malt

Malt is used in brewing. If your symptoms start soon after beginning work and improve at weekends or on holidays, occupational asthma should be suspected.

Type of allergen: inhalant, contact

Symptoms
Anaphylactic shock

Respiratory reactions: asthma (occupational)

Skin reactions: itching, urticaria

Tests
- Blood test: CAP-RAST
- Blood test: ELISA
- Symptom diary (including peak flow meter readings)

Treatments
Avoidance
- In occupational situations, use protective equipment such as gloves and masks
- Check labels carefully and check with a dietitian to ensure that your diet is still nutritionally sound

Prescription medication
- Anaphylactic shock: adrenaline, antihistamines, steroids
- Asthma: anticholinergic drugs, antihistamines (exercise-induced), Beta2 (ß2) adrenoreceptor agonists, cromoglycate,

nedocromil sodium, steroids, xanthine derivatives, zafirlukast
* Itching: antihistamines, emollients
* Urticaria: antihistamines, emollients, steroids

OTC remedies
* Itching: antihistamines, emollients
* Urticaria: calamine lotion, witch hazel

Alternative remedies
* Asthma: acupuncture (mild asthma only), Buteyko method, homeopathy, relaxation techniques, yoga
* Itching: aromatherapy, herbalism
* Urticaria: aromatherapy, herbalism, homeopathy

Self-help tips: for symptom relief see *Asthma, Itching, Urticaria* in the section on *Symptoms*
See also *Yeast*

Mandarin

Mandarin is the fruit of the tree *Citrus reticulata*.

Type of allergen: contact, consumed

Symptoms, tests, treatments and self-help tips, see *Fruit*

Mango

Mango is the fruit of the tree *Mangifera indica*.

Type of allergen: consumed

Symptoms, tests, treatments and self-help tips, see *Fruit*

You might also react to: cashews, pistachios

Mannitol

See *Food additives – emulsifiers, stabilizers and thickeners*

Marjoram

Marjoram is the herb *Origanum majorana*.

Type of allergen: contact

Symptoms, tests, treatments and self-help tips, see *Herbs*

You might also react to: others in the *Labiatae* family, such as mint, oregano, rosemary, sage, thyme

Marrow

Marrow is the vegetable *Cucurbita pepo*.

Symptoms, tests, treatments and self-help tips, see *Vegetables*

You might also react to: others in the *Cucurbitaceae* family, such as courgette, cucumber, melon, pumpkin, squash, watermelon

Mascara

Perfumes and preservatives tend to cause most problems.

Type of allergen: contact

Symptoms, tests, treatments and self-help tips, see *Cosmetics*

Mattresses

See *Dust mite, Latex, Polyurethane*

Matches

See *Chromate, Chromium, Colophony*

Meat and poultry

For further information about the meat itself and cross-reactivity see *Beef, Lamb, Pork, Turkey*

Symptoms

Gastrointestinal reactions
- Abdominal pain – pork
- Diarrhoea – beef, pork
- Gastric upset/irritation – beef
- Nausea – beef, pork
- Vomiting – beef, pork

Headache
- Headache – beef, chicken liver
- Migraine – beef, chicken liver

Mouth, nasal and ear reactions
- Itching mouth/palate – pork
- Rhinitis – pork
- Sneezing – pork

Respiratory reactions
- Asthma – pork
- Breathing problems – beef, pork
- Cough – lamb
- Wheezing – beef, pork, turkey

Skin reactions
- Atopic dermatitis – beef, pork
- Contact dermatitis (occupational) – beef, chicken, duck, goose, horse, lamb, turkey
- Flushing – beef
- Urticaria – beef, pork

Other reactions
- Weight gain – pork

Tests
- Blood test: CAP-RAST (beef, chicken, lamb, mutton, pork, rabbit, turkey)
- Blood test: ELISA (beef, duck, goose, horse, lamb, mutton, pork, rabbit, turkey)
- Skin prick test (beef, chicken, duck, goose, horse, lamb, mutton, pork, turkey)
- Intradermal (beef, chicken, duck, goose, horse, mutton, pork, turkey)

- Elimination diet (beef, chicken liver, lamb, mutton, pork, turkey)
- Food challenge (beef, chicken liver, lamb, mutton, pork, turkey)
- Symptom diary (including peak flow meter readings)

Treatments

Prescription medication

- Abdominal pain and swelling: antacids, anti-spasmodic drugs
- Diarrhoea: antidiarrhoeal drugs
- Gastric upset/irritation: painkillers (use paracetamol rather than aspirin)
- Nausea: antihistamines
- Vomiting: anti-emetics
- Headache: painkillers, non-steroidal anti-inflammatories
- Migraine: painkillers, anti-sickness drugs, ergotamine, 5-HT agonists, beta-blockers, sodium valproate, sumatryptan
- Itching/burning mouth/palate: painkillers
- Rhinitis: antihistamines, decongestants, sodium cromoglycate, immunotherapy
- Sneezing: antihistamines, decongestants, sodium cromogylcate
- Asthma: anticholinergic drugs, antihistamines (exercise-induced), Beta2 (ß2) adrenoreceptor agonists, cromoglycate, nedocromil sodium, steroids, xanthine derivatives, zafirlukast
- Breathing problems: bronchodilators, corticosteroids
- Cough: antihistamines, bronchodilators, corticosteroids
- Wheezing: bronchodilator
- Contact dermatitis: steroids, antihistamines
- Urticaria: antihistamines, emollients, steroids

OTC remedies

- Abdominal pain and swelling: antacids
- Diarrhoea: kaolin and morphine, calcium carbonate, pectin
- Gastric upset/irritation: as prescription medication
- Nausea: antihistamines
- Vomiting: oral rehydration solution
- Headache: as prescription medication
- Migraine: aspirin, ibuprofen, paracetamol
- Itching/burning mouth/palate: painkillers
- Rhinitis: decongestants
- Cough: demulcents, antitussives, expectorants
- Contact dermatitis: coal tar, emollients, steroids
- Urticaria: calamine lotion, witch hazel

Alternative remedies
- Abdominal pain and swelling: aromatherapy, herbalism, homeopathy
- Diarrhoea: aromatherapy, herbalism, homeopathy
- Gastric upset/irritation: aromatherapy, herbalism
- Nausea: aromatherapy, herbalism, homeopathy
- Vomiting: herbalism
- Headache: acupuncture, aromatherapy, herbalism, homeopathy
- Migraine: acupuncture, Alexander technique, aromatherapy, chiropractic, herbalism, homeopathy, hypnosis, osteopathy, reflexology
- Rhinitis: aromatherapy
- Sneezing: acupuncture
- Asthma: acupuncture (mild asthma only), Buteyko method, homeopathy, relaxation techniques, yoga
- Cough: aromatherapy, homeopathy
- Contact dermatitis: aromatherapy, Bach flower remedies, homeopathy
- Flushing: herbalism
- Urticaria: aromatherapy, herbalism, homeopathy

Self-help tips: for symptom relief see *Abdominal pain, Diarrhoea, Gastric upset, Nausea, Vomiting, Headache, Migraine, Itching/burning mouth/palate, Rhinitis, Sneezing, Asthma, Breathing problems, Cough, Wheezing, Contact dermatitis, Flushing, Urticaria* in the section on *Symptoms*

Meat tenderizer
See *Chymopapain*

Megrim
See *Fish*

Melamine
See *Formaldehyde*

Melon
Melon is the fruit of the plant *Cucumin melo spp*. It contains *salicylates*, which have been linked to hyperactivity in children.

Type of allergen: consumed

Symptoms, tests, treatments and self-help tips, see *Fruit*

You might also react to: others in the *Cucurbitaceae* family, such as courgette, cucumber, marrow, pumpkin, squash, watermelon; also ragweed pollen, mugwort pollen, pellitory pollen; and possibly melon if you're allergic to house dust mite or birch/grass/mugwort pollen

Menthol

Menthol is a white, crystalline terpene alcohol, chemical symbol $C_{10}H_{19}OH$. It is extracted from oil of peppermint and is also known as mint camphor or peppermint camphor.

Likely sources of menthol: flavouring agents

Type of allergen: inhalant, contact

Symptoms
Mouth, nasal and ear reactions: burning mouth, mouth ulcers

Respiratory reactions: asthma, breathing problems

Skin reactions: contact dermatitis, allergic contact urticaria

Tests
• Skin patch
• Symptom diary (including peak flow meter readings)

Treatments
Avoidance

Prescription medication
• Mouth ulcers: antiseptic mouthwash, folic acid, hydrocortisone pellets
• Asthma: anticholinergic drugs, antihistamines (exercise-induced), Beta2 (ß2) adrenoreceptor agonists, cromoglycate, nedocromil sodium, steroids, xanthine derivatives, zafirlukast
• Breathing problems: bronchodilators, corticosteroids

- Contact dermatitis: steroids, antihistamines
- Urticaria: antihistamines, emollients, steroids

OTC remedies
- Mouth ulcers: as prescription medication
- Contact dermatitis: coal tar, emollients, steroids
- Urticaria: calamine lotion, witch hazel

Alternative remedies
- Mouth ulcers: aromatherapy, herbalism, homeopathy
- Asthma: acupuncture (mild asthma only), Buteyko method, homeopathy, relaxation techniques, yoga
- Contact dermatitis: aromatherapy, Bach flower remedies, homeopathy
- Urticaria: aromatherapy, herbalism, homeopathy

Self-help tips: for symptom relief see *Mouth ulcers, Asthma, Breathing problems, Contact dermatitis, Urticaria* in the section on *Symptoms*

You might also react to: aspirin, mint

Mercaptobenzothiazole

Mercaptobenzothiazole is an additive in rubber products.

Type of allergen: contact

Likely sources of mercaptobenzothiazole: rubber products – boots, gloves and catheters

Symptoms
Skin reactions: contact dermatitis, itching, skin irritation

Tests
- Skin patch test
- Symptom diary

Treatments
Avoidance
- In occupational situations, use protective equipment and hypoallergenic gloves which don't contain MBT.

Prescription medication
- Contact dermatitis: steroids, antihistamines
- Itching: antihistamines, emollients
- Skin irritation: emollients

OTC remedies
- Contact dermatitis: coal tar, emollients, steroids
- Itching: antihistamines, emollients
- Skin irritation: emollients

Alternative remedies
- Contact dermatitis: aromatherapy, Bach flower remedies, homeopathy
- Itching: aromatherapy, herbalism

Self-help tips: for symptom relief see *Contact dermatitis, Itching, Skin irritation* in the section on *Symptoms*

Mercury

Mercury is a metallic element, chemical symbol Hg.

Type of allergen: contact

Likely sources of mercury: barometers, batteries, dental amalgam, scientific equipment, thermometers, silk

Symptoms, tests, treatments and self-help tips, see *Metals*
See also *Fillings, mercury*

Metals

Many industrial processes involve working with metal; many household items, including clothing fastenings and jewellery, are made of metal, which can cause skin problems. In the form of salts (mainly used in industrial processes), metals can also cause respiratory problems.
See *Antimony, Arsenic, Beryllium, Chromate, Chromium, Cobalt, Copper, Copper sulphate, Gold, Iron, Lead, Mercury, Nickel, Palladium, Platinum salts, Potassium dichromate, Selenium, Silver, tellurium, Vanadium salts, Zinc*

Symptoms
Respiratory reactions
- Asthma (occupational) – chromium, cobalt, nickel, platinum, vanadium salts

Skin reactions
- Contact dermatitis – chromate, chromium, cobalt, copper sulphate, nickel, potassium dichromate
- Occupational dermatitis – antimony, arsenic, beryllium, copper, gold, iron, lead, mercury, palladium, platinum salts, selenium, silver, tellurium, zinc
- Itching – chromate, nickel
- Skin irritation – chromate

Tests
- Blood test: CAP-RAST (platinum salts)
- Skin test: patch test (beryllium, chromate, cobalt, nickel, potassium dichromate)
- Symptom diary (including peak flow meter readings)

Treatments
Avoidance
- In occupational situations, use protective equipment such as gloves or masks; improved ventilation may also help.

Prescription medication
- Asthma: anticholinergic drugs, antihistamines (exercise-induced), Beta2 (ß2) adrenoreceptor agonists, cromoglycate, nedocromil sodium, steroids, xanthine derivatives, zafirlukast
- Itching: antihistamines, emollients
- Dermatitis: steroids, antihistamines
- Skin irritation: emollients

OTC remedies
- Dermatitis: coal tar, emollients, steroids

Alternative remedies
- Asthma: acupuncture (mild asthma only), Buteyko method, homeopathy, relaxation techniques, yoga
- Contact dermatitis: aromatherapy, Bach flower remedies, homeopathy
- Itching: aromatherapy, herbalism

Self-help tips: for symptom relief see *Asthma, Contact dermatitis, Itching, Skin irritation* in the section on *Symptoms*

Methanal
See *Formaldehyde*

Methyl alcohol
Methyl alcohol is a *solvent*.

Type of allergen: inhalant, contact

Likely sources of methyl alcohol: glass cleaners, shellac, stains, dyes, inks, lacquer solvents, fuel additives, an extractant for oils.

Symptoms, tests, treatments and self-help tips, see *Solvents (alcohol solvents)*

Methyl amyl ketone (MAK)
See *Solvents (ketone solvents)*

Methylene chloride (dichloromethane)
See *Solvents (chlorinated hydrocarbons), Solvents (halogenated solvents)*

Methyl ethyl ketone (MEK)
See *Solvents (ketone solvents)*

Methyl 4-hydroxybenzoate
See *Food additives – preservatives*

Methyl isobutyl ketone (MIBK)
See *Solvents – ketone solvents*

Methylnaphthalene
See *Solvents (aromatic hydrocarbons)*

Methyl paraben
See *Food additives – preservatives*

Methylene bisphenyl isocyanate

See *Isocyanates*

Methylene blue

Methylene blue – also known as methylthionine chloride – is used as a dye and an anti-infective agent.

Type of allergen: inhalant, contact

Likely sources of methylene blue: chemical dyes, lipsticks

Symptoms, tests, treatments and self-help tips, see *Dyes*

Mice

See *Pets, Animal hair, Animal protein*

Milk

Milk is one of the most common food allergens. The two parts which are more likely to cause problems are *casein* (the curd that forms when milk is left to sour – this accounts for 80 per cent of the protein in milk, and studies show a high rate of skin test reactions to it; the three casein proteins are alpha, beta and kappa) and *whey* (the watery part left after the curd is removed – it contains the allergens alpha-lactalbumin and beta-lactaglobulin, which studies show as having the highest rate of positive oral challenges).

Most allergy to milk starts at a very young age, and 80 per cent of children outgrow it by the age of six.

Type of allergen: consumed, contact

Symptoms
Anaphylactic shock: rare

Eye reactions: watery or itchy eyes

Gastrointestinal reactions: abdominal pain and swelling, colitis, constipation, diarrhoea (usually very runny), heartburn, nausea, vomiting, wind

Mouth, nasal and ear reactions: ears blocked/painful, rhinitis, sneezing

Psychological problems: irritability (in children)

Respiratory reactions: asthma (particularly childhood), breathing difficulties, coughing, wheezing

Skin reactions: allergic "shiners" (black eyes), angioedema, atopic dermatitis, eczema, urticaria, allergic contact urticaria

Tests
- Blood test: CAP-RAST (including casein, cow's milk (raw and boiled), cows' whey, goat milk, sheep milk, sheep whey, a-lactalbumin, b-lactoglobulin – some experts feel that it is not particularly reliable for children)
- Skin prick test (not particularly reliable for children) – raw and pasteurized cow's milk and casein
- Blood test: ELISA – Enzyme-Linked Immunsorbent Assay. This is a food sensitivity test that measures the amount of the antibody IgG produced by your immune system in response to a specific food group to which you are sensitive. A blood sample is tested for the antibody against each food group; and any raised levels of antibody show you have a sensitivity to that food group. (including cow's milk (raw and boiled), goat's milk, a-lactalbumin, b-lactoglobulin, sheep's milk, whey, yoghurt).
- Challenge test – you avoid milk for up to 28 days, until you no longer have the symptoms of allergy; if symptoms recur when milk is reintroduced to your diet and then abate when you avoid milk again, you're likely to be allergic to cow's milk. In the case of children, your GP may advise yearly testing to see if he or she has grown out of the intolerance. Challenges should always be done under medical supervision, in case there is an anaphylactic reaction.
- Elimination diet
- Symptom diary (including peak flow meter readings)

Treatments
Avoidance
- Check labels carefully and check with a dietitian to ensure that your diet is still nutritionally sound

Prescription medication
- Anaphylactic shock: adrenaline, antihistamines, steroids
- Conjunctivitis: antihistamines, cromoglycate, nedocromil sodium, steroids, sympathomimetics
- Abdominal pain and swelling: antacids, anti-spasmodic drugs
- Colitis: aminosalicylates, immunosuppressants, steroids, sulphasalazine
- Constipation: bulking agents, stimulant laxatives, osmotic laxatives, lubricating agents
- Diarrhoea: antidiarrhoeal drugs
- Gastric upset/irritation: painkillers (use paracetamol rather than aspirin)
- Heartburn: antacids, alginates
- Nausea: antihistamines
- Vomiting: anti-emetics
- Wind: antacids
- Ear problems: sympathomimetics
- Rhinitis: antihistamines, decongestants, sodium cromoglycate, immunotherapy
- Sneezing: antihistamines, decongestants, sodium cromogylcate
- Asthma: anticholinergic drugs, antihistamines (exercise-induced), Beta2 (ß2) adrenoreceptor agonists, cromoglycate, nedocromil sodium, steroids, xanthine derivatives, zafirlukast
- Breathing problems: bronchodilators, corticosteroids
- Cough: antihistamines, bronchodilators, corticosteroids
- Wheezing: bronchodilator
- Angioedema: adrenaline, antihistamines, steroids
- Contact dermatitis: steroids, antihistamines
- Eczema: emollients, immune suppressants, steroids, UVA/UVB light treatment, wet wrapping, antihistamines
- Urticaria: antihistamines, emollients, steroids

OTC remedies
- Conjunctivitis: antihistamines
- Abdominal pain and swelling: antacids
- Constipation: as prescription medication
- Diarrhoea: kaolin and morphine, calcium carbonate, pectin
- Gastric upset/irritation: as prescription medication
- Heartburn: as prescription medication
- Nausea: antihistamines
- Vomiting: oral rehydration solution
- Wind: antacids
- Ear problems: painkillers

- Rhinitis: *decongestants*
- Cough: demulcents, antitussives, expectorants
- Angioedema: *antihistamines*
- Contact dermatitis: coal tar, *emollients*, *steroids*
- Eczema: *emollients*, hydrocortisone cream
- Urticaria: calamine lotion, witch hazel

Alternative remedies
- Conjunctivitis: herbalism, homeopathy
- Abdominal pain and swelling: aromatherapy, herbalism, homeopathy
- Colitis: herbalism
- Constipation: aromatherapy, herbalism, homeopathy
- Diarrhoea: aromatherapy, herbalism, homeopathy
- Gastric upset/irritation: aromatherapy, herbalism
- Heartburn: aromatherapy, homeopathy, herbalism
- Nausea: aromatherapy, herbalism, homeopathy
- Vomiting: herbalism
- Wind: aromatherapy, herbalism, homeopathy
- Ear problems: aromatherapy, herbalism, homeopathy
- Rhinitis: aromatherapy
- Sneezing: acupuncture
- Asthma: acupuncture (mild asthma only), Buteyko method, homeopathy, relaxation techniques, yoga
- Cough: aromatherapy, homeopathy
- Contact dermatitis: aromatherapy, Bach flower remedies, homeopathy
- Eczema: aromatherapy, evening primrose oil, relaxation, herbalism, homeopathy, Chinese herbal medicine, Bach flower remedies
- Urticaria: aromatherapy, herbalism, homeopathy

Self-help tips: check the ingredients on food package labels and ask about the ingredients in foods prepared in restaurants when you eat out – avoid anything on the following list, which may contain milk protein: ammonium, ammonium caseinate, artificial butter, butter, butter solids, calcium, calcium caseinate, caramel colour, caramel flavouring, casein, caseinate, cheese, chocolate (may contain milk solids), cream, curds, delactosed whey, demineralized whey, dried milk, dried milk solids, hydrolyzed casein, hydrolyzed milk protein, iron caseinate, lactaglobulin, lactalbumin, lactalbumin phosphate, lactate, lactic acid, lactoferrin, magnesium, magnesium caseinate, margarine, milk derivative, milk fat, milk potassium caseinate, milk protein, milk solids, rennet casein, skimmed milk, sodium caseinate, sour cream solids, whey, whey powder, whey protein concentrate, yoghurt, zinc caseinate

If milk is implicated, then all sources of milk such as butter, cheese, cottage cheese, buttermilk, chocolate, cream, sour cream, ice-cream, yoghurt, fromage frais, crème fraîche, sauces, milk puddings (e.g. rice pudding) and casein should be avoided and the diet supplemented with calcium and vitamin D; also look out for margarines.

For symptom relief, see *Conjunctivitis, Abdominal pain and swelling, Colitis, Constipation, Diarrhoea, Heartburn, Nausea, Vomiting, Wind, Ear problems, Rhinitis, Sneezing, Asthma, Breathing difficulties, Cough, Wheezing, Angioedema, Dermatitis, Eczema, Urticaria* in the section on *Symptoms*

Alternative products that might not cause a reaction

- Soy-based products or milk-free formula for children who are allergic to milk
- Milk substitutes: sheep's milk, goat's milk, soya milk, creamed coconut, rice milk
- Butter substitutes: margarines (check label), tahini, sunflower spread
- Cheese substitutes: soya-based cheese spread, tofu, humus, gjetost (Norwegian brown cheese made from milk whey)

Alternative sources of calcium, vitamin A and vitamin D to supplement your diet:
- calcium is found in green leafy vegetables, tinned fish that includes soft bones (such as sardines), almonds, sesame seeds, chickpeas, white and brown bread (brown bread is fortified with calcium in the UK, but wholemeal isn't)
- vitamin A is found in dark leafy green vegetables, orange/yellow vegetables, liver
- vitamin D is found in eggs and liver

You might also react to: sheep's or goat's milk (possibly); ragweed pollen, elm pollen, mint

Millet

Millet is a grain.

Type of allergen: contact, consumed

Symptoms, tests, treatments and self-help tips, see *Grain*

Mineral spirits

See *Solvents – aliphatic hydrocarbons*

Mink

See *Animal hair*

Minocycline

See *Antibiotics, Tetracycline, Drugs*

Mint

Mint is an aromatic herb, *Mentha piperita*.

Type of allergen: consumed

Symptoms, tests, treatments and self-help tips, see *Herbs*

You might also react to: others in the *Labiatae* family, such as marjoram, oregano, rosemary, sage, thyme; also ragweed pollen, elm pollen, aspirin, menthol, basil

Moisturizer

Perfumes and preservatives tend to cause most problems.

Type of allergen: contact

Symptoms, tests, treatments and self-help tips, see *Cosmetics*

Monopotassium glutamate
See *Food additives – flavour enhancers*

Monosodium glutamate
Monosodium glutamate is a commonly used flavour enhancer, particularly in Chinese food. A reaction to MSG is known as "Chinese restaurant syndrome" – flushing, pain in the face and back of the neck, headache, tingling/burning sensation in the skin, blurred vision, nausea, vomiting, fast heartbeat, chills and shaking.

Symptoms usually start within two hours of eating the food and resolve themselves.

See also *Food additives – flavour enhancers*

Moth proofing
See *Formaldehyde*

Mould spores (fungi)
Moulds are microscopic plant organisms from the fungus family; they produce spores to reproduce, and the spores become airborne and then grow in house dust.

Mould spores from *Alternaria* can cause asthma in the autumn. The spores of *Aspergillus fumigatus* – often found in rotting vegetation – can also cause asthma.

Mould can also be found indoors: if there is moisture in the house (relative humidity greater than 50 per cent, or leakage from water pipes) and something to grow on, such as wood or fabric. You might not necessarily see mould growing.

Moulds feed on any material containing carbon (such as paper, fabric or hair); they like moist environments and decaying material, such as in compost heaps, dustbins and cut grass.

Type of allergen: inhalant

Likely sources of mould
- Areas with poor air circulation, e.g. cellars and cupboards
- Areas where there has been flooding onto carpets and wallpaper
- Areas with leaky plumbing or poor ventilation – under sinks, washing machines, dishwashers, and in bathrooms, showers

and toilets: you may see mould as the black substance on window frames and pools of condensation, and pinky-grey slime around taps and on tiles
- Air conditioning units and humidifiers
- Garden areas – particularly piled-up leaves, compost heaps and during mowing/raking the lawn

Symptoms

Eye reactions: itchy eyes

Mouth, nasal and ear reactions: rhinitis, sinusitis, sneezing

Respiratory reactions: asthma (including occupational), hypersensitivity pneumonitis, extrinsic allergic alveolitis, breathing problems, cough, wheezing

Skin reactions: angioedema

Tests

- CAP-RAST test (*Alternaria alternata, Alternaria tenuis, Aspergillus fumigatus, Aspergillus niger, Aureobasidium pullulans, Botrytis cinerea, Candida albicans, Cephalosporium acremonium, Chaetomium globosum, Cladosporium herbarum, Curvularia lunata, Epicoccum purpurascens, Fusarium moniliforme, Helminthosporium halodes, Micropolyspora faeni, Mucor racemosus, Penicillium notatum, Phoma betae, Pityrosporum orbiculare, Rhizopus nigricans, Stemphylium botryosum, Trichoderma viride, Trichophyton rubrum*)
- Blood test: ELISA (*Aspergillus amstelodami, Aspergillus clavatus, Aspergillus flavus, Aspergillus fumigatus, Aspergillus nidulans, Aspergillus niger, Aspergillus oryzae, Aspergillus terreus, Aspergillus versicolor, Aspergillus repens, Alternaria tenuis, Aureobasidium pullulans, Botrytis cinerea, Candida albicans, Cephalosporium acremonium, Chaetomium globosum, Cladosporium cladospor, Cladosporium fulvum, Cladosporium herbarum, Curvularia lunata, Curvularia spicifera, epicoccum purpurascens, Fusarium culmorum, Fusarium moniliforme, Fusarium oxysporum, Helminthosporium halodes, Helminthosporium spp, Micropolyspora faeni, Microspora canis, Mucor mucedo, Mucor racemosus, Mucor spinosus, Neurospora sitophila, Paecilomyces spp, Penicillium brevicompactum, Penicillium citrinum, Penicillium commune, Penicillium expansum, Penicillium notatum, Penicillium roqueforti, Penicillium viridicatum, Phoma*

betae, Pullularia pullans, Rhizopus nigricans, Saccharomyces carlsbergensis, Saccharomycescerevisiae, Serpula lacrymans, Sporobolomyces roseus, Stemphylium botryosum, Thermopolyspora, trichoderma viridae, Trichophyton mentagrophytae, Trichophyton rubrum, Urichophyton verrucosum, Ustilago tritici)

- Skin prick test (*Alternaria alternata, Alternaria tenuis, Aspergillus fumigatus, Aspergillus niger, Aureobasidium pullulans, Botrytis cinerea, Candida albicans, Chaetomium globosum, Cladosporium cladosporioides, Cladosporium herbarum, Curvularia lunata, Fusarium culmorum, Fusarium moniliforme, Fusarium roseum, Helminthosporium halodes, Merulius lacrymans, Mucor mucedo, Mucor racemosus, Neurospora sitophila, Penicillium brevicompactum, Penicillium commune, Penicillium notatum, Phoma betae, Pullularia pullulans, Rhizopus nigricans, Saccharomyces carlsbergensis, Saccharomyces cerevisiae, Saccharomyces mellis, Serpula lachrymans, Trichopyton rubrum, Stemphylium botryosum, Trichophyton mentagrophytes, Ustilago tritici)*
- Intradermal – (*Alternaria tenuis, Aspergillus fumigatus, Botrytis cinerea, Candida albicans, Chaetomium globosum, Cladosporium herbarum, Curvularia lunata, Fusarium moniliforme, Helminthosporium halodes, Microsporium canis, Mucor mucedo, Neurospora sitophila, Penicillium notatum, Phoma betae, Pullularia pullulans, Rhizopus nigricans, Saccharomyces cerevisiae, Serpula lacrymans, Sporothrix schenckii, Trichophyton mentagrophytes, Ustilago tritici)*
- Inhalation challenge (*Alternaria alternata, Aspergillus fumigatus, Cladosporium cladosporioides, Penicillium notatum*)
- Symptom diary (including peak flow meter readings)

Treatments
Avoidance
- In occupational situations, use protective equipment such as gloves and masks. Improved ventilation may also help.

Prescription medication
- Conjunctivitis: antihistamines, cromoglycate, nedocromil sodium, steroids, sympathomimetics
- Rhinitis: antihistamines, decongestants, sodium cromoglycate, immunotherapy
- Sneezing: antihistamines, decongestants, sodium cromogylcate
- Asthma: anticholinergic drugs, antihistamines (exercise-induced), Beta2 (ß2) adrenoreceptor agonists, cromoglycate,

nedocromil sodium, steroids, xanthine derivatives, zafirlukast
- Breathing problems: bronchodilators, corticosteroids
- Cough: antihistamines, bronchodilators, corticosteroids
- Wheezing: bronchodilator
- Angioedema: adrenaline, antihistamines, steroids

OTC remedies
- Conjunctivitis: antihistamines
- Rhinitis: decongestants
- Cough: demulcents, antitussives, expectorants
- Angioedema: antihistamines

Alternative remedies
- Conjunctivitis: herbalism, homeopathy
- Rhinitis: aromatherapy
- Sneezing: acupuncture
- Asthma: acupuncture (mild asthma only), Buteyko method, homeopathy, relaxation techniques, yoga
- Cough: aromatherapy, homeopathy

Self-help tips
- Reduce moisture in the house
- Sort out any rising damp – have cracks in the walls fixed and a damp-proof course installed, if needed
- Use silica gel crystals (available in hardware shops) to sort out damp cupboards
- Use an extractor fan in the kitchen and bathroom
- Dry clothes outside and make sure any clothes dryers are ventilated
- Dry damp towels as quickly as possible
- Use showers rather than baths – they produce less steam
- Replace vinyl wallpaper with emulsion paint (vinyl wallpaper keeps moisture on the surface of the paper and encourages mould growth)
- Mop up condensation daily from windows, windowsills and work surfaces
- Ventilate the house, especially if it's a new house or you've had major renovations (drying plaster causes a lot of moisture in the air)
- Keep plugs in sinks, basins and bath plugholes to stop mould spores wafting up
- Reduce mould growth

- Clean rubber seals around fridges and freezers, removing black mould
- Clean mould from windows, bathrooms and kitchens with white spirit, bleach (if you are not sensitive to chlorine) or anti-mould sprays – don't brush with a dry cloth or you'll spread the spores around
- Replace shower curtains regularly
- reduce the number of house plants and regularly replace the top level layer of soil where moulds grow
- Avoid pot pourri
- Moulds dislike relative humidity of less than 65 per cent – having the temperature indoors at roughly 5 degrees higher than outdoors should do this
- Most moulds don't like alkaline environment – wash kitchen work tops, fridges and freezers with a solution of sodium bicarbonate (1 dessertspoon to a bowl of warm water)
- Avoid outdoor moulds
- Avoid piled-up leaves, compost heaps and rotting vegetation
- Ask someone else to mow/rake the lawn
- Avoid barns, stored grain and stacked hay, particularly around harvest time
- Avoid indoor areas where mould concentrations are likely to be high – launderettes, swimming pools, greenhouses, hot kitchens, bathrooms

For symptom relief, see *Conjunctivitis, Rhinitis, Sneezing, Asthma, Breathing difficulties, Cough, Wheezing, Angioedema* in the section on *Symptoms*

You might also react to: foods containing yeast; fungi; antibiotics (based on penicillium or cephalosporium)

Mouthwash

Perfumes and preservatives tend to cause most problems.

Type of allergen: contact

Symptoms, tests, treatments and self-help tips, see *Cosmetics*

Muesli
See *Wheat*

Mushrooms

The common mushroom *Agaricus bisporus* contains benzyl alcohol.

Type of allergen: contact, consumed

Symptoms, tests, treatments and self-help tips, see *Vegetables*
See also *Mould spores, Yeast*

Mushroom compost

Mushroom compost can cause occupational asthma. If symptoms start soon after beginning work and improve at weekends or on holidays, occupational asthma should be suspected.

Type of allergen: inhalant

Symptoms
Respiratory reactions: asthma (occupational)

Tests
• Symptom diary (including peak flow meter readings)

Treatments
Avoidance: in occupational situations, use protective equipment such as gloves and masks. Improved ventilation may also help.

Prescription medication: anticholinergic drugs, antihistamines (exercise-induced), Beta2 (ß2) adrenoreceptor agonists, cromoglycate, nedocromil sodium, steroids, xanthine derivatives, zafirlukast

Alternative remedies: acupuncture (mild asthma only), Buteyko method, homeopathy, relaxation techniques, yoga

Self-help tips: for symptom relief see *Asthma* in the section on *Symptoms*

Mussels
See *Shellfish*

Mustard
Mustard is from the brassica family: white mustard is *Brassica alba*, black mustard is *Brassica nigra*, and wild mustard is *Brassica sinapistrum*.

Type of allergen: inhalant, contact, consumed

Symptoms, tests, treatments and self-help tips, see *Spices*
See also *Curry powder*

You might also react to: cabbage, broccoli, brussel sprouts, cauliflower, horseradish, radish, swede, turnip, watercress

Mutton
See *Lamb, Meat*

Nail varnish
Perfumes and preservatives tend to cause most problems.

Type of allergen: contact

Symptoms, tests, treatments and self-help tips, see *Cosmetics*
See also *Acetate, Acrylate, Formaldehyde, Isocyanates, Phthalic acid, Solvents – esters, Solvents – ketone solvents, Toluenesulphonamide-Formaldehyde resin*

Nail varnish remover
See *Bitter almond oil, Solvents – esters*

Nappies (disposable)
See *Chlorine*

Natamycin

See *Food additives – preservatives; Antibiotics*
Natamycin is a macrolide antibiotic, used for fungal infections.

Nectarines

Nectarines are smooth-skinned varieties of peach. They contain
salicylates, which have been linked to hyperactivity in children

Type of allergen: consumed

Symptoms, tests, treatments and self-help tips, see
Fruit

Needles

See *Nickel, Metals*

Neomycin

Neomycin is an antibiotic produced from *Streptomyces*. Around
1 per cent of people will react with a swollen red rash.

Type of allergen: contact

Likely sources of neomycin: deodorants, creams

Symptoms, tests, treatments and self-help tips, see
Drugs

You might also react to: gentamycin
See also *Antibiotics*

Netilmycin

Netilmycin is an antibiotic of the aminoglycoside group, and is
used against pathogens such as *E Coli* and *Staphylococcus*.

Type of allergen: injected

You might also react to: *gentamycin*
See also *Antibiotics*

Nettles
See *Plants*

Newsprint
The ink used in printing newspapers can cause problems.

Type of allergen: inhalant

Symptoms
Eye reactions: conjunctivitis

Tests
• Symptom diary

Treatments
Avoidance

Prescription medication: antihistamines, cromoglycate, nedo-cromil sodium, steroids, sympathomimetics

OTC remedies: antihistamines

Alternative remedies: herbalism, homeopathy

Self-help tips: for symptom relief see *Conjunctivitis* in the section on *Symptoms*
See also *Inks*

Nickel
Nickel is a silver-white metal, chemical symbol Ni. It is often accompanied by cobalt and is used for plating iron and brass.

Allergy to nickel affects around 14 per cent of the population; it tends to affect more women than men, and can start at any age. Sweat, humidity and high temperatures can also worsen skin reactions as sweat leaches nickel from metallic objects.

Nickel salts can cause occupational asthma for electroplaters. If symptoms start soon after beginning work and improve at weekends or on holidays, occupational asthma should be suspected.

Type of allergen: inhalant, contact

Likely sources of nickel: alloys, cigarette lighters, coins, cosmetics (particularly eye cosmetics), cupboard handles and doorknobs, clasps and studs on clothing, spectacle frames and handbag catches, dyes, glue, hair dyes (nickel sulphate), jewellery, keys and key rings, kitchen utensils and tools, needles, pins, thimbles and scissors, nickel plating (nickel sulphate), paper clips and pens, pocket knives, razors, scissors, stainless steel wire

For symptoms, tests and treatments, see *Metals*

Self-help tips
- If you react to your keys, coat them with several layers of clear nail polish.
- Cover large objects with plastic (e.g. scissors and metal tools)
- Wear gloves when handling metal devices

You might also react to: chromium, cobalt

Alternative products that won't cause a reaction: 18-carat gold, silver, platinum, stainless steel, plastic (e.g. for handles of scissors)

Nitrocellulose
See *Solvents (aromatic hydrocarbons)*

Nitrofurantoin
Nitrofurantoin is an antibiotic used to treat urinary tract infections.

Type of allergen: consumed

Symptoms, tests, treatments and self-help tips, see *Drugs*

Nitrogen dioxide
Nitrogen dioxide (NO_2) is an environmental pollutant which is formed when fuel is burned at high temperatures. It produces inflammation in the airways.

Type of allergen: inhalant

Likely sources of nitrogen dioxide: emissions from vehicles and fuel combustion.

Symptoms, tests, treatments and self-help tips, see *Environmental pollutants*

Nonane
See *Solvents (aliphatic hydrocarbons)*

Nutmeg
Nutmeg is a spice from the fruit of the tree *Myristica fragrans*. Large quantities can cause psychosis (caused by the chemical myristicin, which is structurally similar to mescaline).

Type of allergen: contact

For symptoms, treatments and self-help tips, see *Spices*

Nuts
Nuts are a common allergen and one of the foods that is most likely to cause anaphylactic shock. Nuts are generally distinguished between tree nuts – that is, those grown on trees such as almonds and walnuts – and ground nuts (peanuts).

Likely sources of nuts: sweets, chocolates, nougat, marzipan, praline, bakery products (biscuits and cakes), stuffing mixes, gluten-free bread (ground almonds)

For further information about the nuts themselves and cross-reactivity see *Almond, Brazil nut, Cashew nut, Chestnut, Coconut, Hazelnut, Macadamia, Peanuts, Pecan, Pine nut, Pistachio, Walnut*

Symptoms
Anaphylactic shock
- Almond, Brazil nut, cashew nut, coconut, peanut, pecan, walnut
- Exercise-induced – hazelnut, walnut

Gastrointestinal reactions
- Diarrhoea – Brazil nut
- Vomiting – Brazil nut

Headache
* Migraine – hazelnut

Mouth, nasal and ear reactions
* Itching mouth/palate – coconut
* Rhinitis – hazelnut

Psychological problems
* Hyperactivity – almond

· Respiratory reactions
* Asthma – almond, hazelnut, walnut
* Breathing problems – cashew nut

· Skin reactions
* Angioedema – cashew nut
* Contact dermatitis (including occupational) – almond, cashew nuts, macadamia, pistachio, walnut
* Allergic contact urticaria
* Skin irritation – chestnut, coconut
* Urticaria – cashew nuts, coconut, pine nut

Tests
* Blood test: CAP-RAST (almond, brazil nut, cashew, chestnut, coconut, hazelnut, peanut, pecan, pine nut, pistachio, walnut)
* Blood test: ELISA (almond, brazil nut, cashew, chestnut, cocoa, coconut (including desiccated), hazelnut, peanut, pecan, pine nut, pistachio, walnut)
* Skin prick test (almond, brazil nut, hazelnut, peanut, walnut)
* Intradermal – brazil nut, hazelnut, peanut, walnut
* Symptom diary (including peak flow meter readings)

Treatments
Avoidance
* Check labels carefully for specific nut names and "nut meats"; check with a dietitian
* In an occupational situation, use protective equipment such as gloves

Prescription medication
* Anaphylactic shock: adrenaline, antihistamines, steroids
* Diarrhoea: antidiarrhoeal drugs
* Vomiting: anti-emetics

- Migraine: painkillers, anti-sickness drugs, ergotamine, 5-HT agonists, beta-blockers, sodium valproate, sumatryptan
- Rhinitis: antihistamines, decongestants, sodium cromoglycate, immunotherapy
- Hyperactivity: stimulant drugs
- Asthma: anticholinergic drugs, antihistamines (exercise-induced), Beta2 (ß2) adrenoreceptor agonists, cromoglycate, nedocromil sodium, steroids, xanthine derivatives, zafirlukast
- Breathing problems: bronchodilators, corticosteroids
- Angioedema: adrenaline, antihistamines, steroids
- Contact dermatitis: steroids, antihistamines
- Skin irritation: emollients
- Urticaria: antihistamines, emollients, steroids

OTC remedies
- Diarrhoea: kaolin and morphine, calcium carbonate, pectin
- Nausea: antihistamines
- Migraine: aspirin, ibuprofen, paracetamol
- Rhinitis: decongestants
- Angioedema: antihistamines
- Contact dermatitis: coal tar, emollients, steroids
- Skin irritation: emollients
- Urticaria: calamine lotion, witch hazel

Alternative remedies
- Diarrhoea: aromatherapy, herbalism, homeopathy
- Vomiting: herbalism
- Migraine: acupuncture, Alexander technique, aromatherapy, chiropractic, herbalism, homeopathy, hypnosis, osteopathy, reflexology
- Rhinitis: aromatherapy
- Hyperactivity: herbalism
- Asthma: acupuncture (mild asthma only), Buteyko method, homeopathy, relaxation techniques, yoga
- Contact dermatitis: aromatherapy, Bach flower remedies, homeopathy
- Urticaria: aromatherapy, herbalism, homeopathy

For symptom relief, see *Diarrhoea, Vomiting, Migraine, Itching mouth/palate, Rhinitis, Hyperactivity, Asthma, Breathing problems, Angioedema, Contact dermatitis, Skin irritation, Urticaria* in the section on *Symptoms*

You might also react to: others within the same family of nuts, i.e.
- brazil nuts
- cashews, pistachios (related to mango)
- Macadamia nuts
- walnuts, hickory nuts, pecans
- almonds (related to apricots, cherries, nectarines, peaches, plums)
- hazelnuts

Nylon

Nylon is an artifical fibre made from amide groups, used in textiles, plastics and cosmetics.

Type of allergen: contact

Likely sources of nylon: Contact lenses, cosmetics, filters, textiles

Symptoms
Skin reactions: contact dermatitis

Tests: Symptom diary

Treatments
Avoidance

Prescription medication: steroids, antihistamines

OTC remedies: coal tar, emollients, steroids

Alternative remedies: aromatherapy, Bach flower remedies, homeopathy

Self-help tips: for symptom relief see *Contact dermatitis* in the section on *Symptoms*
See also *Phenol*

Nystatin
See *Antibiotics, Antifungal drugs*

Oak moss
See *Perfumes*

Oats

Oat is the cereal plant *Avena sativa*. The problem with oats is mainly in the gliadin (protein fraction). Oats can also cause asthma in farm workers and bakers. If symptoms start soon after beginning work and improve at weekends or on holidays, occupational asthma should be suspected.

Type of allergen: inhalant, contact, consumed

Likely sources of oats: porridge, bakery goods

Symptoms, tests, treatments and self-help tips, see *Grain*

Octane
See *Solvents – aliphatic hydrocarbons*

Octopamine

Octopamine is a biogenic amine derived from the amino acid tyrosine.

Type of allergen: consumed

Likely sources of octopamine: dairy foods, eggs, fruit juice, salmon, spinach, processed meats, nuts, oranges, plums, tomatoes

Symptoms
Headaches: migraine

Psychological problems: fatigue, mood swings

Skin reactions: flushing

Tests
• Symptom diary

Treatments
Avoidance
* Check labels carefully; check with a dietitian to ensure that your diet is still balanced

Prescription medication
* Migraine: painkillers, anti-sickness drugs, ergotamine, 5-HT agonists, beta-blockers, sodium valproate, sumatryptan

OTC remedies
* Migraine: aspirin, ibuprofen, paracetamol

Alternative remedies
* Migraine: acupuncture, Alexander technique, aromatherapy, chiropractic, herbalism, homeopathy, hypnosis, osteopathy, reflexology
* Fatigue: aromatherapy, Bach flower remedies, homeopathy

Self-help tips: for symptom relief see *Migraine, Fatigue, Flushing* in the section on *Symptoms*

Octopus
See *Fish*

Octyl gallate
See *Food additives – antioxidants*

Oils, cosmetic
For further information about the oils themselves and cross-reactivity see *Balsam of peru, Bitter almond oil, Caraway, Cassia oil, Cedarwood oil, Cinnamon bark, Citronella oil, Coconut oil, Coriander oil, Geranium oil, Lavender oil, Patchouli oil, Petitgrain oil*

Symptoms
Eye reactions
* Conjunctivitis – balsam of Peru

Mouth, nasal and ear reactions
- Hay fever – citronella oil
- Rhinitis – balsam of Peru, bitter almond oil, cassia oil, citronella oil

Respiratory reactions
- Asthma – citronella oil

Skin reactions
- Contact dermatitis – balsam of Peru, bitter almond oil, caraway oil, cassia oil, citronella oil, coconut oil, coriander oil, geranium oil, patchouli oil, petitgrain oil
- Photoallergenic contact dermatitis – cedarwood oil, cinnamon bark, lavender oil, petitgrain oil
- Skin irritation – balsam of Peru
- Contact urticaria – balsam of Peru

Tests
- Blood test: CAP-RAST (balsam of Peru, coconut oil)
- Skin test: skin patch (balsam of Peru, caraway oil, cassia oil, citronella oil, coconut oil, coriander oil, patchouli oil, petitgrain oil)
- Skin test: skin prick (coriander oil)
- Skin test: photopatch test (cedarwood oil, cinnamon bark, lavender oil, petitgrain oil)
- Symptom diary (including peak flow meter readings)

Treatments
Avoidance
- Check labels carefully; in occupational situations, use protective equipment such as gloves and masks

Prescription medication
- Conjunctivitis: antihistamines, cromoglycate, nedocromil sodium, steroids, sympathomimetics
- Hay fever: antihistamines, cromoglycate, decongestants, nedocromil sodium, steroids, sympathomimetics
- Rhinitis: antihistamines, decongestants, sodium cromoglycate, immunotherapy
- Asthma: anticholinergic drugs, antihistamines (exercise-induced), Beta2 (ß2) adrenoreceptor agonists, cromoglycate, nedocromil sodium, steroids, xanthine derivatives, zafirlukast

- Contact dermatitis: steroids, antihistamines
- Photoallergenic Contact dermatitis: emollients, steroids
- Skin irritation: emollients
- Urticaria: antihistamines, emollients, steroids

OTC remedies
- Conjunctivitis: antihistamines
- Hay fever: antihistamines, decongestants
- Rhinitis: decongestants
- Contact dermatitis: coal tar, emollients, steroids
- Skin irritation: emollients
- Urticaria: calamine lotion, witch hazel

Alternative remedies
- Conjunctivitis: herbalism, homeopathy
- Hay fever: aromatherapy, herbalism, homeopathy
- Asthma: acupuncture (mild asthma only), Buteyko method, homeopathy, relaxation techniques, yoga
- Dermatitis: aromatherapy, Bach flower remedies, homeopathy
- Urticaria: aromatherapy, herbalism, homeopathy

Self-help tips: for symptom relief see *Conjunctivitis, Hay fever, Rhinitis, Asthma, Contact dermatitis, Photoallergenic contact dermatitis, Skin irritation, Urticaria* in the section on *Symptoms*

Oil paints
See *Balsam of Peru*

Oil solvent
See *Solvents (chlorinated hydrocarbons)*

Olive
Olive is the fruit of the tree *Olea europaea*.

Type of allergen: contact, consumed

Symptoms, tests, treatments and self-help tips, see *Fruit*

Onion

Onions are the vegetable *Allium cepa*. They are from the same family as shallots, *Allium ascalonicum*.

Onions are one of the most common causes of occupational contact dermatitis.

Type of allergen: contact, consumed

Symptoms, tests, treatments and self-help tips, see *Vegetables*

You might also react to: asparagus, chives, garlic, leek, shallot

Orange

Orange is the fruit of the tree *Citrus aurantium*. It is a common allergenic food in China. It contains tyramine; it also contains *salicylates*, which have been linked to hyperactivity in children.

Type of allergen: contact, consumed

Symptoms, tests, treatments and self-help tips, see *Fruit*
See also *Citrus fruit*

Oregano

Oregano is the herb *Origanum vulgare*. It contains *salicylates*, which have been linked to hyperactivity in children.

Type of allergen: contact, consumed

Symptoms, tests, treatments and self-help tips, see *Herbs*

You might also react to: others in the *Labiatae* family, such as marjoram, mint, rosemary, sage, thyme

Oxytetracycline
See *Antibiotics, Tetracycline, Drugs*

Oyster
See *Shellfish*

Ozone

Ozone is a form of oxygen, also known as O_3. It is colourless or light blue and has an "electrical" smell. It is an environmental pollutant which results from the action of sunlight on hydrocarbons and nitrogen oxide emitted in fuel combustion, so it is more in evidence on warm, sunny days. It produces inflammation in the airways.

Type of allergen: inhalant

Likely sources of ozone: as well as environmental pollution, ozone is generated from air cleaners and photocopying machines

Symptoms, tests, treatments and self-help tips, see *Environmental pollutants*

Paint

The chemical *toluene diisocynate*, used in paint, is the commonest cause of occupational asthma. If symptoms start soon after beginning work and improve at weekends or on holidays, occupational asthma should be suspected.

Paint also contains *benzene* and *phenols*.

Water-based paints contain glycol, glycol ethers, alcohols, and possibly formaldehyde-generating preservatives, amines, volatile plasticizers and free monomers.

Interior and exterior latex or emulsion-based coatings contain glycols (such as ethylene glycol and propylene glycol) which are very slow to evaporate.

Solvent-based paints contain aliphatic and aromatic hydrocarbons, ketoximes, alcohols, free monomers and volatile plasticizers.

General purpose solvent-based paints primarily use the aliphatic hydrocarbons and paraffin naptha as the volatile phase.

Fast-dry paints generally contain faster evaporating solvents such as the aromatic hydrocarbons, (toluene, xylene), ketones, (acetone (C_3H_6O), methyl ethyl ketone), alcohols, (butanol, ethanol) and ester (n-propyl acetate, butyl acetate) solvents.

Type of allergen: inhalant, contact

Symptoms
Respiratory reactions: occupational asthma

Skin reactions: irritant dermatitis

Tests
- Skin patch
- Symptom diary (including peak flow meter readings)

Treatments
Avoidance
- In occupational situations, use protective equipment such as gloves and masks. Improved ventilation may also help.

Prescription medication
- Asthma: anticholinergic drugs, antihistamines (exercise-induced), Beta2 (ß2) adrenoreceptor agonists, cromoglycate, nedocromil sodium, steroids, xanthine derivatives, zafirlukast
- Dermatitis: steroids, antihistamines

OTC remedies
- Dermatitis: coal tar, emollients, steroids

Alternative remedies
- Asthma: acupuncture (mild asthma only), Buteyko method, homeopathy, relaxation techniques, yoga
- Dermatitis: aromatherapy, Bach flower remedies, homeopathy

Self-help tips: for symptom relief see *Asthma, Contact dermatitis* in the section on *Symptoms*
See also *Chlorocresol (preservative), Chromate, Chromium, Cobalt, Colophony, Ethylene diamine, Formaldehyde, Isocyanates, Linseed oil, Phenol, Polyurethane, Potassium dichromate, PVC, Solvents – glycols, thiurams, Volatile organic compounds*

Paint remover/stripper
Paint removers tend to be based on methylene chloride with a blend of *toluene*, wax and some alcohol. Newer forms of non-chloride based products include pine-oil/surfactant blends and phenol-based surfactants, which take longer to dissolve the paint.

Type of allergen: inhalant, contact

See *Amyl alcohol, Chloroform, Isocyanates, Phenol, Solvents – alcohol solvents; Solvents – aromatic hydrocarbons, Solvents – chlorinated hydrocarbons, Solvents – halogenated solvents*

Paint thinner
Type of allergen: contact

Symptoms
Skin reactions: irritant dermatitis
Tests
* Patch test
* Symptom diary

Treatments
Avoidance: in occupational situations, use protective equipment such as gloves.

Prescription medication: steroids, antihistamines

OTC remedies: coal tar, emollients, steroids

Alternative remedies: aromatherapy, Bach flower remedies, homeopathy

Self-help tips: for symptom relief see *Contact dermatitis* in the section on *Symptoms*

See *Chloroform, Isocyanates, Solvents – aliphatic hydrocarbons; Solvents – aliphatic hydrocarbons, Turpentine*

Palladium
Palladium is a white metallic element, symbol Pd.

Type of allergen: contact

Likely sources of palladium: jewellery

Symptoms, tests, treatments and self-help tips, see *Metals*

Pancakes
See *Wheat*

Papain

This is an enzyme that breaks down proteins; it is derived from the papaya fruit (*Carica papaya*) and is used as a meat tenderizer. It can be used to treat herniated lumbar discs instead of surgery; patients are given a skin-test for sensitivity before treatment.

Type of allergen: inhalant, contact, consumed

Symptoms, tests, treatments and self-help tips, see *Enzymes*

Papaya

Papaya or pawpaw is the fruit of the tree *Carica papaya*. The main allergens are *papain* (found in the leaves, stem and fruit) and butanoic acid in the fruit.

Type of allergen: consumed, contact

Symptoms, tests, treatments and self-help tips, see *Fruit*

Paper
See *Chlorine, Cobalt, Colophony, Formaldehyde, mould*

Paper clips
See *Nickel*

Paprika

Paprika is the spice *Capsicum anuum*. It contains *salicylates*, which have been linked to hyperactivity in children

Type of allergen: inhalant, contact, consumed

Symptoms, tests, treatments and self-help tips, see *spices*

You might also react to: other vegetables/plants in the night-shade family such as aubergine, cayenne, chilli, peppers (capsicum), potato, tobacco, tomato

Para-aminobenzoic acid (PABA)

This is a B-complex vitamin used in sunscreen products.

Type of allergen: contact

Symptoms
Skin reactions: photoallergenic contact dermatitis

Tests
- Photopatch testing: the allergen is placed on two skin sites; one is exposed to sunlight after 48 hours, and then both areas are examined for a rash.
- Symptom diary

Treatments
Prescription medication: emollients, steroids

Self-help tips: for symptom relief see *Photoallergenic contact dermatitis* in the section on *Symptoms*

Parabens

Parabens is a chemical derivative of phenol; it includes butyl-paraben, methylparaben and propylparaben, used as a preservative.

Type of allergen: contact

Likely sources of parabens: cosmetics, topical creams, ointments and lotions

Symptoms
Skin reactions: contact dermatitis

Tests
- Skin patch test
- Symptom diary

Treatments

Avoidance: in occupational situations, use protective equipment such as gloves.

Prescription medication: steroids, antihistamines

OTC remedies: coal tar, emollients, steroids

Alternative remedies: aromatherapy, Bach flower remedies, homeopathy

Self-help tips: for symptom relief see *Contact dermatitis* in the section on *Symptoms*

Paracetamol

Paracetamol is a non-narcotic painkiller.

Type of allergen: consumed

Likely sources of paracetamol: dye production and photographic chemicals

Symptoms, tests, treatments and self-help tips, see *Drugs*

Paraphenylenediamine (PPDA)

PPDA is a dark dye used extensively in permanent hair dyes.

Type of allergen: contact

Likely sources of PPDA: dark-coloured cosmetics, black rubber, photocopying and printing inks, oils, greases and gasoline, textile or fur dyes, photographic developer and lithography plates, elastic, shoes

Symptoms

Skin reactions: contact dermatitis

Tests

- Skin patch test
- Symptom diary

Treatments

Avoidance: in occupational situations, use protective equipment such as vinyl or latex gloves. Avoid products containing: paraphenylenediamine (PPDA); 1,4-Benzenediamine; 1,4-Penylenediamine; Para-aminoaniline (p-aminoaniline); Paradiaminobenzene (p-diaminobenzene)

Prescription medication: steroids, antihistamines

OTC remedies: coal tar, emollients, steroids

Alternative remedies: aromatherapy, Bach flower remedies, homeopathy

Self-help tips: for symptom relief see *Contact dermatitis* in the section on *Symptoms*

Alternative products that won't cause a reaction: henna hair dyes; vegetable-based dyes

You might also react to: sunscreens or creams that contain PABA (para-aminobenzoic acid or p-aminobenzoic acid); products containing benzocaine; PABA-based sunscreens or creams; other dye chemicals; semipermanent hair dyes; para-aminosalicylic acid (p-aminosalicylic acid); black rubber products; diaminodiphenylmethane (epoxy hardener); Para-toluenediamine (p-toluenediamine); Para-aminodiphenylamine (p-amino-diphenylamine); 2,4-Diaminoanisole; ortho-amino-phenol (o-aminophenol); benzocaine; Procaine; Sulphonamide drugs; Azo dyes (mainly textile)

Parrot

See *Animal protein, Feathers*

Parsley

Parsley is the herb *Carum Petroselinum*.

Type of allergen: contact, consumed

Symptoms, tests, treatments and self-help tips, see *Herbs*

You might also react to: others in the *Umbelliferae* family, such as aniseed, caraway, carrot, celery, celeriac, cumin, coriander, dill, fennel, parsnip

Parsnip

Parsnip is the root vegetable *Pastinaca sativa*.

Type of allergen: contact, consumed

Symptoms, tests, treatments and self-help tips, see *Vegetables*

You might also react to: others in the *Umbelliferae* family, such as aniseed, caraway, carrot, celery, celeriac, cumin, coriander, dill, fennel, parsley

Passion fruit

Passion fruit is the fruit of the tree *Passiflora edulis*. It contains *salicylates* which have been linked to hyperactivity in children.

Type of allergen: consumed

Symptoms, tests, treatments and self-help tips, see *Fruit*

Pasta
See *Wheat*

Pastry
See *Wheat*

Patchouli oil

An essential oil derived from the leaves of a shrub, *Pogostemon cablin*

Type of allergen: contact

Likely sources of patchouli oil: cosmetics and soaps

Symptoms, tests, treatments and self-help tips, see *Oils, cosmetic*

Patent blue

See *Food additives – colourings*

Pea

Peas are the vegetable *Pisum sativum*. They contain *salicylates*, which have been linked to hyperactivity in children. Immature peas contain fewer albumin proteins, so they are less likely to cause a problem.

Type of allergen: consumed

Symptoms, tests, treatments and self-help tips, see *Vegetables*

You might also react to: beans, chick peas, lentil, liquorice, peanut, senna, soy

Peach

The peach is the fruit of the tree *Prunus persica*. It contains *salicylates*, which have been linked to hyperactivity in children. The allergen may be in the peel; you may react to canned fruit as well as fresh.

Type of allergen: consumed

Symptoms, tests, treatments and self-help tips, see *Fruit*

You might also react to: birch pollen, mugwort or grass; almonds, apricots, cherries, plum

Peanuts

Peanut is one of the "big eight" food allergens and can cause anaphylaxis; if you have asthma and are allergic to peanuts, you need to be particularly careful. If you have a food allergy to peanuts, you may also have a reaction from touching peanuts or even kissing someone who has eaten peanuts. It tends to be a lifelong allergy.

The protein in peanuts is a known food allergen; unless specially prepared, peanut oil also contains the peanut allergens.

The allergens are heat-stable so they are found in roasted nuts as well as raw.

Peanuts also contain oxalates, a derivative of oxalic acid.

As well as food use – in prepared foods, and as a carrier for fat-soluble vitamins and colouring – peanut oil is used in skin care products.

Type of allergen: consumed, contact

Likely sources of peanuts: soups, Chinese foods, marzipan, confectionery, ice cream, desserts; it is also used as a bulking agent in many processed foods; and is an ingredient in soaps, shaving creams and shampoos

Symptoms
Anaphylactic shock

Eye reactions: allergic conjunctivitis

Gastrointestinal reactions: abdominal pain and swelling, diarrhoea, nausea, vomiting

Mouth, nasal and ear reactions: rhinitis

Respiratory reactions: asthma, wheezing

Skin reactions: angioedema, contact dermatitis, eczema, itching, urticaria

Tests
- Blood test: CAP-RAST
- Blood test: ELISA
- Elimination diet
- Food challenge
- Symptom diary (including peak flow meter readings)

Treatments
Avoidance
- Check the ingredients on food package labels and ask about the ingredients in foods prepared in restaurants when you eat out – avoid anything on the following list: peanut, nut meats, arachis oil, arachis hypogaea (peanut oil), groundnuts, groundnut oil, lecithin, mixed nuts

- Check with a dietitian to ensure that your diet is still nutritionally sound

Prescription medication
- Anaphylactic shock: adrenaline, antihistamines, steroids
- Conjunctivitis: antihistamines, cromoglycate, nedocromil sodium, steroids, sympathomimetics
- Abdominal pain and swelling: antacids, anti-spasmodic drugs
- Diarrhoea: antidiarrhoeal drugs
- Nausea: antihistamines
- Vomiting: anti-emetics
- Rhinitis: antihistamines, decongestants, sodium cromoglycate, immunotherapy
- Asthma: anticholinergic drugs, antihistamines (exercise-induced), Beta2 (ß2) adrenoreceptor agonists, cromoglycate, nedocromil sodium, steroids, xanthine derivatives, zafirlukast
- Wheezing: bronchodilator
- Angioedema: adrenaline, antihistamines, steroids
- Contact dermatitis: steroids, antihistamines
- Eczema: emollients, immune suppressants, steroids, UVA/UVB light treatment, wet wrapping, antihistamines
- Itching: antihistamines, emollients
- Urticaria: antihistamines, emollients, steroids

OTC remedies
- Conjunctivitis: antihistamines
- Abdominal pain and swelling: antacids
- Diarrhoea: kaolin and morphine, calcium carbonate, pectin
- Nausea: antihistamines
- Vomiting: oral rehydration solution
- Rhinitis: decongestants
- Angioedema: antihistamines
- Contact dermatitis: coal tar, emollients, steroids
- Eczema: emollients, hydrocortisone cream
- Itching: antihistamines, emollients
- Urticaria: calamine lotion, witch hazel

Alternative remedies
- Conjunctivitis: herbalism, homeopathy
- Abdominal pain and swelling: aromatherapy, herbalism, homeopathy
- Diarrhoea: aromatherapy, herbalism, homeopathy
- Nausea: aromatherapy, herbalism, homeopathy

- Vomiting: herbalism
- Rhinitis: aromatherapy
- Asthma: acupuncture (mild asthma only), Buteyko method, homeopathy, relaxation techniques, yoga
- Contact dermatitis: aromatherapy, Bach flower remedies, homeopathy
- Eczema: aromatherapy, evening primrose oil, relaxation, herbalism, homeopathy, Chinese herbal medicine, Bach flower remedies
- Itching: aromatherapy, herbalism
- Urticaria: aromatherapy, herbalism, homeopathy

Self-help tips: for symptom relief see *Conjunctivitis, Abdominal pain and swelling, Diarrhoea, Nausea, Vomiting, Rhinitis, Asthma, Wheezing, Angioedema, Contact dermatitis, Eczema, Itching, Urticaria* in the section on *Symptoms*

You might also react to: beans (kidney, soya, haricot, navy, baked beans, broad beans, butter beans), carob, chick peas, lentil, liquorice, pea, peanut, senna, soy

Pear
Pear is the fruit of the tree genus *Pyrus*.

Type of allergen: contact, consumed

Symptoms, tests, treatments and self-help tips, see *Fruit*

You might also react to: birch pollen, apple

Pecan
Pecan nuts are the fruit of the tree *Carya illnoensis*.

Type of allergen: consumed

Symptoms, tests, treatments and self-help tips, see *Nuts*

You might also react to: bananas, corn, walnuts

Pectin

Pectin is a fruit sugar, emulsifier and thickener naturally occurring in plants, particularly fruits. It is also used as a treatment for diarrhoea.

Type of allergen: contact, inhalant, consumed

Likely sources of pectin: apples, jam

Symptoms

Gastrointestinal reactions: abdominal pain and swelling, diarrhoea, wind

Mouth, nasal and ear reactions: rhinitis

Respiratory reactions: asthma

Skin reactions: contact dermatitis

Tests
- Blood test: ELISA
- Symptom diary (including peak flow meter readings)

Treatments

Avoidance
- Check the ingredients on food package labels and ask about the ingredients in foods prepared in restaurants when you eat

Prescription medication
- Abdominal pain and swelling: antacids, anti-spasmodic drugs
- Diarrhoea: antidiarrhoeal drugs
- Wind: antacids
- Rhinitis: antihistamines, decongestants, sodium cromoglycate, immunotherapy
- Asthma: anticholinergic drugs, antihistamines (exercise-induced), Beta2 (ß2) adrenoreceptor agonists, cromoglycate, nedocromil sodium, steroids, xanthine derivatives, zafirlukast
- Contact dermatitis: steroids, antihistamines

OTC remedies
- Abdominal pain and swelling: antacids
- Diarrhoea: kaolin and morphine, calcium carbonate, pectin

- Wind: antacids
- Rhinitis: decongestants
- Contact dermatitis: coal tar, emollients, steroids

Alternative remedies
- Abdominal pain and swelling: aromatherapy, herbalism, homeopathy
- Diarrhoea: aromatherapy, herbalism, homeopathy
- Wind: aromatherapy, herbalism, homeopathy
- Rhinitis: aromatherapy
- Asthma: acupuncture (mild asthma only), Buteyko method, homeopathy, relaxation techniques, yoga
- Contact dermatitis: aromatherapy, Bach flower remedies, homeopathy

Self-help tips: for symptom relief see *Abdominal pain and swelling, Diarrhoea, Wind, Rhinitis, Asthma, Contact dermatitis,* in the section on *Symptoms*

Pens
See *Isocyanates, Nickel*

Penicillin
Pencillin is an antibiotic derived from the mould *Penicillum notatum*. It is broken down into penicilloyl in the body; this combines with a carrier protein to become an antigen. Penicillins include: amoxycillin, ampicillin, benzylpenicillin, flucloxacillin, phenyoxymethylpenicillin, procaine penicillin.

An injection of the antibiotic can cause a severe reaction. It is more common in adults than in children. It can also cause occupational contact dermatitis in pharmaceutical workers.

Type of allergen: contact, injected

Symptoms, tests, treatments and self-help tips, see *Drugs*

Alternative products that might not cause a reaction: antibiotics that are not mould-based, such as tetracycline or macrolides

You might also react to: amoxicillin, cephalosporin, moulds (inhalant), moulds in food

Penicillium

Penicillium spores from mouldy cheese can cause occupational asthma in the catering industry. The mould grows on fruits, cheese, bread and cork and some penicillium species are the source of penicillin; however, allergy to penicillium does not necessarily mean allergy to penicillin.

Type of allergen: contact, inhalant

Symptoms
Respiratory reactions: asthma (occupational)

Skin reactions: rash

Tests
- Skin prick test
- Blood test: CAP-RAST
- Symptom diary (including peak flow meter readings)

Treatments
Avoidance
- In occupational situations, use protective equipment such as masks and gloves. Improved ventilation may also help.

Prescription medication
- Asthma: anticholinergic drugs, antihistamines (exercise-induced), Beta2 (ß2) adrenoreceptor agonists, cromoglycate, nedocromil sodium, steroids, xanthine derivatives, zafirlukast
- Dermatitis: steroids, antihistamines

OTC remedies
- Dermatitis: coal tar, emollients, steroids

Alternative remedies
- Asthma: acupuncture (mild asthma only), Buteyko method, homeopathy, relaxation techniques, yoga
- Dermatitis: aromatherapy, Bach flower remedies, homeopathy

Self-help tips: for symptom relief see *Asthma, Contact dermatitis* in the section on *Symptoms*

Pentane

See *Solvents – aliphatic hydrocarbons*

Peppermint oil

This oil is derived from *Mentha piperita*; used as an additive in food and cosmetics; its principal compotent is *menthol*.

Type of allergen: contact, consumed

Symptoms, tests, treatments and self-help tips, see *Herbs*

Peppers

Peppers are the vegetable genus *Capsicum*.
   Capsaicin is found in "hot" peppers; it is a contact irritant. Peppers contain *salicylates*, which have been linked to hyperactivity in children. Green peppers also contain oxalates, a derivative of oxalic acid.

Type of allergen: contact, consumed

Symptoms, tests, treatments and self-help tips, see *Vegetables*

You might also react to: other vegetables/plants in the nightshade family such as aubergine, cayenne, chilli, paprika, potato, tobacco, tomato

Pepper, black and white

Pepper is the condiment derived from the ground berries of the plant *Piper nigrum*.

Type of allergen: inhalant, contact, consumed

Symptoms, tests, treatments and self-help tips, see *Spices*

You might also react to: some plants, i.e. those of the *rhus* family (poison ivy, oak, sumac) and pollen (pigweed)

Perch
See *Fish*

Perchloroethylene
See *Solvents (chlorinated hydrocarbons),*
Solvents (halogenated solvents)

Perfume
There are eight known allergens in perfume: geraniol, cinnamaldehyde, hydroxycitronellal, cinnamic alcohol, eugenol (obtained from clove oil), isoeugenol, amylcinnamaldehyde, and oak moss.

Type of allergen: inhalant, contact

Likely sources of perfume: cosmetics and toiletries; scented household products (such as room fresheners, detergents, cleaning fluids and polishes); foods and toothpastes (some are naturally occurring ingredients); personal hygiene products (tissue, toilet paper, tampons)

Symptoms, tests and treatments, see *Cosmetics*

Self-help tips
• Check labels for all products and avoid those that list: colognes; toilet water; perfumes; masking or unscented perfumes; aroma chemicals; essential oils of plants and animals; cinnamic alcohol; hydroxycitronellal; eugenol; isoeugenol; cinnamic aldehyde; oak moss absolute; amylcinnamic alcohol; anisyl alcohol; benzyl alcohol; benzyl salicylate; coumarin; geraniol; sandalwood oil; musk ambrette; wood tars
• Wear gloves when using detergents and household cleaners.
• Do a patch test on the forearm or behind the ear 24-48 hours before using.

Alternative products that won't cause a reaction: "Unscented" products may contain a masking perfume, so use fragrance-free products

You might also react to: Balsam of Peru, ethylene bassylate, cloves, cinnamon, cassia oil, citronella candles

See also *Acetate, Ammonium dichromate, Balsam of Peru, Benzophenones, Benzyl acetate, Benzyl salicylate (fixing agent), Bitter almond oil, Cassia oil, Cedarwood oil, Cinammon oil, Clove oil, Cosmetics, Geranium oil, Petitgrain oil, Volatile organic compounds*

Perms

See *Ammonium carbonate*

Persimmon

Persimmon is the fruit of the tree *Diospyros kaki*. It is sometimes known as Sharon fruit.

Type of allergen: consumed

Symptoms, tests, treatments and self-help tips, see *Fruit*

Persulphate

Ammonium persulphate, used to speed up the process of hydrogen peroxide bleach on hair, can cause occupational asthma for hairdressers. If symptoms start soon after beginning work and improve at weekends or on holidays, occupational asthma should be suspected.

Type of allergen: inhalant, contact

Symptoms, tests, treatments and self-help tips, see *Chemicals*

Pesticides

See *Phenol, Solvents – aliphatic hydrocarbons*

Petitgrain oil

Petitgrain oil is derived from the bitter orange tree.

Type of allergen: contact

Likely sources of petitgrain oil: cosmetics

Symptoms, tests, treatments and self-help tips, see *Oils, cosmetic*

Petrol
See *Benzene*

Petroleum naptha
See *Solvents – aliphatic hydrocarbons*

Pets

Pets come a close second to dust mites as a cause of allergic disease. Up to 40 per cent of asthmatic children react to the allergens of cats (Fel d1) and dogs (Can f1), which are found in fur, saliva, dander (skin scales), hair and urine. Sufferers may react to some breeds of dogs but not others. Tom cats produce more allergens than female cats; neutering can help reduce the amount of allergens produced.

Budgies and small mammals such as gerbils, hamsters, mice and rats can also cause allergenic asthma; the allergens are contained in the urine, so materials lining the cage will be affected, and allergens are released into the air as the animal moves around and disturbs the cage lining.

Pet allergens tend to be tiny and are easily made airborne; it takes six hours for them to settle in a still room.

Pets may cause occupational allergy for animal handlers and vets.

Type of allergen: inhalant, contact

Symptoms
Eye reactions: conjunctivitis

Mouth, nasal and ear reactions: rhinitis

Respiratory reactions: asthma (especially from cats), hypersensitivity pneumonitis (from birds and droppings)

Skin reactions: eczema

Tests

- Blood test: CAP-RAST – confirm the diagnosis by removing the pet for a few weeks (if possible) and thoroughly cleaning the home to remove dander etc.
- Skin prick test (animal hair – cat, dog, goat, guinea pig, hamster, mouse, rabbit, rat)
- Symptom diary (including peak flow meter readings)

Treatments

- Allergy vaccinations (immunotherapy) – possible for cat or dog allergies – given for at least 3 years – less medication is usually needed after 6 months of weekly injections.

Prescription medication

- Conjunctivitis: antihistamines, cromoglycate, nedocromil sodium, steroids, sympathomimetics
- Rhinitis: antihistamines, decongestants, sodium cromoglycate, immunotherapy
- Asthma: anticholinergic drugs, antihistamines (exercise-induced), Beta2 (ß2) adrenoreceptor agonists, cromoglycate, nedocromil sodium, steroids, xanthine derivatives, zafirlukast
- Eczema: emollients, immune suppressants, steroids, UVA/UVB light treatment, wet wrapping, antihistamines

OTC remedies

- Conjunctivitis: antihistamines
- Rhinitis: decongestants
- Eczema: emollients, hydrocortisone cream

Alternative remedies

- Conjunctivitis: herbalism, homeopathy
- Rhinitis: aromatherapy
- Asthma: acupuncture (mild asthma only), Buteyko method, homeopathy, relaxation techniques, yoga
- Eczema: aromatherapy, evening primrose oil, relaxation, herbalism, homeopathy, Chinese herbal medicine, Bach flower remedies

Self-help tips

- The best advice is to rehome the pet. The allergens will remain in the home for a few months after the pet leaves. Clean up by airing the house thoroughly, then wash all washable items such as bedding, curtains and cushions.

Otherwise:

- Keep pets out of the sufferer's bedroom and, if possible, outdoors – don't let them sleep on the bed
- Don't stroke, hug or kiss pets because of the allergens on the animal's fur or saliva
- Use HEPA filters in a vacuum cleaner to reduce exposure to the pet allergen
- Ventilate the house especially when the pet and the allergic person are indoors
- Washing your pet may help – use pet shampoo
- Wear a mask when changing litter
- Don't let your pet lick you
- Use washable bedding for dogs and cats and wash it frequently

For symptom relief, see *Conjunctivitis, Rhinitis, Asthma, Eczema* in the section on *Symptoms*

You might also react to: clothing made from animal hair (e.g. angora wool, fur coats and hats); old furniture upholstered with horse hair

Phenethyl alcohol

Phenethyl alcohol is a cosmetic preservative and scent; it is derived from oranges, raspberries and tea.

Type of allergen: contact

Likely sources of phenethyl alcohol: cosmetics

Symptoms
Skin reactions: rash

Tests
- Skin patch test
- Symptom diary

Treatments
Avoidance: check labels

Prescription medication: steroids, antihistamines

OTC remedies: coal tar, emollients, steroids

Alternative remedies: aromatherapy, Bach flower remedies, homeopathy

Self-help tips: for symptom relief see *Contact dermatitis* in the section on *Symptoms*

Phenol

Phenol – also known as carbolic acid – is a white crystalline solid, C_6H_5OH, produced by the distillation of organic bodies such as wood or coal, and obtained from coal tar oil.

Type of allergen: contact

Likely sources of phenol: Adhesives, chipboard, cosmetics, creosote, disinfectant, dyes, epoxy resin, explosives, nylon, paint, paint remover, pesticides, pharmaceuticals, plywood, printing ink

Symptoms
Skin reactions: rash, urticaria

Tests
• Skin patch
• Symptom diary

Treatments
Avoidance
• Check labels and avoid where possible; in occupational situations, use protective equipment such as gloves.

Prescription medication
• Contact dermatitis: steroids, antihistamines
• Urticaria: antihistamines, emollients, steroids

OTC remedies
• Contact dermatitis: coal tar, emollients, steroids
• Urticaria: calamine lotion, witch hazel

Alternative remedies
• Contact dermatitis: aromatherapy, Bach flower remedies, homeopathy
• Urticaria: aromatherapy, herbalism, homeopathy

Self-help tips: for symptom relief see *Contact dermatitis, Urticaria* in the section on *Symptoms*
See also *Solvents – aromatic hydrocarbons*

Phenoxymethilpenicillin

Phenoxymethilpenicillin is an antibiotic, usually prescribed for respiratory tract infections.

Type of allergen: consumed

Symptoms, tests, treatments and self-help tips, *see Drugs*
See also *Antibiotics, Penicillin*

Phenylenediamines

Phenylenediamines are a group of chemical substances often used in hair dye; they have been banned in Europe. They are also known as PPD, amino dye, oxidation dye, para dye and peroxide dye.

Type of allergen: contact

Symptoms
Skin reactions: contact dermatitis

Tests
• Skin patch test
• Symptom diary

Treatments
Avoidance: in occupational situations, use protective equipment such as gloves

Prescription medication: steroids, antihistamines

OTC remedies: coal tar, emollients, steroids

Alternative remedies: aromatherapy, Bach flower remedies, homeopathy

Self-help tips: for symptom relief see *Contact dermatitis* in the section on *Symptoms*

Phenylethylamine

Phenylethylamine is a biogenic amine derived from the amino acid phenylalanine, found in grains, nuts, meat, fish, dairy products and beans. If your body does not have enough of the enzyme that breaks phenylethylamine down, you may suffer from migraine and headaches. Its chemical name is $C_8H_{11}N$.

Type of allergen: consumed

Likely sources of phenylethylamine: beans, chocolate, cheese, grains, nuts, salted and pickled fish, meat extracts, liver, sausages, wine, beer

Symptoms
Headache: headache, migraine

Psychological problems: inability to concentrate

Skin reactions: flushing

Other reactions: weight gain

Tests
• Elimination diet
• Food challenge
• Symptom diary

Treatments
Avoidance:
• Avoid trigger foods and check with a dietitian to ensure that it's nutritionally sound

Prescription medication
• Headache: painkillers, non-steroidal anti-inflammatories
• Migraine: painkillers, anti-sickness drugs, ergotamine, 5-HT agonists, beta-blockers, sodium valproate, sumatryptan

OTC remedies
- Headache: as prescription medication
- Migraine: aspirin, ibuprofen, paracetamol

Alternative remedies
- Headache: acupuncture, aromatherapy, herbalism, homeopathy
- Migraine: acupuncture, Alexander technique, aromatherapy, chiropractic, herbalism, homeopathy, hypnosis, osteopathy, reflexology
- Flushing: herbalism

Self-help tips: for symptom relief see *Headache, Migraine, Flushing* in the section on *Symptoms*
See also *Amines*

Phenylmethanol
See *Benzyl alcohol, Solvents*

Photoallergens (cosmetics)
See *Cosmetics*

Photographs
See *Formaldehyde*

Photographic developer
See *Paraphenylenediamine (PPDA)*

Photographic films
See *Solvents – ketone solvents*

Phthalic acid
Phthalic acid is a colourless crystalline dicarboxylic acid and a derivative of benzene, chemical formula $C_6H_4(COOH)_2$, made from *phthalic anhydride*. It is used as a dye.

Type of allergen: inhalant, contact

Likely sources of phthalic acid: cosmetics, nail varnish

Symptoms

Nasal reactions: irritation of mucous membranes

Skin reactions: skin irritation

Tests

- Skin patch test
- Symptom diary

Treatments

Avoidance

- Check labels carefully

Prescription medication

- Irritation of mucous membranes: painkillers
- Skin irritation: emollients

OTC remedies

- Irritation of mucous membranes: painkillers
- Skin irritation: emollients

Alternative remedies

- Irritation of mucous membranes: herbalism

Self-help tips: for symptom relief see *Irritation of mucous membranes, Skin irritation* in the section on *Symptoms*

Phthalic anhydride

Phthalic anhydride is a derivative of naphthalene and is used in making plasticizers and polyester resins.

Type of allergen: inhalant, contact

Likely sources of phthalic anhydride: cosmetic dyes, artificial resins

Symptoms

Nasal reactions: irritation of mucous membranes

Skin reactions: skin irritation

Tests
- Blood test: CAP-RAST
- Blood test: ELISA
- Skin patch test
- Symptom diary

Treatments
Avoidance
- Check labels carefully

Prescription medication
- Skin irritation: emollients

OTC remedies
- Skin irritation: emollients

Self-help tips: for symptom relief see *Irritation of mucous membranes*, *Skin irritation* in the section on *Symptoms*

Pickles
See *Yeast*

Pig bristles
See *Animal hair*

Pigments
See *Cobalt*

Pigeon
See *Animal protein*

Pike
See *Fish*

Pilchard
See *Fish*

Pillows
See *Dust mite, Feathers, Latex, Polyurethane*

Pins
See *Nickel*

Pineapple

Pineapple is the fruit *Ananas comsus* from the *Bromeliaceae* family; it contains vasoactive *amines* which can cause allergic reactions. It also contains *salicylates*, which have been linked to hyperactivity in children, and the enzyme bromelain, which may cross-react with *papain*. Anaphylactic shock can occur from eating or inhaling during processing of fresh pineapple.

Type of allergen: consumed, inhalant

Symptoms, tests, treatments and self-help tips, see *Fruit*

Pine nuts

Pine nuts are the fruit of the tree *Pinus edulis*.

Type of allergen: consumed

Symptoms, tests, treatments and self-help tips, see *Nuts*

Pistachio

Pistachio nuts are the fruit of the tree *Pistacia vera*.

Type of allergen: contact, consumed

Symptoms, tests, treatments and self-help tips, see *Nuts*

You might also react to: cashew, mango

Plaice
See *Fish*

Plants

Common plants causing dermatitis include carrots, celery, chives, chrysanthemums, daisies, daffodils, garlic, hops, hyacinth, ivy, narcissi, nettles, oleander, onion, philodendron, pine trees, poison ivy, poison oak, primrose, primula, pyrethrum, ragweed, *rhus*, tulips, yarrow.

Plants can also cause asthma and occupational asthma; if symptoms start soon after beginning work and improve at weekends or on holidays, occupational asthma should be suspected.

Type of allergen: inhalant, contact

Symptoms
Respiratory reactions: asthma

Skin reactions: itching, irritation, contact dermatitis

Other reactions: more likely to be caused by a reaction to pollen than to the plants themselves

Tests
- Skin prick test – ash, beech, dandelion, dock, English plantain, mugwort, nettle, pine, plane tree, poplar, willow
- Blood test: ELISA – cyclamen, cut grass, pine
- Skin patch test
- Symptom diary (including peak flow meter readings)

Treatments
Avoidance
- In occupational situations, use protective equipment such as gloves and masks. Improved ventilation may also help.

Prescription medication
- Asthma: anticholinergic drugs, antihistamines (exercise-induced), Beta2 (ß2) adrenoreceptor agonists, cromoglycate, nedocromil sodium, steroids, xanthine derivatives, zafirlukast
- Contact dermatitis: steroids, antihistamines
- Itching: antihistamines, emollients
- Skin irritation: cmollients

OTC remedies
- Contact dermatitis: coal tar, emollients, steroids
- Itching: antihistamines, emollients
- Skin irritation: emollients

Alternative remedies
- Asthma: acupuncture (mild asthma only), Buteyko method, homeopathy, relaxation techniques, yoga
- Contact dermatitis: aromatherapy, Bach flower remedies, homeopathy
- Itching: aromatherapy, herbalism

Self-help tips: for symptom relief see *Asthma, Itching, Contact dermatitis, Skin irritation* in the section on *Symptoms*
See also *Pollen*

You might also react to: pork and black pepper, if you suffer from *rhus* allergy (poison ivy, oak, sumac); beef and yeasts if you are allergic to cedars

Plaster
See *Formaldehyde*

Plastics
Plastics are polymeric materials made from *resin*; chemicals involved in the production include fillers, plasticizers, pigments and stabilizers. If plastics are exposed to heat, they may produce gas which includes volatile organic compounds.

Type of allergen: contact

Likely sources of plastic: household and industrial items (e.g. chairs, desktops, wall coverings, tool handles)

Symptoms
Skin reactions: contact dermatitis

Tests
- Skin patch test
- Symptom diary

Treatments

Prescription medication: steroids, antihistamines

OTC remedies: coal tar, emollients, steroids

Alternative remedies: aromatherapy, Bach flower remedies, homeopathy

Self-help tips
- Don't keep food/drink in plastic containers (including mineral water)
- For symptom relief see *Contact dermatitis* in the section on *Symptoms*

See also *anhydrides, epoxy resin, pvc, Solvents – esters, Solvents – ketone solvents*

Plastic bonding
See *Chloroform*

Plasticizers
See *Solvents – glycols*

Plastic laminates
See *Volatile organic compounds*

Plastic solvent
See *Solvents – chlorinated hydrocarbons*

Platinum salts

Platinum salts, used in metal refining, are a major cause of occupational asthma. Up to 50 per cent of people exposed to them are allergic to them; there are regulations on working conditions and if you react to a skin prick test, you will not be allowed to work with platinum salts. If symptoms start soon after beginning work and improve at weekends or on holidays, occupational asthma should be suspected.

Type of allergen: inhalant, contact

Symptoms, tests, treatments and self-help tips, see *Metals*

Plywood

See *Formaldehyde, Phenols*

Plum

Plums are the fruit of the tree *Prunus domestica*. They contain the vasoactive amine tyramine, which causes the blood vessels to widen and may trigger migraines. They also contain *salicylates*, which have been linked to hyperactivity in children.

Type of allergen: contact, consumed

Symptoms, tests, treatments and self-help tips, see *Fruit*

You might also react to: birch pollen, almonds, apricots, cherries, peaches

Poison ivy

See *Plants*

Polish

See *Colophony, Formaldehyde, Perfume, Turpentine, Volatile organic compounds, Wool alcohol*

Pollen

Pollen comprises grains carrying the male gamete of seed plants. It is the most common cause of hay fever.

Type of allergen: inhalant

Symptoms
Eye reactions: allergic conjunctivitis

Nasal reactions: rhinitis, hay fever

Respiratory reactions: asthma, breathing difficulties

Skin reactions: angioedema, urticaria

Tests

• CAP-RAST – acacia (*Acacia longifolia*), American beech (*Fagus grandifolia*), Australian pine (*Casuarina equisetifolia*), bahia grass (*Paspalum notatum*), barley (*Hordeum vulgare*), bent grass or redtop (*Agrostis stolonifera*), Bermuda grass (*Cynodon dactylon*), box elder (*Acer negundo*), Brome grass (*Bromus inermis*), camomile (*Matricaria chamomilla*), canary grass (*Phalaris arundinacea*), cedar (*Libocedrus decurrens*), chestnut (*Castanea sativa*), cocklebur (*Xanthium commune*), cocksfoot grass (*Dactylis glomerata*), common pigweed (*Amaranthus retroflexus*), common ragweed (*Ambrosia elatior*), common reed (*Phragmites communis*), cottonwood (*Populus deltoides*), cypress (*Cupressus sempervirens*), dandelion (*Taraxacum officinale*), date (*Phoenix* canariensis), Douglas fir (*Pseudotsuga taxifolia*), elder (*sambucus nigra*), elm (*Ulmus americana*), English plantain or ribwort (*Plantago lanceolata*), eucalyptus (*Eucalyptus sp*), false oat grass (*Arrhenatherum elatiu*), false ragweed (*Franseria acanticarpa*), firebush or kochia (*Kochia scoparia*), giant ragweed (*Ambrosia trifida*), golden rod (*Solidago virgaurea*), goosefoot or lamb's quarters (*Chenopodium album*), grey alder (*Alnus incana*), hazel (*Corylus avellana*), hornbeam (*Carpinus betulus*), horse chestnut (*Aesculus hippocastanum*), Japanese cedar (*Cryptomeria japonica*), Johnson grass (*Sorghum halepense*), linden (*Tilia cordata*), London plane or maple-leaf sycamore (*Platanus acerifolia*), lupin (*Lupinus sp*), maize (*Zea mays*), meadow fescue (*Festuca elatior*), meadow foxtail (*Alopecurus pratensis*), meadow grass or Kentucky blue (*Poa pratensis*), melaleuca or cajeput tree (*Melaleuca leucadendron*), mesquite (*Prosopis juliflora*), mountain juniper (*Juniperus sabinoides*), mugwort (*Artemisia vulgaris*), mulberry (*Morus alba*), nettle (*Urtica diocia*), oak (*Quercus alba*), oat (*Avena sativa*), olive (*Olea europaea*), oxeye daisy (*Chrysanthemum leucanthemum*), paloverde (*Cercidium floridum*), pecan (*Carya pecan*), pepper tree (*Schinus molle*), pine (*Pinus radiata*), prickly saltwort or Russian thistle (*Salsola kali* and *Salsola pestife*r), privet (*Ligustrum vulgare*), queen palm (*Arecastrum romanzoffianum*), rape (*Brassica napus*), rough marshelder (*Iva ciliata*), rye (*Secale cerale*), rye grass (*Lolium perenne*), salt grass (*Distichlis spicata*), scale or lenscale (*Atriplex lentiformis*), sheep sorrel (*Rumex acetosella*), silver birch (*Betula verrucosa*), spruce (*Picea excelsa*), sugar beet (*Beta vulgaris*), sunflower (*Helianthus annuus*), sweet gum (*liquidambar styracuflua*), timothy grass (*Phleum pratense*), velvet grass (*Holcus lanatus*), vernal grass

(*Anthoxanthum odoratum*), Virginia live oak (*Quercus virginiana*), wall pellitory (*Parietaria officinalis* and *Parietaria judaica*), walnut (*Juglans californica*), western ragweed (*Ambrosia psilostachya*), wheat (*Triticum sativum*), white ash (*Fraxinus americana*), white pine (*Pinus strobus*), wild rye grass (*Elymus triticoides*), willow (*Salox carpea*), wormwood (*Artemisia absinthium*)

- Blood test: ELISA
- GRASS:bahia grass (*Paspalum notatum*), barley (*Hordeum vulgare*), bent grass or redtop (*Agrostis alba*), Bermuda grass (*Cynodon dactylon*), Brome grass (*Bromus inermis*), common reed (*Phragmites communis*), dog's tail grass (*Cynosurus cristatus*), Johnson grass (*Sorghum halapense*), maize (*Zea mays*), meadow fescue (*Festuca elatior*), meadow foxtail (*Alopecurus pratensis*), meadow grass or Kentucky blue (*Poa pratensis*), oat (*Avena sativa*), oat grass tail (*Arrhenatherum elatis*), orchard grass (*Dactylis glomerata*), red top (*Agrostis stolonifera*), rye (*Secale cerale*), rye grass (*Lolium perenne*), salt grass (*Distichlis spicata*), timothy grass (*Phleum pratense*), velvet grass (*Holcus lanatus*), vernal grass (*Anthoxanthum odoratum*), wheat (*Triticum aestivum* and *Triticum sativum*), wheat grass (*Agropyron smithii*), wheat grass (*Agropyron repens*)
- TREES: acacia (*Acacia longifolia*), agave, American beech (*Fagus grandifolia*), Arizona ash (*Fraxinus velutina*), Australian pine (*Casuarina equisetifolia*), bayberry (*Myrica gale*), black walnut (*Juglans nigra*), black willow (*Salix nigra*), box elder (*Acer negundo*), Brazilian pepper , broom (*Genista anglica*), common yew (*Taxus baccata*), cottonwood (*Populus deltoides*), Chinese/Siberian elm (*Ulmus pumila*), daphne (*Daphne mezereum*), elder (*Sambucus nigra*), elm (*Ulmus americana*), eucalyptus (*Eucalyptus spp*), European beech (*Fagus silvatica*), golden chain (*Laburnum spp*), hackberry (*Celtis occidentalis*), hawthorn (*Crataegus spp*), hazel (*Corylus avellana, Corylus americana*), hibiscus (*marshmallow*), horse chestnut (*Aesculus hippocastanum*), Italian cypress (*Cupressus sempervirens*), Japanese cedar (*Cryptomeria japonica*), jasmine (*Jasminum spp*), juniper (*Juniperis monosperma*), lilac (*Syringa vulgaris*), linden (*Tilia cordata*), Loblolly pine (*Pinus taeda*), locust tree (*Robinia pseydoacadia*), London plane or maple-leaf sycamore (*Platanus acerifolia*), magnolia (*Magnolia grandiflora*), melaleuca (*Melaleuca leucadendron*), mesquite (*Prosopis juliflora*), mistletoe (*Viscum album*), mountain cedar (*Juniperus sabinoides/*

sabina), mulberry (*Morus alba*), oak (*Quercus alba*), oleander, olive (*Olea europaea*), orange tree (*Citrus spp*), pecan (*Carya pecan*), pepper tree (*Schinus molle*), privet (*Ligustrum vulgare*), queen palm (*Arecastrum roman, Cocus plumosa*), red alder (*Alnus rubra*), red cedar (*Juniperus virginiana*), red oak (*Quercus rubra*), salt cedar (*Tamarix gallica*), Scotch pine (*Pinus silvestris*), scrub elm (*Ulmus carrisfolia*), smooth alder (*Alnus rugosa*), speckled alder (*Alnus glutinosa*), spruce (*Picea abies*), sweet chestnut (*Castanea sativa*), sweet gum (*Liquidambar styaciflua*), sycamore (*Plantanus occidentalis*), tree of heaven (*Alianthus altissima*), tree of life (*Thuja occidentalis*), Virginia live oak (*Quercus virginiana*), walnut (*Juglans regia*), white ash (*Fraxinus spp*), white bald cypress (*Taxodium distichum*), white birch (*Betula verrucosa/alba, Betula populifolia*), white hickory (*Carya* alba), white pine (*Pinus strobu*s), willow (*Salix carpea*),

– WEEDS: alfalfa (*Medicago sativa*), burrobrush (*Hymenoclea salsola*), careless weed (*Amaranthus palmeri*), cocklebur (*Xanthium commune* and *Xanthium strumarium*), coltsfoot (*Tussilago farfara*), common ragweed (*Ambrosia elatior*), common sagebrush (*Artemisia tridentata*), dandelion (*Taraxacum officinalis*), English plantain or ribwort (*Plantago lanceolata*), false ragweed (*Franseria acanticarpa*), firebush or kochia (*Kochia scoparia*), giant ragweed (*Ambrosia trifida*), golden rod (*Solidago virgaurea*), goosefoot or lamb's quarters (*Chenopodium album*), ironwood (*Ostrya virginiana*), knotgrass (*Polygonum spp*), lenscale (*Atriplex lentiformis*), Mexican tea (*Chenopodium ambrosiodes*), mugwort (*Artemisia* vulgaris), nettle (*Urtica diocia*), oxeye daisy (*Chrysanthemum leucanthemum*), poverty weed (*Iva azillaris*), rabbit bush (*Franseria deltoides*), rough marshelder (*Iva ciliata*), rough pigweed (*Amaranthus retroflexus*), Russian thistle (*Salsola kali*), salt bush (*Atriplex spp*), sheep sorrel (*Rumex acetosella*), spiny pigweed (*Amaranthys spinosus*), sweet clover (*Trifolium pratens*e), wall pellitory (*Parietaria officinale* and *Parietaria judaica*), western ragweed (*Ambrosia psilostachya* and *Ambrosia coronopifolia*), western water hemp (*Acnida tamariscina*), wing scale (*Atriplex canescens*), wormwood (*Artemisia absinthium*), yellow dockweed (*rumex crispus*)

– HERBS/FLOWERS: aster (*Callistephus chinensi*), azalea, balm (Melissa officinalis), cactus, camellia, camomile (*Camomilla*), carnation (*Dianthus spp*), chrysanthemum (*Chrysanthemum spp*), cornflower (*Centaurea cyanus*), dahlia (*Dahlia variabilis*), heather (*Calluna vulgaris*), forsythia (*Forsythia suspensa*), French marigold, gerbera (*Gerbera spp*), geranium (*Geranium spp*), gillyflower (*Matthiola incana*), golden rod (*Solidago spp*), hyacinth (*Hyacinthoides spp*), ivy (*Hedera helix*), lily of the valley (*Convallaria majalis*), lily (*Lilium spp*), lupin (*Lupinus spp*), marigold (*Calendual officinalis*), narcissus (*Narcissus spp*), pansy (*Viola tricolar*), primrose (*Primula variabilis*), rape (*Brassica napus*), rose (*Rosa spp*), St John's wort (*Hypericum spp*), sugar beet (*Beta vulgaris*), sunflower (*Helianthus annuus*), tulip (*Tulipa gesneriana* and *Tulipa spp*), willow herb (*Epilobium angustifolium*), yarrow (*Achillea spp*)

- Skin prick test – alder (*Alnus glutinosa*), ash (*Fraxinus excelsior*), barley (*Hordeum vulgare*), beech (*Fagus sylvatica*), bent grass (*Agrostis stolonifera*), Bermuda grass (*Cynodon dactylon*), black locust (*Robinia pseudoacacia*), daisy (*Chrysanthemum leucanthemum*), dandelion (*Taraxacum officinale*), elderberry (*Sambucus nigra*), elm (*Ulmus campestris*), English plantain (*Plantago lanceolata*), goat willow (*Salix caprea*), goosefoot (*Chenopodium album*), hazel (*Corylus avellana*), horse chestnut (*Aesculus hippocastanum*), linden (*Tilia cordata*), maize (*Zea mays*), maple (*Acer sp*), meadow fescue (*Festuca rubra*), meadow foxtail (*Alopecurus pratensis*), meadow grass (*Poa pratensis*), mugwort (*Artemisia vulgaris*), nettle (*Urtica dioica*), oak (*Quercus robur*), oat (*Arrhenatherum elatius* and *Avena sativa*), olive (*Olea europea*), orchard (*Dactylis glomerata*), pellitory (*Parietaria*), poplar (*Populus sp*), ragweed (*Ambrosia elatior*), red sorrel (*Rumex acetosella*), rye (*Secale cerale*), rye grass (*Lolium perenne*), silver birch (*Betula verrucosa*), sweet vernal (*Anthoxanthum odoratum*), sycamore (*Platanus acerifolia*), timothy grass (*Phleum pratense*), velvet (*Holcus lanatus*), wheat (*Triticum satium*)
- Intradermal: acacia, alder (*Alnus glutinosa*), ash (*Fraxinus excelsior*), barley (*Hordeum vulgare*), beech (*Fagus sylvatica*), birch (*Betula verrucosa*), dandelion (*Taraxacum officinale*), elderberry (*Sambucus nigra*), elm (*Ulmus campestris*), grass, English plantain (*Plantago lanceolata*), hazel (*Corylus avellana*), linden (*Tilia cordata*), mugwort (*Artemisia vulgaris*), nettle (*Urtica dioica*), oak (*Quercus robur*), oat (*Avena sativa*), plane, poplar (*Populus sp*), red sorrel (*Rumex acetosella*), rye (*Secale cerale*), sallow, silver birch (*Betula verrucosa*), wheat (*Triticum satium*)
- Nasal challenge: alder (*Alnus glutinosa*), English plantain (*Plantago lanceolata*), goosefoot (*Chenopodium album*), hazel (*Corylus avellana*), mugwort (*Artemisia vulgaris*), red sorrel

(*Rumex acetosella*), silver birch (*Betula verrucosa*), timothy grass (*Phleum pratense*)
- Symptom diary (including peak flow meter readings)

Treatments
Avoidance

Prescription medication
- Conjunctivitis: antihistamines, cromoglycate, nedocromil sodium, steroids, sympathomimetics
- Hay fever: antihistamines, cromoglycate, decongestants, nedocromil sodium, steroids, sympathomimetics
- Rhinitis: antihistamines, decongestants, sodium cromoglycate, immunotherapy
- Asthma: anticholinergic drugs, antihistamines (exercise-induced), Beta2 (ß2) adrenoreceptor agonists, cromoglycate, nedocromil sodium, steroids, xanthine derivatives, zafirlukast
- Breathing problems: bronchodilators, corticosteroids
- Angioedema: adrenaline, antihistamines, steroids
- Urticaria: antihistamines, emollients, steroids

OTC remedies
- Conjunctivitis: antihistamines
- Hay fever: antihistamines, decongestants
- Rhinitis: decongestants
- Angioedema: antihistamines
- Urticaria: calamine lotion, witch hazel

Alternative remedies
- Conjunctivitis: herbalism, homeopathy
- Hay fever: aromatherapy, herbalism, homeopathy
- Rhinitis: aromatherapy
- Asthma: acupuncture (mild asthma only), Buteyko method, homeopathy, relaxation techniques, yoga
- Urticaria: aromatherapy, herbalism, homeopathy

Self-help tips
Personal care:
- wear sunglasses to stop pollen getting in your eyes
- wear a mask over your nose and mouth
- shower and wash your hair every night to keep pollen from getting on your pillows and bedding.

In the home:
- keep windows closed as much as possible, especially in your bedroom
- cover bedding with a spare sheet to keep pollen from getting on your pillows and bedding – roll the sheet up carefully at night
- damp dusting
- regular vacuuming, particularly with a HEPA filter
- keep pets out of the house in the pollen season (they bring pollen in on their fur) or ask someone not allergic to pollen to brush them thoroughly before they come indoors

In the garden:
- don't mow the lawn, rake up leaves or cut hay, and stay inside while it's being done
- don't hang washing out to dry, as pollens and moulds may collect in them
- wear a hat when gardening to prevent pollen getting in your hair
- don't use organic mulches in the garden (e.g. tree bark and mushroom compost)

In the car:
- keep car windows closed
- use HEPA pollen filters in your car

Timing:
- check pollen counts (often included in radio, TV and newspaper reports), and try to avoid going out when the count is high; if you do have to go out, avoid grassy and leafy areas
- note that there's likely to be more pollen around first thing in the morning, in the early evening, on windy days and during thunderstorms

For symptom relief, see *Conjunctivitis, Rhinitis, Hay fever, Asthma, Breathing difficulties, Angioedema, Urticaria* in the section on *Symptoms*

You might also react to
- bananas, camomile tea, egg, honey, lettuce, milk products, mint, melons, sunflower seeds if you are allergic to ragweed pollen
- apple, camomile tea, carrot, celery, melon, potato, tobacco,

tomato, watermelon if you are allergic to mugwort pollen
- black pepper and pork if you are allergic to pigweed pollen
- milk products and mint if you are allergic to elm pollen
- egg and apple if you are allergic to oak pollen
- apple, buckwheat, carrot, cherry, fennel, honey, pear, peach, plum, potato, spinach, walnut, wheat if you are allergic to birch pollen
- cherry and melon if you are allergic to pellitory pollen

Polyester

Polyester is a polymer formed by the interaction of polyhydric alcohol and polybasic acid. The problem is more likely to be in the materials used than the polyester itself, although polyester may give off volatile materials in gas form (see *Plastic*).

Type of allergen: inhalant, contact

Likely sources of polyester: fibres, including fabric, coatings containers and synthetic panelling.
See also *Cobalt, Phthalic anhydride, Resin, Solvent*

Polyethylene
See *Colophony*

Polyoxyetheylene (8) Stearate
See *Food additives – emulsifiers, Stabilizers and thickeners*

Polystyrene

Polystyrene compounds – chemical symbol C_8H_8 – are the third largest production plastics in use. They are formed by polymerization of styrene (phenylethene) and benzoyl peroxide.

Type of allergen: contact

Likely sources of polystyrene: food packaging materials (egg cartons, coffee cups, trays and other disposable products); electrical insulation
See *Plastics*

Polyurethane

Polyurethane is a polymer; its production involves *isocyanates*.

Type of allergen: contact

Likely sources of polyurethane: Paint, plastic, varnish, rubber, foam
See *Isocyanates*

Poppy seed

Poppy seed – botanical name *Papaver somniferum* – is often used to decorate bread and other bakery goods.
Type of allergen: consumed

Symptoms
Anaphylactic shock

Gastrointestinal reactions: diarrhoea, vomiting

Respiratory reactions: asthma

Skin reactions: angioedema, atopic dermatitis, urticaria

Tests
• Blood test: CAP-RAST
• Elimination diet
• Food challenge
• Symptom diary (including peak flow meter readings)

Treatments
Avoidance
• Check labels carefully and check with a dietitian to ensure that your diet is still nutritionally sound

Prescription medication
• Anaphylactic shock: adrenaline, antihistamines, steroids
• Diarrhoea: antidiarrhoeal drugs
• Vomiting: anti-emetics
• Asthma: anticholinergic drugs, antihistamines (exercise-induced), Beta2 (ß2) adrenoreceptor agonists, cromoglycate, nedocromil sodium, steroids, xanthine derivatives, zafirlukast

- Angioedema: adrenaline, antihistamines, steroids
- Contact dermatitis: steroids, antihistamines
- Urticaria: antihistamines, emollients, steroids

OTC remedies
- Diarrhoea: kaolin and morphine, calcium carbonate, pectin
- Vomiting: oral rehydration solution
- Angioedema: antihistamines
- Contact dermatitis: coal tar, emollients, steroids
- Urticaria: calamine lotion, witch hazel

Alternative remedies
- Diarrhoea: aromatherapy, herbalism, homeopathy
- Vomiting: herbalism
- Asthma: acupuncture (mild asthma only), Buteyko method, homeopathy, relaxation techniques, yoga
- Contact dermatitis: aromatherapy, Bach flower remedies, homeopathy
- Urticaria: aromatherapy, herbalism, homeopathy

Self-help tips: for symptom relief see *Diarrhoea, Vomiting, Asthma, Angioedema, Dermatitis, Urticaria* in the section on *Symptoms*

Pork

The allergen in pork is an *albumin protein*.

Type of allergen: consumed

Symptoms, tests, treatments and self-help tips, see *Meat and poultry*

You might also react to: some plants, i.e. those of the *rhus* family (poison ivy, oak, sumac) and pollen (pigweed)

Postage stamps
See *Colophony*

Potassium benzoate
See *Food additives – preservatives*

Potassium chloride

See *Food additives – anti-caking agents*

Potassium dichromate

Potassium dichromate is a salt of the metal *Chromium*.

Type of allergen: contact

Likely sources of potassium dichromate: bleaches, cement, leather goods, photographic supplies, plating dyes, tanning agents, yellow paint

Symptoms, tests, treatments and self-help tips, see *Metals*
See also *Chromium salts*

Potassium metabisulphite

See *Food additives – preservatives*

Potassium nitrite

See *Food additives – preservatives*

Potassium polyphosphates

See *Food additives – emulsifiers, stabilizers and thickeners*

Potassium propionate

See *Food additives – preservatives*

Potato

Potato is the edible tuber of the plant *Solanum tuberosum*. The protein is heat-labile so cooked potato is usually tolerated. In ready-prepared foods, the problem is often with the preservative used: *sodium metabisulphite*. You may have an itching mouth/palate during the pollen season.

Type of allergen: contact, consumed

Likely sources of potato: chips, crisps, ready-made meals, savoury snack foods, soups, vegetarian pasties, potato flour

Symptoms, tests, treatments and self-help tips, see *Vegetables*

Alternative products that won't cause a reaction: Yams, sweet potatoes, cassava, millet

You might also react to: other vegetables/plants in the nightshade family such as aubergine, cayenne, chilli, peppers (capsicum), paprika, potato, tobacco, tomato; also physalis (cape gooseberry), sage, birch tree pollen, mugwort pollen

Pottery
See *Cobalt*

Powder
See *Cosmetics, Talc*

Prawns
See *Shellfish*

Prescription medication
See *Drugs*

Preservative agents (cosmetics)
See *Ammonia, Benzyl alcohol, Formaldehyde*

Preservatives
For further information about the preservatives themselves and cross-reactivity see *Chlorocresol*.

Symptoms
Skin reactions: contact dermatitis – chlorocresol

Tests
• Patch test chlorocresol

Treatments
Avoidance: in an occupational situation, use protective equipment such as gloves.

Prescription medication
• Contact dermatitis: steroids, antihistamines

OTC remedies
• Contact dermatitis: coal tar, emollients, steroids

Alternative remedies
• Contact dermatitis: aromatherapy, Bach flower remedies, homeopathy

Self-help tips: for symptom relief see *Contact dermatitis* in the section on *Symptoms*
See also *Volatile organic compounds*

Primula
See *Plants*

Printing
See *Cobalt, Colophony*

Procaine
See *Anaesthetic, Drugs*

Promethazine hydrochloride
See *Antihistamines, Drugs*

2-propanone
See *Solvents – ketone solvents*

Propellants
See *Chloroform*

Propylene glycol
See *Solvents – glycols*

Propylene glycol methyl ether (PGME)
See *Solvents – glycol ether*

Propylene glycol n-butyl ether (PnB)
See *Solvents – glycol ether*

Propyl gallate
See *Food additives – antioxidants*

Propyl4-hydroxybenzoate
See *Food additives – preservatives*

Propyl4-hydroxybenzoate sodium salt
See *Food additives – preservatives*

Propylene glycol
See *Cosmetics*

Prunes
Prunes are dried plums. They contain the vasoactive amine *tyramine*, which causes the blood vessels to widen and may trigger migraines. They also contain *salicylates*, which have been linked to hyperactivity in children.

Type of allergen: consumed

Symptoms, tests, treatments and self-help tips, see *Fruit*

Pumpkin
Pumpkin is the gourd *Cucurbita pepo*.

Symptoms, tests, treatments and self-help tips, see *Vegetables*

Type of allergen: consumed

You might also react to: others in the *Cucurbitaceae* family, such as courgette, cucumber, marrow, melon, squash, watermelon

PVC
Polyvinyl chloride (PVC – chemical symbol $C_2H_3C_l$) is a common resin used extensively in plastic manufacture and as a rubber substitute. It can cause occupational asthma; if symptoms

start soon after beginning work and improve at weekends or on holidays, occupational asthma should be suspected.

Type of allergen: inhalant

Likely sources of PVC: Fabric, flexible coatings, floor tiles, plastic wrapping, water-based emulsion paints, wire coatings

Symptoms
Respiratory reactions: asthma (occupational)

Tests
• Symptom diary (including peak flow meter readings)

Treatments
Avoidance: in occupational situations, use protective equipment such as gloves and masks

Prescription medication: anticholinergic drugs, antihistamines (exercise-induced), Beta2 (ß2) adrenoreceptor agonists, cromoglycate, nedocromil sodium, steroids, xanthine derivatives, zafirlukast

Alternative remedies: acupuncture (mild asthma only), Buteyko method, homeopathy, relaxation techniques, yoga

Self-help tips: for symptom relief see *Asthma* in the section on *Symptoms*
See also *Epoxy resin, Plastic*

Quinine

Quinine is an alkaloid obtained from the bark of the *cinchona* tree. It is used as an antimalarial drug and also to relieve night cramps.

Type of allergen: contact

Likely sources of quinine: Hair care products, bitter lemon, tonic water

Symptoms
Skin reactions: photoallergenic contact dermatitis
Tests

- Photopatch testing (the allergen is placed on two skin sites; one is exposed to sunlight after 48 hours, and then both areas are examined for a rash)
- Symptom diary

Treatments

Avoidance: check labels; use protective equipment such as gloves in an occupational situation

Prescription medication: emollients, steroids

Self-help tips: for symptom relief see *Photoallergenic contact dermatitis* in the section on *Symptoms*

Quinoline Yellow
See *Food additives – colourings*

Rabbits
See *Pets, Animal hair*

Radish
Radish is the salad vegetable *Raphanus sativus*.

Type of allergen: contact, consumed

Symptoms, tests, treatments and self-help tips, see *Vegetables*

Raisin
Raisins are grapes that have been dried either in the sun or by artificial heat. They contain *salicylates*, which have been linked to hyperactivity in children.

Type of allergen: consumed

Symptoms, tests, treatments and self-help tips, see *Fruit*

Rape seed

Rape seed is from the plant *Brassica rapa*. The pollen and the flour are allergens. If symptoms start soon after beginning work and improve at weekends or on holidays, occupational asthma should be suspected.

Type of allergen: contact, inhalant

Likely sources of rape seed: fields of rape seed

Symptoms

Eye reactions: conjunctivitis

Mouth, nasal and ear reactions: rhinitis, sneezing

Respiratory reactions: asthma (occupational), cough, wheezing

Skin reactions: dermatitis

Tests
- Blood test: CAP-RAST
- Skin prick test (rape seed oil)
- Symptom diary

Treatments

Avoidance: in occupational situations, use protective equipment such as gloves and masks. Improved ventilation may also help.

Prescription medication
- Conjunctivitis: antihistamines, cromoglycate, nedocromil sodium, steroids, sympathomimetics
- Rhinitis: antihistamines, decongestants, sodium cromoglycate, immunotherapy
- Sneezing: antihistamines, decongestants, sodium cromogylcate
- Asthma: anticholinergic drugs, antihistamines (exercise-induced), Beta2 (ß2) adrenoreceptor agonists, cromoglycate, nedocromil sodium, steroids, xanthine derivatives, zafirlukast
- Cough: antihistamines, bronchodilators, corticosteroids
- Wheezing: bronchodilator
- Contact dermatitis: steroids, antihistamines

OTC remedies
- Conjunctivitis: antihistamines

- Rhinitis: decongestants
- Cough: demulcents, antitussives, expectorants
- Contact dermatitis: coal tar, emollients, steroids

Alternative remedies
- Conjunctivitis: herbalism, homeopathy
- Rhinitis: aromatherapy
- Sneezing: acupuncture
- Asthma: acupuncture (mild asthma only), Buteyko method, homeopathy, relaxation techniques, yoga
- Cough: aromatherapy, homeopathy
- Contact dermatitis: aromatherapy, Bach flower remedies, homeopathy

Self-help tips: for symptom relief see *Conjunctivitis, Rhinitis, Sneezing, Asthma, Cough, Contact dermatitis* in the section on *Symptoms*

Raspberry
Raspberries are the fruit of the plant *Rubus idaeus*. They contain *salicylates*, which have been linked to hyperactivity in children.

Type of allergen: consumed

Symptoms, tests, treatments and self-help tips, see *Fruit*

You might also react to: blackberries, strawberries

Rats
See *Pets, Animal hair, Animal protein*

Razors
See *Nickel*

Redcurrant
Redcurrants are the fruit of the plant *Ribes sylvestre*. They contain oxalates, a derivative of oxalic acid.

Type of allergen: consumed

Symptoms, tests, treatments and self-help tips, see *Fruit*

Refrigerants
See *Chloroform*

Resin

Amino resins are thermoset materials that are generally used in adhesives, coatings and some insulating products. They are cured with formaldehyde, which may be released as a gas from the product over a long period of time. Phenolic resins are used as coatings and adhesives in particle board, plywood and other composite wood products.

Type of allergen: inhalant, contact

Likely sources of resin: adhesives, coatings, insulating products
See *Benzene*.

Resin, artificial
See *Phthalic anhydride*

Resin solvent
See *Solvents – aromatic hydrocarbons,*
Solvents – chlorinated hydrocarbons

Rhubarb

Rhubarb is the plant *Rheum rhaponticum*. It contains oxalates, a derivative of oxalic acid.

Type of allergen: consumed

Symptoms, tests, treatments and self-help tips, see *Fruit*

You might also react to: buckwheat

Rice

Rice is the grain *Oryza sativa*. The allergic component, albumin, is heat-stable, but is very weak and allergy to rice is rare. Rice is often included in a hypoallergenic diet.

The dust may cause occupational asthma; if symptoms start soon after beginning work and improve at weekends or on holidays, occupational asthma should be suspected.

Type of allergen: inhalant, consumed, contact

Likely sources of rice: as well as rice dishes, watch for Indian/Japanese sweetmeats (which use rice flour), spring rolls (the pastry is made from rice flour) and rice noodles

Symptoms
Anaphylactic shock: very rare; likely to be exercise-induced

Eye reactions: conjunctivitis

Gastrointestinal reactions: gastric upset/irritation

Mouth, nasal and ear reactions: rhinitis, sneezing

Respiratory reactions: occupational asthma (to dust)

Skin reactions: angioedema, contact dermatitis, eczema, flushing, itching, urticaria

Tests
- Blood test: CAP-RAST
- Blood test: ELISA
- Skin prick test
- Elimination diet
- Food challenge
- Symptom diary (including peak flow meter readings)
- Exercise challenge

Treatments
Avoidance
- Check labels carefully (including rice flour) and check with a dietitian to ensure that your diet is still nutritionally sound. In occupational situations, use protective equipment such as gloves and masks; improved ventilation may also help.

Prescription medication
- Anaphylactic shock: adrenaline, antihistamines, steroids
- Conjunctivitis: antihistamines, cromoglycate, nedocromil sodium, steroids, sympathomimetics
- Gastric upset/irritation: painkillers (use paracetamol rather than aspirin)
- Rhinitis: antihistamines, decongestants, sodium cromoglycate, immunotherapy
- Sneezing: antihistamines, decongestants, sodium cromogylcate
- Asthma: anticholinergic drugs, antihistamines (exercise-induced), Beta2 (ß2) adrenoreceptor agonists, cromoglycate, nedocromil sodium, steroids, xanthine derivatives, zafirlukast
- Angioedema: adrenaline, antihistamines, steroids
- Contact dermatitis: steroids, antihistamines
- Eczema: emollients, immune suppressants, steroids, UVA/UVB light treatment, wet wrapping, antihistamines
- Itching: antihistamines, emollients
- Urticaria: antihistamines, emollients, steroids

OTC remedies
- Conjunctivitis: antihistamines
- Gastric upset/irritation: as prescription medication
- Rhinitis: decongestants
- Angioedema: antihistamines
- Contact dermatitis: coal tar, emollients, steroids
- Eczema: emollients, hydrocortisone cream
- Itching: antihistamines, emollients
- Urticaria: calamine lotion, witch hazel

Alternative remedies
- Conjunctivitis: herbalism, homeopathy
- Gastric upset/irritation: aromatherapy, herbalism
- Rhinitis: aromatherapy
- Sneezing: acupuncture
- Asthma: acupuncture (mild asthma only), Buteyko method, homeopathy, relaxation techniques, yoga
- Contact dermatitis: aromatherapy, Bach flower remedies, homeopathy
- Eczema: aromatherapy, evening primrose oil, relaxation, herbalism, homeopathy, Chinese herbal medicine, Bach flower remedies
- Itching: aromatherapy, herbalism

- Flushing: herbalism
- Urticaria: aromatherapy, herbalism, homeopathy

Self-help tips: for symptom relief see *Conjunctivitis, Gastric upset/Irritation, Rhinitis, Sneezing, Asthma, Angioedema, Contact dermatitis, Eczema, Flushing, Itching, Urticaria* in the section on *Symptoms*

Alternative products that might not cause a reaction: sorghum, millet, buckwheat, barley

You might also react to: wild rice; wheat; corn

Room fragrancers
See *Perfume*

Rose Bengal
Rose Bengal is a dipotassium salt which is used as a dye and biological stain.

Type of allergen: contact

Likely sources of rose Bengal: chemical dyes, lipsticks

Symptoms, tests, treatments and self-help tips, see *Dyes*

Rosemary
Rosemary is the herb *Rosmarinus officinalis*. It contains *salicylates*, which have been linked to hyperactivity in children.

Type of allergen: contact, consumed

Symptoms, tests, treatments and self-help tips, see *Herbs*

You might also react to: others in the *Labiatae* family, such as marjoram, mint, oregano, sage, thyme; also basil

Rosin

See *Colophony*

Rubber

See *Benzene, Latex*

Rubber cement thinners

See *Solvents – aliphatic hydrocarbons*

Rye

Rye is the grain *Secale cereale*. Its salt-soluble proteins are indicated in baker's asthma. If symptoms start soon after beginning work and improve at weekends or on holidays, occupational asthma should be suspected.

Type of allergen: inhalant, contact, consumed

Likely sources of rye: bread, baked foods

Symptoms, tests, treatments and self-help tips, see *Grain*

You might also react to: wheat

Saffron

Saffron is the spice derived from the dried, powdered stigmas of the crocus *Crocus sativus*.

Type of allergen: consumed

Symptoms, tests, treatments and self-help tips, see *Spices*

Sage

Sage is the herb *Salvia officinalis*.

Type of allergen: contact

Symptoms, tests, treatments and self-help tips, see *Herbs*

You might also react to: others in the *Labiatae* family, such as marjoram, mint, oregano, rosemary, thyme; also basil, celery, potato, tobacco, tomato

Salicylamides

Salicylamides are the amid of salicylic acid.

Type of allergen: contact

Likely sources of salicylanides: antiseptic soaps, cosmetics

Symptoms
Skin reactions: photoallergenic contact dermatitis

Tests
• Photopatch testing: the allergen is placed on two skin sites; one is exposed to sunlight after 48 hours, and then both areas are examined for a rash
• Symptom diary

Treatments
Avoidance: check labels

Prescription medication: emollients, steroids

Self-help tips: for symptom relief see *Photoallergenic contact dermatitis* in the section on *Symptoms*

Salicylates

Salicylates are the salts of salicylic acid, or the salicylate esters of an organic acid. One of the best-known forms of *salicylates* is *aspirin*, which is acetylsalicylic acid.

Salicylates occur naturally in many foods; a lethal dose is 20g (roughly equivalent to 40 x 500mg aspirins). Salicylates are produced by plants, including willow bark and meadowsweet (*Spiraea ulmaria*).

Type of allergen: consumed

Likely sources of salicylates: almond, aniseed, apple, apricot, asparagus, banana, blackberry, blackcurrant, blueberry, cherry, cider, cider vinegar, cloves, citrus fruit, cranberry, cucumber, cumin, curry powder, currants, dates, dill, gooseberries, grape, liquorice, mace, melon, nectarines, orange, oregano, paprika, passion fruit, peach, peas, peppers (capsicum), pineapple, plum, prunes, raisin, raspberry, rosemary, strawberry, tarragon, thyme, tomatoes, turmeric, wine vinegar, Worcestershire sauce

Symptoms
Gastrointestinal reactions: diarrhoea, gastric upset/irritation

Mouth, nasal and ear reactions: swollen lips and tongue, rhinitis

Psychological problems: hyperactivity

Respiratory reactions: asthma, wheezing

Skin reactions: angioedema, itching, urticaria (this has been dismissed by some experts)

Tests
- Elimination diet
- Food challenge
- Symptom diary
- Exercise challenge

Treatments
Avoidance

Prescription medication
- Diarrhoea: antidiarrhoeal drugs
- Gastric upset/irritation: painkillers (use paracetamol rather than aspirin)
- Rhinitis: antihistamines, decongestants, sodium cromoglycate, immunotherapy
- Hyperactivity: stimulant drugs
- Asthma: anticholinergic drugs, antihistamines (exercise-induced), Beta2 (ß2) adrenoreceptor agonists, cromoglycate, nedocromil sodium, steroids, xanthine derivatives, zafirlukast
- Wheezing: bronchodilator
- Angioedema: adrenaline, antihistamines, steroids

- Itching: antihistamines, emollients
- Urticaria: antihistamines, emollients, steroids

OTC remedies
- Diarrhoea: kaolin and morphine, calcium carbonate, pectin
- Gastric upset/irritation: as prescription medication
- Rhinitis: decongestants
- Angioedema: antihistamines
- Itching: as prescription medication
- Urticaria: calamine lotion, witch hazel

Alternative remedies
- Diarrhoea: aromatherapy, herbalism, homeopathy
- Gastric upset/irritation: aromatherapy, herbalism
- Rhinitis: aromatherapy
- Hyperactivity: herbalism
- Asthma: acupuncture (mild asthma only), Buteyko method, homeopathy, relaxation techniques, yoga
- Itching: aromatherapy, herbalism
- Urticaria: aromatherapy, herbalism, homeopathy

Self-help tips: for symptom relief see *Diarrhoea, Gastric upset/ irritation, Rhinitis, Hyperactivity, Asthma, Wheezing, Angioedema, Itching, Urticaria* in the section on *Symptoms*

Alternative products that won't cause a reaction
Foods which contain no salicylate include:
- Fruit – banana, pear (peeled)
- Vegetables – green cabbage, celery, lentils, lettuce, potato (peeled)
- Cereals – oats, wheat
- Dairy products – cheese, milk, yoghurt, eggs
- Meats and fish – beef, chicken, salmon, tuna

You might also react to: aspirin, oil of wintergreen (*methyl salicylate*)

Salmon
See *Fish*

Sanitary products

Perfumed sanitary pads can cause skin problems.

Type of allergen: contact

Symptoms, tests, treatments and self-help tips, see *Cosmetics*
See also *Chlorine*

Sardine

See *Fish*

Sauerkraut

Histamine can be found in sauerkraut.

Type of allergen: consumed

Symptoms
Headaches: migraine

Skin reactions: angioedema, flushing, urticaria

Tests
* Elimination diet
* Food challenge
* Symptom diary

Treatments
Avoidance: check labels carefully and check with a dietitian to ensure that your diet is still nutritionally sound

Prescription medication
* Migraine: painkillers, anti-sickness drugs, ergotamine, 5-HT agonists, beta-blockers, sodium valproate, sumatryptan
* Angioedema: adrenaline, antihistamines, steroids
* Urticaria: antihistamines, emollients, steroids

OTC remedies
* Migraine: aspirin, ibuprofen, paracetamol
* Flushing: herbalism
* Urticaria: calamine lotion, witch hazel

Alternative remedies
- Migraine: acupuncture, Alexander technique, aromatherapy, chiropractic, herbalism, homeopathy, hypnosis, osteopathy, reflexology
- Flushing: herbalism
- Urticaria: aromatherapy, herbalism, homeopathy

Self-help tips: for symptom relief see *Migraine, Angioedema, Flushing, Urticaria* in the section on *Symptoms*

Sauces
See *Wheat*

Sausages

Histamine – produced by bacteria – can be found in sausages such as pepperoni and salami. Salami also contains the vasoactive amines *tyramine* and *phenylethylamine*, which cause the blood vessels to widen and may trigger migraines.

Type of allergen: consumed

Symptoms
Headache: migraine

Skin reactions: angioedema, flushing, urticaria

Tests
- Elimination diet
- Food challenge
- Symptom diary

Treatments
Avoidance
- Check labels carefully and check with a dietitian to ensure that your diet is still nutritionally sound

Prescription medication
- Headache: painkillers, non-steroidal anti-inflammatories
- Migraine: painkillers, anti-sickness drugs, ergotamine, 5-HT agonists, beta-blockers, sodium valproate, sumatryptan

- Angioedema: adrenaline, antihistamines, steroids
- Urticaria: antihistamines, emollients, steroids

OTC remedies
- Headache: as prescription medication
- Migraine: aspirin, ibuprofen, paracetamol
- Urticaria: calamine lotion, witch hazel

Alternative remedies
- Headache: acupuncture, aromatherapy, herbalism, homeopathy
- Migraine: acupuncture, Alexander technique, aromatherapy, chiropractic, herbalism, homeopathy, hypnosis, osteopathy, reflexology
- Flushing: herbalism
- Urticaria: aromatherapy, herbalism, homeopathy

Self-help tips: for symptom relief see *Migraine, Angioedema, Flushing, Urticaria* in the section on *Symptoms*

Scallops
See *Shellfish*

Scissors
See *Nickel*

Seafood
See *Fish, Shellfish*

Sedatives
Chlormethiazole – a sedative used for short-term treatment of insomnia – may cause eye irritation, nasal congestion, rash and anaphylaxis.

Type of allergen: consumed

Symptoms, tests, treatments and self-help tips, see *Drugs*

Selenium

Selenium is a metallic element, chemical symbol Se.

Type of allergen: contact

Likely sources of selenium: photocells

Symptoms, tests, treatments and self-help tips, see *Metals*

Semen

Seminal plasma protein allergy (SPPA) is a rare immune response to human semen; sufferers often have recurrent vaginitis associated with intercourse and do not respond to traditional therapies. Prevalence is difficult to determine because of the sensitive nature of the symptoms and resultant underreporting.

Type of allergen: contact

Symptoms
Skin reactions: angioedema, blisters, contact dermatitis, inflammation, itching, skin irritation

Tests
- CAP-RAST
- Symptom diary

Treatments
- Cromolyn vaginal cream for local reactions
- Immunotherapy with human seminal plasma

Semolina
See *Wheat*

Senna

Senna is the leaves of the plant *Cassia acutifolia*, used as a laxative.

Type of allergen: consumed

Symptoms
Mouth, nasal and ear reactions: itching mouth/palate

Tests
• Symptom diary

Treatments
Prescription medication: painkillers

OTC remedies: painkillers

You might also react to: beans, chick peas, lentil, liquorice, pea, peanut, soy

For symptom relief, see *Itching/burning mouth/palate* in the section on *Symptoms*

Serotonin
Serotonin (5-hydroxy-tryptamine) is a biogenic amine derived from the amino acid tryptophan, which is found in fish, meat, herbs, dairy products. It is a neurotransmitter which is associated with mood, appetite, sex and sleep.

It is present in the platelets in the blood; when it is released, it is involved with blood clotting and inflammation.

Too much tryptophan-rich protein can cause problems such as migraine and joint problems.

Type of allergen: consumed

Likely sources of serotonin: avocado, banana, cheese, chocolate, pickled fish, octopus, pineapple, plums, tomatoes, wines. Processing the foods can increase the concentration.

Symptoms
Headache: migraine

Other reactions: joint pain and swelling, weight gain

Tests
• Elimination diet
• Food challenge
• Symptom diary

Treatments
Avoidance: check labels carefully and check with a dietitian to ensure that your diet is still nutritionally sound

Prescription medication
- Migraine: painkillers, anti-sickness drugs, ergotamine, 5-HT agonists, beta-blockers, sodium valproate, sumatryptan
- Joint pain and swelling: anti-inflammatory drugs, painkillers, steroids

OTC remedies
- Migraine: aspirin, ibuprofen, paracetamol
- Joint pain and swelling: aspirin, paracetamol

Alternative remedies
- Migraine: acupuncture, Alexander technique, aromatherapy, chiropractic, herbalism, homeopathy, hypnosis, osteopathy, reflexology
- Joint pain and swelling: acupuncture, aromatherapy, herbalism, homeopathy

Self-help tips: for symptom relief see *Migraine, Joint pain* in the section on *Symptoms*

Sesame
Sesame is the plant *Sesamum indicum*. Its seeds are used as a food and also for producing oil. Sesame oil contains sesamolin, sesamin and sesamol, which can cause contact dermatitis.

Type of allergen: contact, consumed

Likely sources of sesame: halva, tahini, sesame seed oil, rolls, bread, bagels, breadsticks, crackers, poppadoms, vegeburgers, rice cakes, sesame bars

Symptoms
Anaphylactic shock

Headache

Skin reactions: contact dermatitis (including occupational)

Tests
- Blood test: CAP-RAST test
- Blood test: ELISA
- Elimination diet
- Food challenge
- Symptom diary

Treatments
Avoidance
- Check labels carefully for sesame and sesame oil and check with a dietitian to ensure that your diet is still nutritionally sound. In occupational situations, use protective equipment such as gloves.

Prescription medication
- Anaphylactic shock: adrenaline, antihistamines, steroids
- Headache: painkillers, non-steroidal anti-inflammatories
- Contact dermatitis: steroids, antihistamines

OTC remedies
- Headache: as prescription medication
- Contact dermatitis: coal tar, emollients, steroids

Alternative remedies
- Headache: acupuncture, aromatherapy, herbalism, homeopathy
- Contact dermatitis: aromatherapy, Bach flower remedies, homeopathy

Self-help tips: for symptom relief see *Headache, Contact dermatitis* in the section on *Symptoms*

Shallot
Shallot is a type of onion, *Allium ascalonicum*.

Type of allergen: consumed

Symptoms, tests, treatments and self-help tips, see *Onion*

You might also react to: asparagus, chives, garlic, leek, onion

Shampoos
Type of allergen: contact

Symptoms, tests, treatments and self-help tips, see
Cosmetics
See also *Butyl alcohol, Formaldehyde*

Shaving products
Type of allergen: contact

Symptoms, tests, treatments and self-help tips, see
Cosmetics
See also *Linseed oil*

Sheepskin
See *Wool, Animal hair*

Shellac
Shellac is a thermoplastic resin material dissolved in methyl
alcohol. See *Resin, Formaldehyde, Methyl alcohol, Solvents –
alcohol solvents*

Type of allergen: inhalant

Shellac thinner
See *Amyl alcohol, Solvents – alcohol solvents*

Shellfish
Shellfish is the third most common food allergy after *eggs* and
milk.

Shellfish can cause occupational asthma in fish and shellfish
workers, particularly if automatic gutting machines are used; if
symptoms start soon after beginning work and improve at
weekends or on holidays, occupational asthma should be
suspected.

You're most likely to react to shrimp, crab, crayfish, lobster,
oysters, clams, scallops, mussels, squid, and snails; the major
allergens in shellfish are tropomyosin. Shrimp, lobster and

crayfish have common allergens so you may react to all three.

Reactions usually appear within two hours but may be delayed up to twenty-four.

Type of allergen: inhalant, contact, consumed

Symptoms
Anaphylactic shock

Gastrointestinal reactions: abdominal pain, diarrhoea, gastric upset, heartburn, nausea, vomiting, wind

Headache: migraine

Mouth, nasal and ear reactions: rhinitis

Respiratory reactions: asthma (including occupational), wheezing

Skin reactions: angioedema, dermatitis, eczema, flushed face, itching, urticaria

Tests
• Blood test: CAP-RAST
• Blood test: ELISA – clam, crab, langoustines (spiny lobster), lobster, mussel, oyster, shrimp, snail
• Elimination diet
• Food challenge
• Symptom diary (including peak flow meter readings)

Treatments
Avoidance
• Avoid eating fish and any dish that may contain fish (or has been cooked in the same pan as fish, if your reaction is severe) – check labels and check with a dietitian to ensure that your diet is still nutritionally sound
• In an occupational situation, use protective equipment such as gloves and masks. Improved ventilation may also help.

Prescription medication
• Anaphylactic shock: adrenaline, antihistamines, steroids
• Abdominal pain and swelling: antacids, anti-spasmodic drugs
• Diarrhoea: antidiarrhoeal drugs

- Gastric upset/irritation: painkillers (use paracetamol rather than aspirin)
- Heartburn: antacids, alginates
- Nausea: as prescription medication
- Vomiting: anti-emetics
- Wind: as prescription medication
- Migraine: painkillers, anti-sickness drugs, ergotamine, 5-HT agonists, beta-blockers, sodium valproate, sumatryptan
- Rhinitis: antihistamines, decongestants, sodium cromoglycate, immunotherapy
- Asthma: anticholinergic drugs, antihistamines (exercise-induced), Beta2 (ß2) adrenoreceptor agonists, cromoglycate, nedocromil sodium, steroids, xanthine derivatives, zafirlukast
- Wheezing: bronchodilator
- Angioedema: adrenaline, antihistamines, steroids
- Contact dermatitis: steroids, antihistamines
- Eczema: emollients, immune suppressants, steroids, UVA/UVB light treatment, wet wrapping, antihistamines
- Itching: antihistamines, emollients
- Urticaria: antihistamines, emollients, steroids

OTC remedies
- Abdominal pain and swelling: antacids
- Diarrhoea: kaolin and morphine, calcium carbonate, pectin
- Gastric upset/irritation: as prescription medication
- Heartburn: as prescription medication
- Nausea: antihistamines
- Vomiting: oral rehydration solution
- Wind: antacids
- Migraine: aspirin, ibuprofen, paracetamol
- Rhinitis: decongestants
- Angioedema: antihistamines
- Contact dermatitis: coal tar, emollients, steroids
- Eczema: emollients, hydrocortisone cream
- Itching: antihistamines, emollients
- Urticaria: calamine lotion, witch hazel

Alternative remedies
- Abdominal pain and swelling: aromatherapy, herbalism, homeopathy
- Diarrhoea: aromatherapy, herbalism, homeopathy
- Gastric upset/irritation: aromatherapy, herbalism
- Heartburn: aromatherapy, homeopathy, herbalism

- Nausea: aromatherapy, herbalism, homeopathy
- Vomiting: herbalism
- Wind: aromatherapy, herbalism, homeopathy
- Migraine: acupuncture, Alexander technique, aromatherapy, chiropractic, herbalism, homeopathy, hypnosis, osteopathy, reflexology
- Rhinitis: aromatherapy
- Asthma: acupuncture (mild asthma only), Buteyko method, homeopathy, relaxation techniques, yoga
- Contact dermatitis: aromatherapy, Bach flower remedies, homeopathy
- Eczema: aromatherapy, evening primrose oil, relaxation, herbalism, homeopathy, Chinese herbal medicine, Bach flower remedies
- Flushing: herbalism
- Itching: aromatherapy, herbalism
- Urticaria: aromatherapy, herbalism, homeopathy

Self-help tips: for symptom relief see *Abdominal pain, Diarrhoea, Gastric upset, Heartburn, Nausea, Vomiting, Wind, Migraine, Rhinitis, Asthma, Wheezing, Angioedema, Eczema, Flushing, Itching, Urticaria* in the section on *Symptoms*

Shock absorber fluids
See *Solvents – glycol ether*

Shoes
See *Latex, Leather, Paraphenylenediamine (PPDA)*

Shoe polish
See *Chromium*

Silk
See *Mercury*

Silk screen poster inks
See *Solvents – aliphatic hydrocarbons*

Silver
Silver is a metallic element, chemical symbol Ag.

Type of allergen: contact

Likely sources of silver: jewellery, photographic chemicals

Symptoms, tests, treatments and self-help tips, see *Metals*

Silver nitrate
See *Hair dyes*

Skincare products (creams, lubricants, preparations)
Perfumes and preservatives tend to cause most problems.

Type of allergen: contact

Symptoms, tests, treatments and self-help tips, see *Cosmetics*
See also *Camphor oil*

Snail
See *Shellfish*

Soap
Soap contains an alkaline irritant. Perfumes and preservatives may also cause problems.

Type of allergen: contact

Symptoms, tests, treatments and self-help tips, see *Cosmetics*

Alternative products that won't cause a reaction: Soap substitute: preferably aqueous cream, or emulsifying ointment.
See also *Benzophenones, Benzyl acetate, Bithionol, Bitter almond oil, Caraway, Cedarwood oil, Coconut oil, Colophony, Cosmetics, Dichlorophen, Digalloyl trioleate, Hexachlorophene, Isopropanol, Linseed oil, Patchouli oil, Salicylanides, Solvents – alcohol solvents, Thiurams*

Sodium benzoate, Sodium bisulphite
See *Food additives – preservatives*

Sodium carbonates
See *Food additives – anti-caking agents*

Sodium guanylate
See *Food additives – flavour enhancers*

Sodium metabisulphite, Sodium nitrite, Sodium propionate
See *Food additives – preservatives*

Sodium pyrophosphate
See *Food additives – emulsifiers, stabilizers and thickeners*

Sodium sulphite
See *Food additives – preservatives*

Sodium 5'-inosinate, Sodium 5'-ribonucleotide
See *Food additives – flavour enhancers*

Soft furnishings
See *Dust mites*

Soldering fumes
See *Colophony*

Sole
See *Fish*

Solvents

Solvents are liquids that clean, dissolve or thin other materials. If the materials are not soluble in water (e.g. grease, resins, oils, varnish, paint and laquers), you'll need to use organic solvents. They can cause occupational asthma; if symptoms start soon after beginning work and improve at weekends or on holidays, occupational asthma should be suspected.

The lower the boiling point of the solvent, the more volatile they are and the more quickly they evaporate and accumulate as vapours in the air.

Type of allergen: inhalant, contact

Alcohol solvents

Alcohol solvents are used as base materials for further processing of other chemicals such as esters, plasticizers and synthetic lubricants. The most common types are ethanol, isoamyl alcohol, isobutyl alcohol, isooctanol, isopropanol, methanol, methyl alcohol, methyl cyclohexanol, methyl isobutyl carbinol, n-butanol and cyclohexanol.

Aliphatic hydrocarbons

Aliphatic hydrocarbons – also called petroleum distillates – are common components of oil and alkyd-based coatings and adhesives. The most common types are cyclohexane, mineral spirits, nonane, paint thinner, pentane, petroleum naptha, octane. They can cause occupational asthma; if symptoms start soon after beginning work and improve at weekends or on holidays, occupational asthma should be suspected.

Likely sources of aliphatic hydrocarbons include carpet cleaning fluids, cosmetics, dry cleaning fluids, glues, paint thinners, pesticides, rubber cement thinners, silk screen poster inks, white spirit (paint thinner)

Aromatic hydrocarbons

Aromatic hydrocarbons are components and reducer solvents for industrial and fast dry alkyd enamels, spray enamels, many specialty coatings and adhesives; they are produced by distillation of petroleum or coal tar. The most common types are benzene, diethylbenzene, ethylbenzene, methylnaphthalene, phenol, styrene, toluene, xylene. They can cause occupational asthma; if symptoms start soon after beginning work and improve at weekends or on holidays, occupational asthma should be suspected.

Likely sources of aromatic hydrocarbons include: aerosol spray cans, engine cleaners, fluorescent dye solvent, furniture made from particle board, lacquer thinners, nitrocellulose and acrylic lacquer coatings and reducers, paint strippers, paint and varnish remover, resin solvent

Chlorinated hydrocarbons

Chlorinated hydrocarbons include tetracloroethane (acetylene tetrachloride), chloroform, ethylene dichloride, methylene chloride (dichloromethane), perchloroethylene and trichloroethylene. They can cause occupational asthma; if symptoms start soon after beginning work and improve at weekends or on holidays, occupational asthma should be suspected.

Likely sources of chlorinated hydrocarbons include: wax, oil, resin, grease and plastics solvent; paint stripper.

Esters

Esters are the reaction products of acids with monohydric or polyhydric alcohols. The most common types are n-amyl acetate, ethyl acetate, n-propyl acetate, isobutyl acetate, n-butyl acetate, vinyl acetate, ethyl acrylate, diethyl maleate and ethyl silicate.

They can cause occupational asthma; if symptoms start soon after beginning work and improve at weekends or on holidays, occupational asthma should be suspected.

Likely sources of esters include lacquer coatings and solvents, nail polishes and removers, vinyl coatings, adhesives. latex emulsion polymers, thermoplast and thermoset plastics.

Glycols

Glycols are colourless hygroscopic liquids made by hydrolysis of epoxyethane. The most common types are diethylene glycol, ethylene glycol, glycerol, hexylene glycol, propylene glycol. They can cause occupational asthma; if symptoms start soon after beginning work and improve at weekends or on holidays, occupational asthma should be suspected.

Likely sources of glycols include antifreeze (ethylene glycol and propylene glycol), cosmetics, lubricants, plastisizers, water-based emulsion paints (ethylene glycol).

Glycol ether solvents

The most common types of glycol ether solvents are diethylene glycol monobutyl ether (DGMBE), ethylene glycol monobutyl ether (EGMBE), ethylene glycol monoethyl ether (EGEE), propylene glycol methyl ether (PGME), propylene glycol n-butyl ether (PnB). They can cause occupational asthma; if symptoms start soon after beginning work and improve at weekends or on holidays, occupational asthma should be suspected.

Likely sources of glycol ether solvents include coatings, chemical processes, hydraulic brake fluids, shock absorber fluids, hydraulic fluids, stains, inks, some insecticides and dry cleaning solvents.

Halogenated solvents

Halogenated solvents dissolve oils and evaporate rapidly. The most common types are carbon tetrachloride, chloroform, dichlorobenzene, ethylene dichloride, methylene chloride, perchloroethylene, propylene dichloride, 1,1,1-trichloroethane, trichloroethylene. They can cause occupational asthma; if symptoms start soon after beginning work and improve at weekends or on holidays, occupational asthma should be suspected.

Likely sources of halogenated solvents include aerosol propellants, dry cleaning fluids, degreasing solvents, electrical cleaning solvents, inks, paint strippers.

Ketone solvents

Ketone solvents are used in lacquer, cement, nail polish and vinyl coatings

The most common types are acetone, cyclohexanone, dimethyl ketone, isophorone, methyl amyl ketone (MAK), methyl ethyl ketone (MEK), methyl isobutyl ketone (MIBK), and 2-propanone.

They can cause occupational asthma; if symptoms start soon after beginning work and improve at weekends or on holidays, occupational asthma should be suspected.

Likely sources of ketone solvents include the production of plastics, photographic films and synthetic materials; dewaxing of lubricating oils; furniture made from particle board.

Symptoms

Eye reactions
• Conjunctivitis – alcohol solvents, aliphatic hydrocarbons, esters, ketone solvents

Gastrointestinal reactions
• Nausea – alcohol solvents, aliphatic hydrocarbons
• Vomiting – alcohol solvents, aliphatic hydrocarbons

Mouth, nasal and ear reactions
• Rhinitis – esters, ketone solvents

Respiratory reactions
• Occupational asthma (alcohol solvents, aliphatic hydrocarbons, aromatic hydrocarbons, chlorinated hydrocarbons, esters, glycols, glycol ether solvents, halogenated solvents)

- Breathing problems – alcohol solvents, aromatic hydrocarbons, chlorinated hydrocarbons, esters, glycol ether solvents, halogenated solvents, ketone solvents

Skin reactions
- Irritant dermatitis (alcohol solvents, aliphatic hydrocarbons, aromatic hydrocarbons, chlorinated hydrocarbons, esters, glycols, glycol ether solvents, halogenated solvents, ketone solvents)
- Skin irritation (alcohol solvents, aliphatic hydrocarbons, aromatic hydrocarbons, chlorinated hydrocarbons, esters, glycols, glycol ether solvents, halogenated solvents, ketone solvents)
- Inflammation (alcohol solvents, aliphatic hydrocarbons, aromatic hydrocarbons, chlorinated hydrocarbons, esters, glycols, glycol ether solvents, halogenated solvents, ketone solvents)

Tests
- Skin patch
- Symptom diary (including peak flow meter readings)

Treatments

Avoidance
- In occupational situations, use protective equipment such as gloves, goggles and masks. Improved ventilation may also help.

Prescription medication
- Conjunctivitis: antihistamines, cromoglycate, nedocromil sodium, steroids, sympathomimetics
- Nausea: antihistamines
- Vomiting: anti-emetics
- Rhinitis: antihistamines, decongestants, sodium cromoglycate, immunotherapy
- Asthma: anticholinergic drugs, antihistamines (exercise-induced), Beta2 (ß2) adrenoreceptor agonists, cromoglycate, nedocromil sodium, steroids, xanthine derivatives, zafirlukast
- Breathing problems: bronchodilators, corticosteroids
- Irritant dermatitis: steroids, antihistamines
- Inflammation: antihistamines, emollients, steroids
- Skin irritation: emollients

OTC remedies
- Conjunctivitis: antihistamines
- Nausea: as prescription medication
- Vomiting: oral rehydration solution
- Rhinitis: decongestants
- Irritant dermatitis: coal tar, emollients, steroids
- Inflammation: antihistamines, emollients
- Skin irritation: as prescription medication

Alternative remedies
- Conjunctivitis: herbalism, homeopathy
- Nausea: aromatherapy, herbalism, homeopathy
- Vomiting: herbalism
- Rhinitis: aromatherapy
- Asthma: acupuncture (mild asthma only), Buteyko method, homeopathy, relaxation techniques, yoga
- Irritant dermatitis: aromatherapy, Bach flower remedies, homeopathy

Self-help tips
- Wash hands with a mild soap and water after exposure to solvents, and apply a fragrance-free skin moisturizer. Never wash hands in solvents. Baby oil or vegetable oils can remove paint from the skin
- For symptom relief, see *Conjunctivitis, Nausea, Vomiting, Rhinitis, Asthma, Breathing problems, Contact dermatitis, Skin irritation, Inflammation* in the section on *Symptoms*

Sorbic acid
See *Food additives – preservatives*

Sorbitol
See *Food additives – emulsifiers, stabilizers and thickeners*

Soy sauce
Soy sauce contains the vasoactive amine *tyramine*, which causes the blood vessels to widen and may trigger migraines.

Type of allergen: consumed

Symptoms
Headache: migraine

Skin reactions: flushing, urticaria

Tests
- Elimination diet
- Food challenge
- Symptom diary

Treatments
Avoidance
- Check labels carefully and check with a dietitian to ensure that your diet is still nutritionally sound

Prescription medication
- Headache: painkillers, non-steroidal anti-inflammatories
- Migraine: painkillers, anti-sickness drugs, ergotamine, 5-HT agonists, beta-blockers, sodium valproate, sumatryptan
- Angioedema: adrenaline, antihistamines, steroids
- Urticaria: antihistamines, emollients, steroids

OTC remedies
- Headache: as prescription medication
- Migraine: aspirin, ibuprofen, paracetamol
- Urticaria: calamine lotion, witch hazel

Alternative remedies
- Headache: acupuncture, aromatherapy, herbalism, homeopathy
- Migraine: acupuncture, Alexander technique, aromatherapy, chiropractic, herbalism, homeopathy, hypnosis, osteopathy, reflexology
- Flushing: herbalism
- Urticaria: aromatherapy, herbalism, homeopathy

Self-help tips: for symptom relief see *Headache, Migraine, Flushing, Urticaria* in the section on *Symptoms*
See also *Yeast*

Soya

Soya comes from the leguminous plant *soja hispida*. It is most widely used as an oil; it also used as flour, and is the protein in textured vegetable protein or TVP. Reactions tend to be more in small children than in adults. The problem is with soya protein, though you may also react if it's genetically modified soya that contains brazil nut protein.

* Soya can also cause asthma if the dust or flour is inhaled.
* Soya protein: found in infant milk formulas, baked foods, canned tuna, soups and sauces – is another allergen encountered. Peanut and soya oils are generally non-allergenic and safe to use in the diet.

Type of allergen: consumed

Likely sources of soya: vegetarian ready meals, burgers, gluten-free products – also bread, breakfast cereals, confectionery, desserts, meat products

Symptoms
Anaphylactic shock: rarely

Eye reactions: conjunctivitis

Gastrointestinal reactions: abdominal pain and swelling, colitis, diarrhoea, gastric upset/irritation, vomiting

Headaches

Mouth, nasal and ear reactions: rhinitis

Psychological problems: irritability (in children)

Respiratory reactions: asthma, breathing problems, cough, wheezing

Skin reactions: angioedema, atopic dermatitis, contact dermatitis, eczema, itching, urticaria

Other reactions: weight loss

Tests
* Blood test: CAP-RAST
* Blood test: ELISA

- Skin prick test
- Elimination diet
- Food challenge
- Symptom diary (including peak flow meter readings)

Treatments
Avoidance
- Check labels carefully and check with a dietitian to ensure that your diet is still nutritionally sound. Check labels for soya flour, soya meat, soy sauce, soya meal, soya milk, soya yoghurts, soya cheese; avoid anything on the following list: emulsifiers, hydrolyzed plant protein (HPP), hydrolyzed vegetable protein (HVP), lecithin, miso, modified food starch, mono-diglyceride soy, soy, soya, stabilizers, tempeh, textured vegetable protein (TVP), tofu, vegetable gum, vegetable oil, vegetable paste, vegetable protein concentrate, vegetable starch

Prescription medication
- Anaphylactic shock: adrenaline, antihistamines, steroids
- Conjunctivitis: antihistamines, cromoglycate, nedocromil sodium, steroids, sympathomimetics
- Abdominal pain and swelling: antacids, anti-spasmodic drugs
- Colitis: aminosalicylates, immunosuppressants, steroids, sulphasalazine
- Diarrhoea: antidiarrhoeal drugs
- Gastric upset/irritation: painkillers (use paracetamol rather than aspirin)
- Vomiting: anti-emetics
- Headache: painkillers, non-steroidal anti-inflammatories
- Rhinitis: antihistamines, decongestants, sodium cromoglycate, immunotherapy
- Asthma: anticholinergic drugs, antihistamines (exercise-induced), Beta2 (ß2) adrenoreceptor agonists, cromoglycate, nedocromil sodium, steroids, xanthine derivatives, zafirlukast
- Breathing problems: bronchodilators, corticosteroids
- Cough: antihistamines, bronchodilators, corticosteroids
- Wheezing: bronchodilator
- Angioedema: adrenaline, antihistamines, steroids
- Contact dermatitis: steroids, antihistamines
- Eczema: emollients, immune suppressants, steroids, UVA/UVB light treatment, wet wrapping, antihistamines
- Itching: antihistamines, emollients
- Urticaria: antihistamines, emollients, steroids

OTC remedies
- Conjunctivitis: antihistamines
- Abdominal pain and swelling: antacids
- Diarrhoea: kaolin and morphine, calcium carbonate, pectin
- Gastric upset/irritation: as prescription medication
- Vomiting: oral rehydration solution
- Headache: as prescription medication
- Rhinitis: decongestants
- Cough: demulcents, antitussives, expectorants
- Angioedema: antihistamines
- Contact dermatitis: coal tar, emollients, steroids
- Eczema: emollients, hydrocortisone cream
- Itching: as prescription medication
- Urticaria: calamine lotion, witch hazel

Alternative remedies
- Conjunctivitis: herbalism, homeopathy
- Abdominal pain and swelling: aromatherapy, herbalism, homeopathy
- Colitis: herbalism
- Diarrhoea: aromatherapy, herbalism, homeopathy
- Gastric upset/irritation: aromatherapy, herbalism
- Vomiting: herbalism
- Headache: acupuncture, aromatherapy, herbalism, homeopathy
- Rhinitis: aromatherapy
- Asthma: acupuncture (mild asthma only), Buteyko method, homeopathy, relaxation techniques, yoga
- Cough: aromatherapy, homeopathy
- Contact dermatitis: aromatherapy, Bach flower remedies, homeopathy
- Eczema: aromatherapy, evening primrose oil, relaxation, herbalism, homeopathy, Chinese herbal medicine, Bach flower remedies
- Itching: aromatherapy, herbalism
- Urticaria: aromatherapy, herbalism, homeopathy

Self-help tips: for symptom relief see *Conjunctivitis, Abdominal pain and swelling, Colitis, Diarrhoea, Gastric upset/Irritation, Vomiting, Headache, Rhinitis, Weight loss, Asthma, Breathing problems, Cough, Wheezing, Angioedema, Contact dermatitis, Eczema, Itching, Urticaria* in the section on *Symptoms*

Alternative products that won't cause a reaction: sesame oil

You might also react to: beans, beansprouts, carob, chick peas, lentil, liquorice, pea, peanut, soy

Spelt

Spelt is a type of wheat, *Triticum spelta*.

Type of allergen: contact, consumed

Likely sources of spelt: bakery goods, flour

Symptoms, tests, treatments and self-help tips, see *Grain*

Spices

For further information about the spices themselves and cross-reactivity, see *Allspice, Anise, Aniseed, Caraway, Cardamom, Cayenne pepper, Chilli pepper, Cinnamon, Clove, Cumin, Curry Powder, Fenugreek, Ginger, Horseradish, Juniper berry, Mace, Mustard, Nutmeg, Paprika, Pepper, Saffron, Turmeric, Vanilla*
    Spicy food can also cause cystitis.

Symptoms
Anaphylactic shock
• Anise, cumin, curry powder, mustard, saffron

Eye reactions
• Stinging – cinnamon

Gastrointestinal reactions
• Abdominal pain – cayenne pepper, pepper (black and white), saffron
• Gastric upset/irritation – cinnamon, horseradish, mustard
• Nausea – anise
• Vomiting – horseradish, mustard

Mouth, nasal and ear reactions
• Itching mouth/palate – clove, mustard

- Rhinitis – mustard, pepper (black and white)
- Sneezing – mustard

Psychological problems
Hyperactivity – aniseed, clove, cumin, curry powder, mace, paprika, turmeric

Respiratory reactions
- Asthma (occupational) – anise, cinnamon, fenugreek, mace
- Asthma – aniseed, cumin
- Wheezing – aniseed, clove, cumin, curry powder, fenugreek, mace, paprika, turmeric

Skin reactions
- Angioedema – anise, aniseed, clove, cumin, curry powder, horseradish, mace, mustard, paprika, saffron, turmeric
- Atopic dermatitis – allspice, caraway, cardamom, cayenne pepper, cinnamon, clove, fenugreek, ginger, mace, pepper (black and white)
- Contact dermatitis, including occupational – allspice, caraway, cardamom, cayenne pepper, cinnamon, clove, cumin, curry powder, ginger, horseradish, juniper berry, mace, mustard, nutmeg, paprika, pepper (black and white), turmeric, vanilla
- Eczema – allspice, cardamom, clove, ginger, mace, pepper (black and white)
- Flushing – nutmeg
- Skin irritation – aniseed, clove oil, cumin, mace
- Urticaria (this has been dismissed by some experts) – aniseed, clove, cumin, curry powder, horseradish, mustard, mace, paprika, saffron, turmeric

Other reactions: weight loss – cinnamon

Tests
- Blood test: CAP-RAST (allspice, anise, caraway, cardamom, chilli pepper, cinnamon, curry powder, fenugreek, ginger, mace, mustard, nutmeg, paprika, pepper (black and white), saffron, vanilla)
- Blood test: ELISA (allspice, aniseed, cumin, curry powder, ginger, juniper, mustard, nutmeg, paprika, pepper – black and white, saffron, turmeric, vanilla)
- Skin test: skin prick (anise, aniseed, caraway, cardamom, cayenne pepper, cumin, curry powder, fenugreek, horseradish, mustard, paprika, pepper – black and white)

- Skin test: intradermal (paprika)
- Skin test: patch test (cayenne pepper, cinnamon, cumin, curry powder, ginger, nutmeg)
- Elimination diet (anise, aniseed, cayenne pepper, chilli pepper, cinnamon, cumin, curry powder, ginger, horseradish, mace, mustard, paprika, pepper – black and white, saffron, turmeric, vanilla)
- Food challenge (anise, aniseed, cayenne pepper, chilli pepper, cinnamon, cumin, curry powder, ginger, horseradish, mace, mustard, paprika, pepper – black and white, saffron, turmeric, vanilla)
- Symptom diary (including peak flow meter readings)

Treatments
Avoidance
- In occupational situations, use protective equipment such as gloves or masks; improved ventilation may also help.
- Check labels carefully and check with a dietitian to ensure that your diet is still nutritionally sound

Prescription medication
- Anaphylactic shock: adrenaline, antihistamines, steroids
- Abdominal pain and swelling: antacids, anti-spasmodic drugs
- Gastric upset/irritation: painkillers (use paracetamol rather than aspirin)
- Nausea: antihistamines
- Vomiting: anti-emetics
- Itching/burning mouth/palate: painkillers
- Rhinitis: antihistamines, decongestants, sodium cromoglycate, immunotherapy
- Hyperactivity: stimulant drugs
- Asthma: anticholinergic drugs, antihistamines (exercise-induced), Beta2 (ß2) adrenoreceptor agonists, cromoglycate, nedocromil sodium, steroids, xanthine derivatives, zafirlukast
- Wheezing: bronchodilator
- Angioedema: adrenaline, antihistamines, steroids
- Dermatitis: steroids, antihistamines
- Eczema: emollients, immune suppressants, steroids, UVA/UVB light treatment, wet wrapping, antihistamines
- Skin irritation: emollients
- Urticaria: antihistamines, emollients, steroids

OTC remedies
- Abdominal pain and swelling: antacids
- Gastric upset/irritation: as prescription medication
- Nausea: as prescriptin medication
- Vomiting: oral rehydration solution
- Itching/burning mouth/palate: as prescriptin medication
- Rhinitis: decongestants
- Dermatitis: coal tar, emollients, steroids
- Eczema: emollients, hydrocortisone cream
- Urticaria: calamine lotion, witch hazel

- **Alternative remedies**
- Abdominal pain and swelling: aromatherapy, herbalism, homeopathy
- Gastric upset/irritation: aromatherapy, herbalism
- Nausea: aromatherapy, herbalism, homeopathy
- Vomiting: herbalism
- Rhinitis: aromatherapy
- Angioedema: antihistamines
- Contact dermatitis: aromatherapy, Bach flower remedies, homeopathy
- Eczema: aromatherapy, evening primrose oil, relaxation, herbalism, homeopathy, Chinese herbal medicine, Bach flower remedies
- Flushing: herbalism
- Urticaria: aromatherapy, herbalism, homeopathy

Self-help tips: for symptom relief see *Conjunctivitis, Abdominal pain and swelling, Gastric upset/Irritation, Nausea, Vomiting, Itching/burning mouth/palate, Rhinitis, Sneezing, Asthma, Wheezing, Angioedema, Contact dermatitis, Eczema, Flushing, Skin irritation, Urticaria* in the section on *Symptoms*
See also *Aromatherapy oils*

Spinach
Spinach is the vegetable *Spinacia oleracea*. It contains the vasoactive amine tyramine, which causes the blood vessels to widen and may trigger migraines. It also contains high levels of *histamine* and contains oxalates, a derivative of oxalic acid. Spinach powder is used as a food dye.

Type of allergen: contact, consumed

Symptoms, tests, treatments and self-help tips, see *Vegetables*

You might also react to: latex, birch pollen

Spiny lobster
See *Shellfish*

Spirits
See *Yeast*

Spores
See *Moulds*

Squash

Squash is a pumpkin-like fruit from genus *Cucurbita*.

Type of allergen: consumed

Symptoms, tests, treatments and self-help tips, see *Vegetables*

You might also react to: others in the *Cucurbitaceae* family, such as courgette, cucumber, marrow, melon, pumpkin, watermelon

Squid
See *Shellfish*

Stains
See *Solvents – glycol ether*

Stain proofing
See *Volatile organic compounds*

Stain remover
See *Benzene, Isocyanates*

Steel, chrome
See *Chromium*

Steel, stainless
See *Chromium*

Sterilizers
See *Chlorine*

Sterilizing fluid
See *Glutaraldehyde*

Stock cubes
See *Yeast*

Strawberries

Strawberries are the fruit of the plant *Fragaria vesca*. They contain *salicylates*, which have been linked to hyperactivity in children, and oxalates, a derivative of oxalic acid. Strawberries trigger the production of *histamine* and there may also be a link with sensitivity to acetylsalicylic acid. Strawberry seeds may irritate colitis.

Type of allergen: contact, consumed

Symptoms, tests, treatments and self-help tips, see *Fruit*

You might also react to: blackberries, raspberries

Streptomycin

Streptomycin is an antibiotic, also used as an anti-tuberculosis drug.

Type of allergen: contact, consumed

Symptoms, tests, treatments and self-help tips, see *Drugs*

You might also react to: *gentamycin*

Styrene

Styrene is used in the production of styrene polymers such as polystyrene plastics, styrene butadiene latex emulsions and rubber, acrylonitrile butadiene-styrene (ABS), and styrenated alkyd coatings; it is also used as a reactive solvent in polyester compositions.

Type of allergen: inhalant
See *Solvents – aromatic hydrocarbons*

Sugar

Sugar is thought to cause hyperactivity but is not an allergen as such.

Symptoms
Gastrointestinal reactions: heartburn

Psychological problems: hyperactivity

Tests
- Blood test: ELISA
- Elimination diet
- Food challenge
- Symptom diary

Treatments
Avoidance
- Check labels carefully and check with a dietitian to ensure that your diet is still nutritionally sound

Prescription medication
- Heartburn: antacids, alginates
- Hyperactivity: stimulant drugs

OTC remedies
- Heartburn: as prescription medication

Alternative remedies
- Heartburn: aromatherapy, homeopathy, herbalism
- Hyperactivity: herbalism

Self-help tips: for symptom relief see *Heartburn, Hyperactivity* in the section on *Symptoms*

Sulfamethoxazol

Sulfamethoxazol is an antibiotic used for urinary tract and respiratory tract infections.

Type of allergen: contact, consumed

Symptoms, tests, treatments and self-help tips, see *Drugs*

Sulphadiazine, Sulphadimidine, Sulphametopyrazine

See *Drugs, Sulphonamides*

Sulphonamides

Sulphonamides are a group of drugs that are antibacterial. Although they have been superseded by newer antibiotics, they are still sometimes prescribed for urinary tract infections. They include: co-trimoxazole, sulphametopyrazine, sulphadiazine and sulphadimidine.

Type of allergen: contact, consumed

Symptoms, tests, treatments and self-help tips, see *Drugs*

Sulphur dioxide

Sulphur dioxide, chemical symbol SO_2, is an environmental pollutant. It is formed by the burning of sulphur-containing fuels such as coal and by petroleum processing or refining. Other sources are metal refining, paper manufacture and Portland cement manufacturing.

If your body doesn't have enough of the enzyme sulphite oxidase, which metabolizes the active sulphites into inactive sulphites, you may react badly to sulphites (see *Food additives*).

Symptoms, treatments and self-help tips, see *Environmental pollutants*

Tests
To test sensitivity to sulphite, a double-blind test with potassium metabisulphite solution and a placebo (swilled around the mouth and spat out) will be made; your lung function will be tested through total body plethysmography which will show whether the size of your airways have changed. In body plethysmography, the patient sits inside an airtight box, inhales or exhales to a particular volume (usually FRC), and then a shutter drops across their breathing tube. The patient then tries to breathe against the closed shutter (panting), which causes their chest volume to expand and decompresses the air in their lungs. The increase in their chest volume causes an increase in pressure in the airtight box and the measurement of this shows residual volume, functional residual capacity, and total lung capacity.
See also *Food additives – preservatives*

Type of allergen: inhalant

Sunburn preparations
See *Benzocaine, Para-aminobenzoic acid (PABA)*

Suncreams
Perfumes and preservatives tend to cause most problems.

Symptoms, tests, treatments and self-help tips, see *Cosmetics*
See also *Benzophenones, Benzyl salicylate (fixing agent), Cosmetics, paba*

Sunflower seeds
Sunflower seeds are the seeds of the plant *Helianthus annus*.

Type of allergen: contact, consumed

Likely sources of sunflower seeds or oil: salad oil, resin, soap manufacture

Symptoms

Anaphylactic shock

Gastrointestinal reactions: diarrhoea, gastric upset/irritation, nausea, vomiting

Headache

Respiratory reactions: wheezing

Skin reactions: angioedema, itching, urticaria

Tests
• Blood test: ELISA

Treatments

Avoidance

Prescription medication
• Anaphylactic shock: adrenaline, antihistamines, steroids
• Diarrhoea: antidiarrhoeal drugs
• Gastric upset/irritation: painkillers: (use paracetamol rather than aspirin)
• Nausea: antihistamines
• Vomiting: anti-emetics
• Headache: painkillers, non-steroidal anti-inflammatories
• Wheezing: bronchodilator
• Angioedema: adrenaline, antihistamines, steroids
• Itching: antihistamines, emollients
• Urticaria: antihistamines, emollients, steroids

OTC remedies
• Diarrhoea: kaolin and morphine, calcium carbonate, pectin
• Gastric upset/irritation: as prescription medication
• Nausea: as prescription medication
• Vomiting: oral rehydration solution
• Headache: as prescription medication
• Angioedema: antihistamines
• Itching: as prescription medication
• Urticaria: calamine lotion, witch hazel

Alternative remedies
- Diarrhoea: aromatherapy, herbalism, homeopathy
- Gastric upset/irritation: aromatherapy, herbalism
- Nausea: aromatherapy, herbalism, homeopathy
- Vomiting: herbalism
- Headache: acupuncture, aromatherapy, herbalism, homeopathy
- Itching: aromatherapy, herbalism
- Urticaria: aromatherapy, herbalism, homeopathy

Self-help tips: for symptom relief see *Diarrhoea, Gastric upset/ Irritation, Nausea, Vomiting, Headache, Wheezing, Angioedema, Itching, Urticaria* in the section on *Symptoms*

You might also react to: ragweed pollen; artichoke, chicory, dandelion, endive, lettuce, tarragon

Sunlight

Fair-skinned people are more prone to this problem which can be triggered even in relatively weak sun. It usually starts when the skin is first exposed, and the reaction then subsides with further exposure.

Symptoms
Skin reactions: urticaria

Tests
- Symptom diary

Treatments
Prescription medication: antihistamines, emollients, steroids

OTC remedies: calamine lotion, witch hazel

Alternative remedies: aromatherapy, herbalism, homeopathy

Self-help tips
- You may be able to prevent it by using a total sunblock, but remember to apply it before going out into the sun, and top up regularly. Some people find the special anti-allergy sun

protection products effective, although they are relatively expensive

• For symptom relief, see *Urticaria* in the section on *Symptoms*

Sunset Yellow
See *Food additives – colourings*

Swede
Swede is the root vegetable *Brassica napus*. It is also known as rutabaga.

Type of allergen: contact, consumed

Symptoms, tests, treatments and self-help tips, see *Vegetables*

You might also react to: cabbage, broccoli, Brussels sprouts, cauliflower, horseradish, mustard, radish, turnip, watercress

Swimming pools
See *Chlorine*

Swordfish
See *Fish*

Synephrine
See *Citrus fruit*

Synthetic foams
See *Volatile organic compounds*

Synthetic materials
See *Solvents (ketone solvents)*

Talc
Talc – a mineral form of magnesium silicate – is used as a lubricant and filler in paper, paints and rubber, and the production of ceramics. It can cause asthma; if symptoms start soon after beginning work and improve at weekends or on holidays, occupational asthma should be suspected. It can also cause irritant contact dermatitis in rubber workers.

Type of allergen: inhaled, contact

Likely sources of talc: cosmetics, rubber

Symptoms
Respiratory reactions: asthma (including occupational)
Skin reactions: contact dermatitis

Tests
* Symptom diary (including peak flow meter readings)
* Skin patch

Treatments
Avoidance
* In occupational situations, use protective equipment such as gloves and masks. Improved ventilation may also help.

Prescription medication
* Asthma: anticholinergic drugs, antihistamines (exercise-induced), Beta2 (ß2) adrenoreceptor agonists, cromoglycate, nedocromil sodium, steroids, xanthine derivatives, zafirlukast
* Contact dermatitis: steroids, antihistamines

OTC remedies
* Contact dermatitis: coal tar, emollients, steroids

Alternative remedies
* Asthma: acupuncture (mild asthma only), Buteyko method, homeopathy, relaxation techniques, yoga
* Contact dermatitis: aromatherapy, Bach flower remedies, homeopathy

Self-help tips: for symptom relief see *Asthma, Contact dermatitis* in the section on *Symptoms*

Tampons
See *Cosmetics, Perfume, Sanitary products*

Tangerine
See *Fruit*

Tarragon

Tarragon is the herb *Artemisia dracunclus*. It contains *salicylates*, which have been linked to hyperactivity in children.

Type of allergen: consumed

Symptoms, tests, treatments and self-help tips, see *Herbs*

You might also react to: artichoke, chicory, dandelion, endive, lettuce, sunflower seeds

Tartrazine
See *Food additives – colourings*

Tattoos
See *Cobalt*

Tea

Tea – *Camellia sinensis* – contains *salicylates*, which have been linked to hyperactivity in children. It also contains oxalates, a derivative of oxalic acid.

Type of allergen: consumed

Symptoms
Gastrointestinal reactions: abdominal pain, diarrhoea, vomiting

Other reactions: cystitis

Psychological problems: hyperactivity

Respiratory reactions: asthma, wheezing

Skin reactions: angioedema, skin irritation, urticaria (this has been dismissed by some experts)

Tests
• Blood test: CAP-RAST
• Blood test: ELISA
• Elimination diet

- Food challenge
- Symptom diary (including peak flow meter readings)

Treatments
Avoidance
- Check labels carefully

Prescription medication
- Abdominal pain and swelling: antacids, anti-spasmodic drugs
- Diarrhoea: antidiarrhoeal drugs
- Vomiting: anti-emetics
- Cystitis: antibiotics (for infection)
- Hyperactivity: stimulant drugs
- Asthma: anticholinergic drugs, antihistamines (exercise-induced), Beta$_2$ (β_2) adrenoreceptor agonists, cromoglycate, nedocromil sodium, steroids, xanthine derivatives, zafirlukast
- Wheezing: bronchodilator
- Angioedema: adrenaline, antihistamines, steroids
- Skin irritation: emollients
- Urticaria: antihistamines, emollients, steroids

OTC remedies
- Abdominal pain and swelling: antacids
- Diarrhoea: kaolin and morphine, calcium carbonate, pectin
- Vomiting: oral rehydration solution
- Cystitis: potassium citrate
- Angioedema: antihistamines
- Skin irritation: as prescription medication
- Urticaria: calamine lotion, witch hazel

Alternative remedies
- Abdominal pain and swelling: aromatherapy, herbalism, homeopathy
- Diarrhoea: aromatherapy, herbalism, homeopathy
- Vomiting: herbalism
- Cystitis: aromatherapy, herbalism, homeopathy
- Asthma: acupuncture (mild asthma only), Buteyko method, homeopathy, relaxation techniques, yoga
- Urticaria: aromatherapy, herbalism, homeopathy

Self-help tips: for symptom relief see *Abdominal pain, Diarrhoea, Vomiting, Cystitis, Hyperactivity, Asthma, Wheezing, Skin irritation, Urticaria* in the section on *Symptoms*

Teicoplanin

Teicoplanin is an *antibiotic* used for respiratory tract infections, peritonitis and joint infections.

Type of allergen: consumed

Symptoms, tests, treatments and self-help tips, see *Drugs*

Tellurium

Tellurium is a metallic element, chemical symbol Te. It is used in semiconductors and steel making.

Type of allergen: contact

Symptoms, tests, treatments and self-help tips, see *Metals*

Temperature

Exposure to cold water or ice can cause "essential cold urticaria". A variation is "cold-induced cholinergic urticaria", caused by exercising in a cold environment; this can lead to anaphylactic shock.

Symptoms
Anaphylactic shock

Respiratory reactions: breathing problems

Skin reactions: angioedema, urticaria

Tests
- "Ice-cube test" – an ice cube is placed on your arm for five minutes; if you have a positive reaction, urticaria appears as the skin warms.
- Symptom diary

Treatments
Prescription medication
- Anaphylactic shock: adrenaline, antihistamines, steroids
- Breathing problems: bronchodilators, corticosteroids

- Angioedema: adrenaline, antihistamines, steroids
- Urticaria: antihistamines, emollients, steroids

OTC remedies
- Angioedema: antihistamines
- Urticaria: calamine lotion, witch hazel

Alternative remedies
- Urticaria: aromatherapy, herbalism, homeopathy

Self-help tips: for symptom relief see *Breathing problems, Angioedema, Urticaria* in the section on *Symptoms*

Terbinafine
See *Antifungal drugs, Drugs*

Tert-Butylhydroquinone
See *Food additives – antioxidants*

Tetracloroethane (acetylene tetrachloride)
See *Solvents – chlorinated hydrocarbons*

Tetracycline
Tetracycline is a broad-spectrum *antibiotic*, used for infections such as bronchitis, chest infections that can't be treated by penicillin, pelvic inflammatory disease and some skin conditions. They work by inhibiting the production of protein in bacteria, which stops them multiplying.

Tetracyclines include: demeclocycline, doxycycline, lymecycline, minocycline, oxytetracycline, tetracycline.

Type of allergen: consumed

Symptoms, tests, treatments and self-help tips, see *Drugs*

You might also react to: amoxycillin, cephalosporin, moulds (inhalant), moulds in food
See also *Antibiotics*

Textiles
See *Wool alcohol*

Thermometers
See *Mercury*

Thimbles
See *Nickel*

Thiurams
Thiurams are an additive to rubber.

Type of allergen: contact

Likely sources of thiurams: rubber products, fungicides in paint and soap

Symptoms
Skin reactions: contact dermatitis, itching, skin irritation

Tests
- Skin patch test
- Symptom diary

Treatments
Avoidance
- In occupational situations, wear protective clothing such as hypoallergenic gloves

Prescription medication
- Contact dermatitis: steroids, antihistamines
- Itching: antihistamines, emollients
- Skin irritation: emollients

OTC remedies
- Contact dermatitis: coal tar, emollients, steroids
- Itching: as prescription medication
- Skin irritation: as prescription medication

Alternative remedies
- Contact dermatitis: aromatherapy, Bach flower remedies, homeopathy
- Itching: aromatherapy, herbalism

Self-help tips: for symptom relief see *Contact dermatitis, Itching, Skin irritation* in the section on *Symptoms*

You might also react to: mercaptobenzothiazole

Thyme

Thyme is the herb *Thymus vulgaris*. It contains *salicylates*, which have been linked to hyperactivity in children.

Type of allergen: consumed

Symptoms, tests, treatments and self-help tips, see *Herbs*

You might also react to: others in the *Labiatae* family, such as marjoram, mint, oregano, rosemary, sage

Tiles

See *Adhesives*

Tissues

See *Chlorine, Perfume*

Tobacco

Cigarette smoke is a source of benzene.

Type of allergen: consumed, inhalant

You might also react to: other vegetables/plants in the nightshade family: aubergine, cayenne, chilli, peppers (capsicum), paprika, potato, tomato; also sage, mugwort pollen

Tobramycin

Tobramycin is a broad-spectrum antibiotic produced by the bacterium streptomyces tenebraria; it is used for gastric infections, meningitis, septicaemia and infections of the respiratory tract.

Type of allergen: consumed

Symptoms, tests, treatments and self-help tips, see *Drugs*

You might also react to: *gentamycin*
See also *Antibiotics*

Toilet bowl cleaners
See *Alkalis*

Toilet paper
See *Chlorine, Perfume*

Toiletries
See *Benzocaine, Citronella oil, Coconut oil, Cosmetics, Geranium oil, Perfume, Wool alcohol*

Toluene
A hydrocarbon, $C_6H_5CH_3$, of the aromatic series; it is a light colourless liquid obtained by distilling tolu balsam, coal tar, etc.

Type of allergen: inhalant
See *Solvents – aromatic hydrocarbons*

Toluene diisocyanate
See *Isocyanates*

Toluenesulphonamide-formaldehyde resin
This chemical is found in nail varnish but the skin reaction is likely to affect the eyelids, sides of the neck and around the mouth rather than the hands – see *Nail varnish*.

Type of allergen: inhalant/contact

Tomato
Tomatoes are the fruit *Lycopersicon lycopersicum*. They contain *histamine* and the vasoactive amine *tyramine*, which causes the blood vessels to widen and may trigger migraines. They also contain *salicylates*, which have been linked to hyperactivity in children, *tryptamine* and *serotonin*.

Type of allergen: contact, consumed

You might also react to: other vegetables/plants in the nightshade family: aubergine, cayenne, chilli, peppers (capsicum), paprika, potato, tobacco; also sage, mugwort pollen

Tools
See *Cobalt*

Toothpaste

Perfumes and preservatives tend to cause most problems.

Type of allergen: contact

Symptoms, tests, treatments and self-help tips, see *Cosmetics*

Alternative products that might not cause a reaction: bicarbonate of soda and salt
See also *Ammonia, Cinnamon oil, Formaldehyde, Perfume*

Toys
See *Latex*

Trees
See *Plants*

Traffic fumes
See *Environmental pollutants, Ozone, Sulphur dioxide*

Tragacanth
See *Food additives – emulsifiers, stabilizers and thickeners*

1,1,1-trichloroethane
See *Solvents – halogenated solvents*

Trichloroethylene
See *Solvents – chlorinated hydrocarbons,*
Solvents – halogenated solvents

Trout

See *Fish*

Tryptamine

Tryptamine is a biogenic *amine* derived from the amino acid tryptophan, found in grains, nuts, meat, fish, dairy products and beans. If your body does not have enough of the enzyme that breaks tryptamine down, you may suffer from migraine and headaches.

Type of allergen: consumed

Likely sources of tryptamine: Beans, dairy products, grains, nuts, fish, meat

Symptoms
Joint pain and stiffness

Tests
• Elimination diet
• Food challenge
• Symptom diary

Treatments
Avoidance: avoid trigger foods and check with a dietitian to ensure that it's nutritionally sound

Prescription medication: anti-inflammatory drugs, painkillers, steroids

OTC remedies: aspirin, paracetamol

Alternative remedies: acupuncture, aromatherapy, herbalism, homeopathy

Self-help tips: for symptom relief see *Joint pain and swelling* in the section on *Symptoms*
See also *Amines*

Tuna

See *Fish*

Turkey

Type of allergen: contact, consumed

Symptoms, tests, treatments and self-help tips, see *Meat and poultry*

You might also react to: chicken.

Turmeric

Turmeric is the spice *Curcuma longa*, also known as curcumin. It contains *salicylates*, which have been linked to hyperactivity in children

Type of allergen: inhalant, contact, consumed

Symptoms, tests, treatments and self-help tips, see *Spices*

You might also react to: ginger, cardamom

Turpentine

Turpentine is an oily liquid extracted from pine resin; it is also produced synthetically. It contains pinene and other terpenes and is used as a *solvent*, particularly for oil paint and varnish.

Type of allergen: inhalant, contact

Likely sources of turpentine: cosmetics, polishes, varnishes, paint thinners, pine-scented cleaners

Symptoms
Eye reactions: conjunctivitis

Gastrointestinal reactions: gastric upset

Headaches

Mouth, nasal and ear reactions: rhinitis

Psychological problems: anxiety

Skin reactions: contact dermatitis

Tests
* Patch test
* Symptom diary

Treatments
Avoidance
* Use protective equipment such as gloves and masks.

Prescription medication
* Conjunctivitis: antihistamines, cromoglycate, nedocromil sodium, steroids, sympathomimetics
* Gastric upset/irritation: painkillers (use paracetamol rather than aspirin)
* Headache: painkillers, non-steroidal anti-inflammatories
* Rhinitis: antihistamines, decongestants, sodium cromoglycate, immunotherapy
* Anxiety: benzodiazepenes, beta-blockers
* Contact dermatitis: steroids, antihistamines

OTC remedies
* Conjunctivitis: antihistamines
* Gastric upset/irritation: as prescription medication
* Headache: as prescription medication
* Rhinitis: decongestants
* Contact dermatitis: coal tar, emollients, steroids

Alternative remedies
* Conjunctivitis: herbalism, homeopathy
* Gastric upset/irritation: aromatherapy, herbalism
* Headache: acupuncture, aromatherapy, herbalism, homeopathy
* Rhinitis: aromatherapy
* Anxiety: aromatherapy, Bach flower remedies, herbalism, homeopathy
* Contact dermatitis: aromatherapy, Bach flower remedies, homeopathy

Self-help tips: for symptom relief see *Conjunctivitis, Gastric upset, Headaches, Rhinitis, Anxiety, Contact dermatitis* in the section on *Symptoms*

You might also react to: balsam of Peru, benzoin, chrysanthemums, citrus fruit peel

Tyramine

Tyramine is a biogenic amine derived from the amino acid tyrosine, which is found in dairy foods, eggs, salmon, spinach, processed meats and nuts. Its function in the body is to support blood pressure. It is thought to trigger migraines because people who are susceptible to it lack the enzymes in their body to remove it quickly; it affects the blood vessels, causing high blood pressure, and the effect is directly in proportion to the amount consumed. Levels of tyramine increase in spoiled food.

Type of allergen: consumed

Likely sources of tyramine: aubergines, avocado, bananas, beef, beer, bread (home-made), broad beans, canned meats, cheese, chicken liver, chocolate, eggs, figs, game that's been hung, gravy (commercial), oranges, pickled fish, prunes, plums, raisins, salami, sour cream, soy sauce, spinach, tomatoes, wine (especially red), vermouth, yeast, yeast extract (Marmite), yoghurt

Symptoms
Gastrointestinal reactions: nausea, vomiting

Headache: headache, migraine

Psychological problems: fatigue, mood swings

Tests
- Elimination diet
- Food challenge
- Symptom diary

Treatments
Avoidance
- Check labels

Prescription medication
- Nausea: antihistamines
- Vomiting: anti-emetics
- Headache: painkillers, non-steroidal anti-inflammatories

- Migraine: painkillers, anti-sickness drugs, ergotamine, 5-HT agonists, beta-blockers, sodium valproate, sumatryptan

OTC remedies
- Nausea: as prescription medication
- Vomiting: oral rehydration solution
- Headache: as prescription medication
- Migraine: aspirin, ibuprofen, paracetamol

Alternative remedies
- Nausea: aromatherapy, herbalism, homeopathy
- Vomiting: herbalism
- Headache: acupuncture, aromatherapy, herbalism, homeopathy
- Migraine: acupuncture, Alexander technique, aromatherapy, chiropractic, herbalism, homeopathy, hypnosis, osteopathy, reflexology

Self-help tips: for symptom relief see *Nausea, Vomiting, Headaches, Migraine, Fatigue* in the section on *Symptoms*

Tyres
See *Latex*

Utensils, kitchen
See *Chromium, Nickel*

Vanadium salts
Vanadium is a silvery-white metallic element, chemical symbol V. It is used in the production of steel alloy, and can cause occupational asthma in steelworkers. If symptoms start soon after beginning work and improve at weekends or on holidays, occupational asthma should be suspected.

Type of allergen: inhalant

Likely sources of vanadium salts: steel alloy manufacturing

Symptoms, tests, treatments and self-help tips, see *Metals*

Vanilla

Vanilla is the spice *Vanilla planifola*.

Type of allergen: contact

Symptoms, tests, treatments and self-help tips, see *Spices*

Varnish

The chemical toluene diisocynate, used in varnish, is the commonest cause of occupational asthma. If symptoms start soon after beginning work and improve at weekends or on holidays, occupational asthma should be suspected. Varnish is also a source of benzene.

Type of allergen: inhalant

Symptoms
Respiratory reactions: occupational asthma

Tests
• Symptom diary (including peak flow meter readings)

Treatments
Avoidance: in occupational situations, use protective equipment such as gloves and masks. Improved ventilation may also help

Prescription medication: anticholinergic drugs, antihistamines (exercise-induced), Beta2 (ß2) adrenoreceptor agonists, cromoglycate, nedocromil sodium, steroids, xanthine derivatives, zafirlukast

Alternative remedies: acupuncture (mild asthma only), Buteyko method, homeopathy, relaxation techniques, yoga

Self-help tips: for symptom relief see *Asthma* in *Symptoms*
See also *Colophony, Isocyanates, Linseed oil, Turpentine*

Varnish remover
See *Amyl alcohol, Solvents*
(alcohol solvents, aromatic hydrocarbons)

Vegetables

See *Artichoke, Asparagus, Aubergine, Bamboo shoot, Bean (pinto, white), Bean (red kidney), Beetroot, Broad beans, Broccoli, Brussels sprouts, Cabbage (red, Chinese, pickled, savoy), Carrot, Cauliflower (boiled and raw), Celery, Courgette, Cress, Cucumber, Endive, Green bean, Kohlrabi, Leek, Lettuce, Mushroom (oyster), Mushroom, Onion, Parsnip, Pea, Peppers, Potato, Pumpkin, Radish (giant), Spinach, Squash (summer), Swede, Sweetcorn, Sweet potato, Tomato*

Symptoms

Anaphylactic shock
- Cabbage, carrot, celery, lettuce, parsnip, tomato
- Exercise-induced – celery, courgette, mushroom, potato

Eye reactions
- Conjunctivitis – asparagus, celery, onion, potato

Gastrointestinal reactions
- Abdominal pain and swelling – beetroot, carrot, celery, cress, leek, pea, pepper, spinach
- Colic – broccoli
- Diarrhoea – beetroot, carrot, leek, pea, pepper, spinach
- Gastric upset/irritation – celery, onion, potato
- Heartburn – onion
- Nausea – carrot, pea
- Vomiting – beetroot, carrot, leek, pea, pepper, spinach
- Wind – Brussels sprouts, cabbage, cauliflower

Headaches
- Aubergine, broad beans, spinach, tomato, migraine – aubergine, broad beans, bean (pinto, white), kidney bean, spinach, tomato

Mouth, nasal and ear reactions
- Ears blocked – tomato
- Itching/burning mouth/palate – carrot, celery, lettuce, parsnip, pea, potato, spinach, swede
- Rhinitis – asparagus, bamboo shoots, carrot, celery, lettuce, onion, parsnip, pea, potato, swede
- Sneezing – potato

Psychological problems
- Hyperactivity – asparagus, cucumber, pea, pepper, tomato

Respiratory reactions
- Asthma – asparagus, bamboo shoots, carrot, celery, pea, potato (tends to be more in childhood)
- Breathing problems – asparagus, celery
- Cough – asparagus, squash
- Wheezing – asparagus, celery, cucumber, pea, pepper, pumpkin, spinach, tomato

Skin reactions
- Angioedema – asparagus, cabbage, carrot, celery, cucumber, lettuce, mushroom, parsnip, pea, pepper, potato, spinach, tomato
- Atopic dermatitis – carrot, celery, pea, pumpkin
- Contact dermatitis, including occupational – bamboo shoots, broccoli, carrot, endive, lettuce, mushroom, onion, parsnip, pepper, potato, radish, squash, swede, tomato
- Photoallergenic contact dermatitis – carrot, celery, parsnip, spinach
- Eczema – celery, tomato
- Eczema (occupational) – artichoke, carrot, onion, potato (raw)
- Flushing – aubergine, bean (pinto, white), broad beans, mushroom, spinach, tomato
- Itching – celery, tomato
- Inflammation – mushroom
- Urticaria (this has been dismissed by some experts) – asparagus, aubergine, bean (pinto, white), broad beans, carrot, celery, cucumber, lettuce, mushroom, pea, pepper, potato, spinach, tomato

Other reactions
- Cystitis – carrot
- Faintness – celery
- Fever – cress, shiitake mushroom
- Joint pain – cress

Tests
- Blood test: CAP-RAST – asparagus, aubergine, bamboo shoots, bean (green, white, red kidney), beetroot, broccoli, Brussels sprouts, cabbage, carrot, cauliflower, celery, cucumber, lettuce, onion, pea, pepper (green), potato, pumpkin (vegetable and seeds), spinach, sweet potato, tomato
- Blood test: ELISA – artichoke, asparagus, aubergine, bamboo shoots, bean (green, pinto, red kidney, white), beetroot,

broccoli, Brussels sprouts, courgette, cress, kohlrabi, leek, lettuce, onion, pea, pepper (green, red), potato, radish (giant), spinach, squash, sweetcorn, sweet potato, tomato
- Skin test: skin prick – asparagus, carrot, cauliflower, celery (including root), cucumber, onion, pea, pepper, potato (with peel), radish, spinach, tomato
- Skin test: Intradermal – asparagus, cauliflower, pea, potato, spinach, tomato
- Elimination diet – asparagus, aubergine, bean (pinto, white), beetroot, broad beans, broccoli, Brussels sprouts, cabbage, carrot, cauliflower, celery, courgette, cucumber, leek, lettuce, parsnip, pea, pepper, potato, pumpkin, radish, spinach, swede, sweet potato, tomato)
- Food challenge – asparagus, aubergine, bean (pinto, white), beetroot, broad beans, broccoli, Brussels sprouts, cabbage, carrot, cauliflower, celery, courgette, cucumber, leek, lettuce, parsnip, pea, pepper, potato, pumpkin, radish, spinach, swede, sweet potato, tomato
- Symptom diary (including peak flow meter readings)
- Exercise challenge

Treatments
Avoidance
- In occupational situations, use protective equipment such as gloves or masks; improved ventilation may also help.
- Check labels carefully and check with a dietitian to ensure that your diet is still nutritionally sound

Prescription medication
- Anaphylactic shock: adrenaline, antihistamines, steroids
- Abdominal pain and swelling: antacids, anti-spasmodic drugs
- Diarrhoea: antidiarrhoeal drugs
- Gastric upset/irritation: painkillers (use paracetamol rather than aspirin)
- Heartburn: antacids, alginates
- Nausea: antihistamines
- Vomiting: anti-emetics
- Wind: antacids
- Headache: painkillers, non-steroidal anti-inflammatories
- Migraine: painkillers, anti-sickness drugs, ergotamine, 5-HT agonists, beta-blockers, sodium valproate, sumatryptan
- Ear problems: sympathomimetics

- Itching/burning mouth/palate: painkillers
- Rhinitis: antihistamines, decongestants, sodium cromoglycate, immunotherapy
- Hyperactivity: stimulant drugs
- Asthma: anticholinergic drugs, antihistamines (exercise-induced), Beta2 (ß2) adrenoreceptor agonists, cromoglycate, nedocromil sodium, steroids, xanthine derivatives, zafirlukast
- Breathing problems: bronchodilators, corticosteroids
- Cough: antihistamines, bronchodilators, corticosteroids
- Wheezing: bronchodilator
- Angioedema: adrenaline, antihistamines, steroids
- Itching: antihistamines, emollients
- Dermatitis: steroids, antihistamines
- Photoallergenic contact dermatitis: emollients, steroids
- Eczema: emollients, immune suppressants, steroids, UVA/UVB light treatment, wet wrapping, antihistamines
- Inflammation: antihistamines, emollients, steroids
- Urticaria: antihistamines, emollients, steroids
- Cystitis: antibiotics (for infection)
- Fever: aspirin, ibuprofen, paracetamol
- Joint pain and swelling: anti-inflammatory drugs, painkillers, steroids
- Faintness: adrenaline (as part of anaphylaxis)

OTC remedies
- Conjunctivitis: antihistamines
- Abdominal pain and swelling: antacids
- Diarrhoea: kaolin and morphine, calcium carbonate, pectin
- Gastric upset/irritation: as prescription medication
- Heartburn: as prescription medication
- Nausea: as prescription medication
- Vomiting: oral rehydration solution
- Wind: as prescription medication
- Headache: as prescription medication
- Migraine: aspirin, ibuprofen, paracetamol
- Itching/burning mouth/palate: painkillers
- Rhinitis: decongestants
- Cough: demulcents, antitussives, expectorants
- Dermatitis: coal tar, emollients, steroids
- Eczema: emollients, hydrocortisone cream
- Inflammation: antihistamines, emollients
- Urticaria: calamine lotion, witch hazel

- Cystitis: potassium citrate
- Fever: aspirin, ibuprofen, paracetamol
- Joint pain and swelling: aspirin, paracetamol

Alternative remedies
- Conjunctivitis: herbalism, homeopathy
- Abdominal pain and swelling: aromatherapy, herbalism, homeopathy
- Diarrhoea: aromatherapy, herbalism, homeopathy
- Gastric upset/irritation: aromatherapy, herbalism
- Heartburn: aromatherapy, homeopathy, herbalism
- Nausea: aromatherapy, herbalism, homeopathy
- Vomiting: herbalism
- Wind: aromatherapy, herbalism, homeopathy
- Headache: acupuncture, aromatherapy, herbalism, homeopathy
- Migraine: acupuncture, Alexander technique, aromatherapy, chiropractic, herbalism, homeopathy, hypnosis, osteopathy, reflexology
- Faintness: aromatherapy, Bach flower remedies
- Ear problems: aromatherapy, herbalism, homeopathy
- Rhinitis: aromatherapy
- Cystitis: aromatherapy, herbalism, homeopathy
- Fever: herbalism, homeopathy
- Joint pain and swelling: acupuncture, aromatherapy, herbalism, homeopathy
- Asthma: acupuncture (mild asthma only), Buteyko method, homeopathy, relaxation techniques, yoga
- Cough: aromatherapy, homeopathy
- Angioedema: antihistamines
- Contact dermatitis: aromatherapy, Bach flower remedies, homeopathy
- Eczema: aromatherapy, evening primrose oil, relaxation, herbalism, homeopathy, Chinese herbal medicine, Bach flower remedies
- Flushing: herbalism
- Itching: aromatherapy, herbalism
- Urticaria: aromatherapy, herbalism, homeopathy

Self-help tips: for symptom relief see *Conjunctivitis, Abdominal pain and swelling, Diarrhoea, Gastric upset/Irritation, Heartburn, Nausea, Vomiting, Headaches, Faintness, Ear problems, Itching/burning mouth/palate, Rhinitis, Sneezing, Cystitis, Fever,*

Hyperactivity, Asthma, Breathing problems, Cough, Wheezing, Angioedema, Contact dermatitis, Photoallergenic contact dermatitis, Eczema, Flushing, Itching, Inflammation, Urticaria in the section on *Symptoms*

Vinegar
See *Yeast*

Vinegar, cider
See *Cider vinegar*

Vinegar, wine
See *Wine vinegar*

Vinyl
See *Epoxy resin*

Vinyl acetate
See *Solvents (esters)*

Vinyl coatings
See *Solvents (esters, ketone solvents)*

Vitamins

Vitamins B, E and K can cause occupational contact dermatitis in pharmaceutical workers.

Type of allergen: contact

Symptoms
Skin reactions: occupational contact dermatitis

Tests
• Skin patch test
• Symptom diary

Treatments
Avoidance
• In occupational situations, use protective equipment such as gloves.

Prescription medication: steroids, antihistamines

OTC remedies: coal tar, emollients, steroids

Alternative remedies: aromatherapy, Bach flower remedies, homeopathy

Self-help tips: for symptom relief see *Contact dermatitis* in the section on *Symptoms*

Vitamin supplements containing B-vitamins
See *Yeast*

Volatile organic compounds (VOCs)

Volatile organic compounds are materials that can form a gas at room temperature or when heated – for example, paint is a liquid whose volatile component (solvent) becomes a gas, leaving the non-volatile material behind.

Type of allergen: inhalant, contact

Likely sources of VOCs: Aerosols (hydrocarbon propellants), acrylic sealant (window and door frames), adhesives, asphalt sealant, carpet backings, creosote, furniture oils, furniture stuffing, household cleaners, insect repellents, paint, perfume, plastic laminates, polishes, preservatives, stain proofing, synthetic foams

Symptoms
Eye reactions: conjunctivitis

Gastrointestinal reactions: gastric upset/irritation, nausea, vomiting

Headache

Mouth, nasal and ear reactions: irritation of mucous membranes

Respiratory reactions: breathing problems, wheezing

Skin reactions: angioedema, inflammation, itching

Tests
* Skin patch
* Symptom diary

Treatments
Avoidance
* Use protective equipment such as masks, goggles and gloves. Ventilation may also help.

Prescription medication
* Conjunctivitis: antihistamines, cromoglycate, nedocromil sodium, steroids, sympathomimetics
* Gastric upset/irritation: painkillers (use paracetamol rather than aspirin)
* Nausea: antihistamines
* Vomiting: anti-emetics
* Headache: painkillers, non-steroidal anti-inflammatories
* Irritation of mucous membranes: painkillers
* Breathing problems: bronchodilators, corticosteroids
* Wheezing: bronchodilator
* Angioedema: adrenaline, antihistamines, steroids
* Inflammation: antihistamines, emollients, steroids
* Itching: antihistamines, emollients

OTC remedies
* Conjunctivitis: antihistamines
* Gastric upset/irritation: as prescription medication
* Nausea: as prescription medication
* Vomiting: oral rehydration solution
* Headache: as prescription medication
* Irritation of mucous membranes: as prescription medication
* Angioedema: antihistamines
* Inflammation: antihistamines, emollients
* Itching: antihistamines, emollients

Alternative remedies
* Conjunctivitis: herbalism, homeopathy
* Gastric upset/irritation: aromatherapy, herbalism

- Nausea: aromatherapy, herbalism, homeopathy
- Vomiting: herbalism
- Headache: acupuncture, aromatherapy, herbalism, homeopathy
- Irritation of mucous membranes: herbalism
- Itching: aromatherapy, herbalism

Self-help tips
- Allow time for volatiles to disperse before entering the room
- Store in a separate, well-ventilated area
- For symptom relief, see *Conjunctivitis, Gastric upset/irritation, Nausea, Vomiting, Headache, Irritation of mucous membranes, Breathing problems, Wheezing, Angioedema, Inflammation, Itching* in the section on *Symptoms*.

Wall panel coverings
See *Epoxy resin*

Wallpaper
Wall-coverings may contain free vinyl acetate, styrene, vinyl chloride, acrylic and plasticizers which may release gas.

Type of allergen: inhalant

See *Volatile organic compounds, Adhesives*

Walnut
Walnuts are the fruit of the tree *Juglans spp*.

Type of allergen: contact, consumed

Symptoms, tests, treatments and self-help tips, see *Nuts*

You might also react to: birch pollen, pecan

Washing powders
See *Enzymes, Soap*

Water
See *Chlorine*

Watermelon
See *Melon, Fruit*

Waxes
See *Colophony, Formaldehyde, Wool alcohol*

Wax solvent
See *Solvents – chlorinated hydrocarbons*

Wheat

The problem area with wheat is often *gluten*, which is formed of gliadin and glutenin.

Symptoms may occur within minutes or up to three days after eating wheat.

There are four main groups of proteins in wheat that can be allergens: water-soluble, salt-soluble, alcohol-soluble and alcohol-insoluble. It can can cause occupational asthma in bakers; if symptoms start soon after beginning work and improve at weekends or on holidays, occupational asthma should be suspected.

Type of allergen: inhalant, contact, consumed

Likely sources of wheat: breads, flour, cakes, biscuits, pancakes, semolina, pastry, sauces, gravy, pasta, cereals, muesli, couscous, bulgar wheat

Symptoms, tests, treatments and more self-help tips, see *Grain*

Self-help tips: check the ingredients on food package labels and ask about the ingredients in foods prepared in restaurants when you eat out – avoid anything on the following list: bran, bread, cereal binder, cereal extract, cereal filler, cereal protein, cereal starch, coucous, durum, edible starch, farina, flour, food starch, gluten, graham, hydrolysates, malt, modified food starch, modified starch, semolina, starch, vegetable starch, vegetable gum, wheat, wheat germ, whole wheat flour

Alternative products that won't cause a reaction:
Wheat-allergic children can usually tolerate oats, rye, barley and corn; replace breads and flours based on wheat starch by products made from naturally gluten-free foods such as maize, potato, rice or soya, sweet potato, cassava, sago, tapioca

You might also react to: rye, barley, oats (rye most likely to react); possibly also corn, rice and millet; birch pollen

White spirit
See Solvents – aliphatic hydrocarbons

Window and door frames
See Volatile organic compounds

Wine
Red wine contains *histamine*. It also contains the vasoactive amines *tyramine* and *phenylethylamine*, which cause the blood vessels to widen and may trigger migraines.

Type of allergen: consumed

Symptoms
Headache: migraine

Skin reactions: flushing, urticaria

Tests
• Blood test: ELISA (white and red)
• Elimination diet
• Food challenge
• Symptom diary

Treatments
Avoidance
• Check labels carefully and check with a dietitian to ensure that your diet is still nutritionally sound

Prescription medication
• Migraine: painkillers, anti-sickness drugs, ergotamine, 5-HT agonists, beta-blockers, sodium valproate, sumatryptan

• Urticaria: antihistamines, emollients, steroids

OTC remedies
• Migraine: aspirin, ibuprofen, paracetamol
• Urticaria: calamine lotion, witch hazel

Alternative remedies
• Migraine: acupuncture, Alexander technique, aromatherapy, chiropractic, herbalism, homeopathy, hypnosis, osteopathy, reflexology
• Flushing: herbalism
• Urticaria: aromatherapy, herbalism, homeopathy

Self-help tips: for symptom relief see *Migraine, Flushing, Urticaria* in the section on *Symptoms*.
See also *Yeast*

Wine vinegar

Contains *salicylates*, which have been linked to hyperactivity in children

Type of allergen: consumed

Symptoms
Psychological problems: hyperactivity

Respiratory reactions: wheezing

Skin reactions: angioedema, urticaria (this has been dismissed by some experts)

Tests
• Blood test: ELISA
• Elimination diet
• Food challenge
• Symptom diary

Treatments
Avoidance
• Check labels carefully and check with a dietitian to ensure that your diet is still nutritionally sound

Prescription medication
- Hyperactivity: stimulant drugs
- Wheezing: bronchodilator
- Angioedema: adrenaline, antihistamines, steroids
- Urticaria: antihistamines, emollients, steroids

OTC remedies
- Angioedema: antihistamines
- Urticaria: calamine lotion, witch hazel

Alternative remedies
- Hyperactivity: herbalism
- Urticaria: aromatherapy, herbalism, homeopathy

Self-help tips: for symptom relief see *Hyperactivity, Wheezing, Angioedema, Urticaria* in the section on *Symptoms*

Wires
See *Epoxy resin, Copper*

Wood dust

Wood dust can cause occupational asthma for carpenters, sawmill workers, forest workers and cabinetmakers. The most common woods affecting people are oak, boxwood and cedar – 5 per cent of people exposed to it get asthma, caused by the plicatic acid in the wood. If symptoms start soon after beginning work and improve at weekends or on holidays, occupational asthma should be suspected

You may also have contact dermatitis from the following woods:
- iroko (*Chlorophora excelsa*)
- mansonia (*Mansonia altissima*)
- African mahogany (*Khaya anthotheca*)
- rosewood (*Dalbergia sp*)
- western red cedar (*Thuja plicata*)
- false rosewood (*Machaerium scleroxylon*)
- white peroba (*Paratecoma peroba*)
- teak (*Tectona grandis*)

Type of allergen: inhalant, contact

Symptoms
Respiratory reactions: occupational asthma

Skin reactions: contact dermatitis

Tests
- Blood test: ELISA – abechi wood (dust), ash, beech, birch, red cedar, cherry wood, kambala wood, limba, mahogany, makore, maple, meranti, white pine, oak, ramin, silver fir, spruce, teak, walnut
- Patch test
- Symptom diary (including peak flow meter readings)

Treatments
Avoidance
- In occupational situations, use protective equipment such as gloves and masks. Improved ventilation may also help.

Prescription medication
- Asthma: anticholinergic drugs, antihistamines (exercise-induced), Beta2 (ß2) adrenoreceptor agonists, cromoglycate, nedocromil sodium, steroids, xanthine derivatives, zafirlukast
- Contact dermatitis: steroids, antihistamines

OTC remedies
- Contact dermatitis: coal tar, emollients, steroids

Alternative remedies
- Asthma: acupuncture (mild asthma only), Buteyko method, homeopathy, relaxation techniques, yoga
- Contact dermatitis: aromatherapy, Bach flower remedies, homeopathy

Self-help tips: for symptom relief see *Asthma, Contact dermatitis* in the section on *Symptoms*

Wood preservative
See *Chromium*

Wood pulp

Can cause occupational asthma; if symptoms start soon after beginning work and improve at weekends or on holidays, occupational asthma should be suspected

Type of allergen: inhalant

Symptoms
Respiratory reactions: occupational asthma

Tests
• Symptom diary (including peak flow meter readings)

Treatments
Avoidance: in occupational situations, use protective equipment such as masks. Improved ventilation may also help.

Prescription medication: anticholinergic drugs, antihistamines (exercise-induced), Beta2 (ß2) adrenoreceptor agonists, cromoglycate, nedocromil sodium, steroids, xanthine derivatives, zafirlukast

Alternative remedies: acupuncture (mild asthma only), Buteyko method, homeopathy, relaxation techniques, yoga

Self-help tips: For symptom relief see *Asthma* in the section on *Symptoms*

Wool

It tends to be the *lanolin* in wool that causes allergic reactions.

Type of allergen: contact

Likely sources of wool: carpets, knitwear, sheepskin coats or rugs

Symptoms
Headaches

Mouth, nasal and ear reactions: rhinitis

Respiratory reactions: breathing problems

Skin reactions: itching, rash

Other reactions: joint pain and swelling

Tests
- Skin prick test
- Blood test: ELISA (treated and untreated wool)
- Symptom diary

Treatments
Avoidance

Prescription medication
- Headache: painkillers, non-steroidal anti-inflammatories
- Rhinitis: antihistamines, decongestants, sodium cromoglycate, immunotherapy
- Breathing problems: bronchodilators, corticosteroids
- Contact dermatitis: steroids, antihistamines
- Itching: antihistamines, emollients
- Joint pain and swelling: anti-inflammatory drugs, painkillers, steroids

OTC remedies
- Headache: as prescription medication
- Rhinitis: decongestants
- Joint pain and swelling: aspirin, paracetamol
- Contact dermatitis: coal tar, emollients, steroids
- Itching: as prescription medication

Alternative remedies
- Headache: acupuncture, aromatherapy, herbalism, homeopathy
- Rhinitis: aromatherapy
- Joint pain and swelling: acupuncture, aromatherapy, herbalism, homeopathy
- Contact dermatitis: aromatherapy, Bach flower remedies, homeopathy
- Itching: aromatherapy, herbalism

Self-help tips: for symptom relief see *Headache, Rhinitis, Joint pain, Breathing problems, Itching, Contact dermatitis* in the section on *Symptoms*

You might also react to: angora, cashmere, mohair, sheepskin products

Wool alcohol

Wool alcohol or lanolin occurs naturally in the fleece of sheep.

Type of allergen: contact

Likely sources of wool alcohol: cosmetics, ink, leather goods, lubricants, polish, skin medications, textiles, toiletries, wax

Symptoms
Skin reactions: contact dermatitis

Tests
- Blood test: ELISA
- Skin patch test
- Symptom diary

Treatments
Avoidance: check labels of cosmetics, toiletries and medicines and avoid those that contain lanolin or wool alcohol. It may be listed as: lanolin, wool fat, wool wax, wool grease, adeps lanae anhydrous, aloholes lanae, lanolin acid, lanolic acid, lanolin alcohol, lanolin oil, lanolin wax

Prescription medication: steroids, antihistamines

OTC remedies: coal tar, emollients, steroids

Alternative remedies: aromatherapy, Bach flower remedies, homeopathy

Self-help tips: for symptom relief see *Contact dermatitis* in the section on *Symptoms*

You might also react to: wool, which contains lanolin

Worcestershire sauce
Contains *salicylates*, which have been linked to hyperactivity in children.

Type of allergen: consumed

Symptoms
Psychological problems: hyperactivity

Respiratory reactions: wheezing

Skin reactions: angioedema, urticaria (this has been dismissed by some experts)

Tests
- Elimination diet
- Food challenge
- Symptom diary

Treatments
Avoidance: check labels carefully and check with a dietitian

Prescription medication
- Hyperactivity: stimulant drugs
- Wheezing: bronchodilator
- Angioedema: adrenaline, antihistamines, steroids
- Urticaria: antihistamines, emollients, steroids

OTC remedies
- Angioedema: antihistamines, emollients
- Urticaria: calamine lotion, witch hazel

Alternative remedies
- Hyperactivity: herbalism
- Urticaria: aromatherapy, herbalism, homeopathy

Self-help tips: for symptom relief see *Hyperactivity, Wheezing, Angioedema, Urticaria* in the section on *Symptoms*

Xylene
See Solvents – aromatic hydrocarbons

Yeast

Reactions to yeast are more likely to be intolerance than allergy. Yeast also contains the vasoactive amine tyramine, which causes the blood vessels to widen and may trigger migraines.

Type of allergen: consumed

Likely sources of yeast: leavened bread, pitta bread, pizza; yeast extract spread (Marmite, vegemite); stock cubes; beer, wine, cider, ginger beer, fortified wine, some spirits; vinegar and pickles; malt products, including whisky, some breakfast cereals, some drinks; vitamin supplements containing B-vitamins; fruit – dried, overripe, unpeeled, fruit juices; soy sauce; ready meals; mushrooms.

Yeast is also an occupational allergen in vineyards, breweries and food processing

Symptoms
Anaphylactic shock

Headache: headache, migraine

Mouth, nasal and ear reactions: rhinitis

Respiratory reactions: asthma

Skin reactions: eczema, flushing, urticaria

Tests
- Blood test: CAP-RAST
- Blood test: ELISA (brewer's, baker's and wine)
- Elimination diet
- Food challenge
- Symptom diary (including peak flow meter readings)

Treatments
Avoidance
- Check labels carefully and check with a dietitian to ensure that your diet is still nutritionally sound; avoid anything on the following list: hydrolyzed protein, hydrolyzed vegetable protein, leavening

Prescription medication
- Anaphylactic shock: adrenaline, antihistamines, steroids
- Headache: painkillers, non-steroidal anti-inflammatories
- Migraine: painkillers, anti-sickness drugs, ergotamine, 5-HT agonists, beta-blockers, sodium valproate, sumatryptan
- Rhinitis: antihistamines, decongestants, sodium cromoglycate, immunotherapy
- Asthma: anticholinergic drugs, antihistamines (exercise-induced), Beta2 (ß2) adrenoreceptor agonists, cromoglycate, nedocromil sodium, steroids, xanthine derivatives, zafirlukast
- Eczema: emollients, immune suppressants, steroids, UVA/UVB light treatment, wet wrapping, antihistamines
- Urticaria: antihistamines, emollients, steroids

OTC remedies
- Headache: as prescription medication
- Migraine: aspirin, ibuprofen, paracetamol
- Rhinitis: decongestants
- Eczema: emollients, hydrocortisone cream
- Urticaria: calamine lotion, witch hazel

Alternative remedies
- Headache: acupuncture, aromatherapy, herbalism, homeopathy
- Migraine: acupuncture, Alexander technique, aromatherapy, chiropractic, herbalism, homeopathy, hypnosis, osteopathy, reflexology
- Rhinitis: aromatherapy
- Asthma: acupuncture (mild asthma only), Buteyko method, homeopathy, relaxation techniques, yoga
- Eczema: aromatherapy, evening primrose oil, relaxation, herbalism, homeopathy, Chinese herbal medicine, Bach flower remedies
- Flushing: herbalism
- Urticaria: aromatherapy, herbalism, homeopathy

Self-help tips: for symptom relief see *Headache, Migraine, Rhinitis, Asthma, Eczema, Flushing, Urticaria* in the section on *Symptoms*

Alternative products that won't cause a reaction: soda bread, matzo, chapatti

You might also react to: mould spores, mushrooms, edible fungi, cheese (such as Brie and camembert), Quorn, mycoproteins, cedar pollen

Yeast extract spread (Marmite, Vegemite)
See *Yeast*

Yellow 2G
See *Food additives – colourings*

Zinc
Zinc is a metallic element, chemical symbol Zn. It is used in alloys and galvanizing.

Type of allergen: contact

Symptoms, tests, treatments and self-help tips, see *Metals*

Zips
See *Cobalt*

Appendix 1: Glossary of terms

Acetylcholine – chemical that carries messages from the nerves which make the airway muscles tighten

Adrenaline – naturally occurring hormone released by the adrenal gland; increases the heart rate, dilates the airways and narrows blood vessels in the skin. Used for treatment of anaphylaxis

Allergy – the reaction of the immune system to substances that are harmless to most people

Allergen – a substance that causes the immune system to produce IgE and triggers an allergic reaction

Allergic crease – horizontal line that developes across the nose as a result of an "allergic salute"

Allergic salute – when the nose is wiped upwards to stop it itching or running

Allergic shiner – dark rings under the eyes caused by allergy

Anaphylaxis – a medical emergency where the whole body has an allergic reaction. Also known as anaphylactic shock

Antibody – a protein (also called an immunoglobulin) manufactured by lymphocytes in the blood to neutralize an antigen

Antibody-mediated cytotoxic hypersensitivity – when antibodies lodge in the body's cells, bind to them and destroy them; also known as Type II antibody-mediated, non-IgE hypersensitivity

Anticholinergic – bronchodilator that works by neutralizing the effect of acetylcholine

Antigen – a substance (usually a protein not found naturally in the body) that triggers the immune system to produce antibodies

Antihistamine – medication that blocks the effects of histamine; it reduces itching, sneezing, and a runny nose

Anti-inflammatory medication – drugs which reduce the symptoms and signs of inflammation

Atopy – allergic condition of people who have asthma, eczema, rhinitis and urticaria

B-cells – see *Lymphocyte*

Basophils – part of the cells which release histamine during an allergic reaction

Beta2-agonist – drugs that bind to beta-receptors in the muscle surrounding the airways; they are also known as bronchodilators

Bronchodilator – a drug that widens the airways in the lungs

Bronchi – large air passages that connect the windpipe (trachea) to the lungs

Bronchioles – small air passages in the lungs

CAP-RAST (Radio AllergoSorbent Test) – it tests for the presence of IgE antibodies in your blood

Chemoattractants – chemicals released by a mast cell which cause inflammation

Cilia – hair-like projections in the mucous membrane of the nose that help the nasal passages remain clear

Consumed allergen – allergen that causes a reaction when eaten or drunk

Contact allergen – allergen that causes a reaction when it touches the skin

Corticosteroids – anti-inflammatory drugs similar to the natural corticosteroid hormones produced by the adrenal glands

Cross-sensitivity – where people who are allergic to one allergen also react to another

Cytokines – protein molecules released by cells in response to activation or injury and cause inflammation

Dander – small scales from animal skin; it is a common allergen.

Degranulation – the release of chemicals (histamine, leukotriene and chemoattractants) from the mast cells

Delayed hypersensitivity (DTH) – when symptoms take between 24 and 72 hours to appear; also known as type IV hypersensitivity. Tends to be contact allergens

Desensitization – also known as immunotherapy, where you are given minute substances of the allergen by injection and the dose is gradually increased over a number of months

ELISA test – Enzyme-Linked ImmunoSorbent Assay, used to detect IgE antibodies to specific allergens

Eosinophils – white blood cells which are attracted to broken mast cells and cause inflammation

Histamine blocking agents – drugs which impede the stimulation of cells by histamine

Histamine – chemical released by a mast cell which causes an allergic reaction

IgE – *see* Immunoglobulin E

Immediate onset reaction – a very fast response to specific allergens following repeated exposure; also known as Type I IgE-mediated allergic hypersensitivity

Immune-complex-mediated hypersensitivity – when antibodies and antigens are too large to be destroyed by leukocytes and migrate to tissues such as the lungs and skin, causing inflammation; also known as Type III antibody-mediated, non-IgE hypersensitivity

Immune system – a collection of cells and proteins that protects the body from potentially harmful or infectious microscopic life-forms such as bacteria, viruses and fungi

Immunoglobulin – antibody produced by the body to attack potentially harmful attackers:

- Immunoglobulin A (IgA) found in tears and saliva; protects respiratory and digestive systems
- Immunoglobulin M (IgM) – "temporary" antibody which is formed when your body is invaded by a new attacker
- Immunoglobulin G (IgG) – takes over from IgM as a permanent antibody
- Immunoglobulin D (IgD) –

currently not known what it does, only that it exists

- **Immunoglobulin E (IgE)** – allergy antibody, produced in very small amounts by people who do not have allergies and in large amounts by those who do

Inflammation – swelling following injury

Inhalant allergen – allergen (either fumes or very small particles) that enters your body through the cells lining the eyes, nose, sinuses and bronchial tubes

Injectant allergen – allergen that enters your body through injection (either drugs or insect stings)

Intolerance – unpleasant body reaction caused when the body doesn't produce enough of the right enzyme to break a substance down

Leukotriene – chemical released by a mast cell which causes an allergic reaction by constricting the smooth muscle in the bronchioles

Lymphocyte – white blood cells which are attracted to broken mast cells and cause inflammation; also known as B-cells

Mast cell – cells to which antibodies attach themselves – found mainly in connective tissue (such as the dermis or innermost layer of skin) – and which then release histamine

Mucus – clear, sticky film on the surface of the lining of the nose and lungs

PEFR – Peak Expiry Flow Rate, or the maximum flow of air from the lungs when it's forced out after a deep breath in

PGE2 – Prostaglandin E2, which causes inflammation

Phagocytes – scavenging cells in the body which destroy the invading protein

Pollen – male fertilizing agent of flowering plants, trees, grasses, and weeds – major cause of allergic reactions

Prostaglandin – hormone-like substances metabolized from dietary fats and activated when the mast cells burst; some prosta-glandins (such as PGE2) cause inflammation and some relieve it

Protein – the part of a living organism that includes hydrogen, oxygen and nitrogen.

RAST Test – RadioAllergoSorbent Test, used to detect IgE antibodies to specific allergens

Respiratory system – group of organs which carry oxygen from the air to the bloodstream and expel carbon dioxide

Sensitization – repeated exposure to an antigen that results in the production of IgE, making the sufferer more likely to have an allergic reaction

Sensitivity – the body's reaction similar to a normal side-effect produced by that substance, but exaggerated

Sinus – air cavities within the facial bones, lined by mucous membranes

Appendix 2: Further reading

Allergies, general
✦ *ABC of Work-Related Disorders*;
ed. David Snashall, BMJ
publishing group, London 1997,
ISBN 0-7279-1154-6
All about Asthma and Allergy;
Dr H Morrow Brown,
The Crowood Press,
Marlborough 1990,
ISBN 1-85223-324-9
✦ *Allergies A-Z*; Myron A
Lipkowitz and Tova Navarra;
Facts on File, New York 1997;
ISBN 0-8160-3654-3
✦ *Allergies at Your Fingertips*;
Dr Joanne Clough; Class
Publishing, London 1997;
ISBN 1-872362-52-4
✦ *Allergies – the Complete Guide
to Diagnosis, Treatment and Daily
Management*; Stuart H Young;
Plume (Penguin), New York
1999, ISBN 0-452-27966-6
✦ *Allergies, How your Diet can
Help*; Stephen Terrass,
Thorsons, London 1994,
ISBN 0-7225-2984-8
✦ *The Allergy Survival Guide*;
Jane Houlton, Vermilion,
London 1993, ISBN 009-177505-1
✦ *Allergy, the Facts*; Robert Davies
and Susan Ollier, Oxford
University Press, Oxford 1992
(Reprint); ISBN 0-19-261858-X
✦ *The Complete Allergy Book*;
June Engel, Firefly Books, New
York 1998, ISBN 1-55209-203-8
✦ *The Complete Book of
Children's Allergies*, Dr B Robert
Feldman with David Carroll,
Aurum Press, London 1988,
ISBN 948149-83-3
✦ *The Natural Way: Allergies*;
Moira Crawford,
Element Books, Dorset 1997,
ISBN 1-86204-114-8

Anaphylactic shock
✦ *Life-threatening Allergic
Reactions: Understanding and
Coping with Anaphylaxis*;
Dr Deryk Williams, Anna
Williams & Laura Croker,
Piatkus, London 1997,
ISBN 0-7499-1700-8

Asthma
✦ *Alternative Answers to Asthma
and Allergies*; Barbara Rowlands,
Marshall Publishing, London
1999; ISBN 1-84028-104-9
✦ *Asthma at your Fingertips*;
Dr Mark Levy, Prof Sean Hilton
and Greta Barnes, second ed,
Class Publishing, London 1997,
ISBN 1-872362-67-4
✦ *Asthma, the CompleteGuide*;
Dr Jonathan Brostoff and Linda
Gamlin, Bloomsbury, London
1999, ISBN 0-7475-4043-8
✦ *Asthma, the Complete Guide
for Sufferers and Carers*;
Dr Deryk Williams, Anna
Williams and Laura Croker,
Piatkus, London 1996,
ISBN 0-7499-1606-0
✦ *Asthma, the Facts, third edition*;
Donald J Lane, Oxford
University Press, Oxford 1996,
ISBN 0-19-262151-3
✦ *The BMA Family Doctor Guide
to Asthma*; Professor Jon Ayres,
Dorling Kindersley, London
1999, ISBN 07513-0676 2
✦ *Coping Successfully with your
Child's Asthma*; Dr Paul Carson,

Sheldon Press, London 1987,
ISBN 0-85969-553-0
✦ *Family Health Guide,
Asthma & Allergies*; Ann Kent,
Ward Lock, London 1995;
ISBN 0-7063-7252-2
✦ *Living with Asthma*;
Dr Robert Youngson,
Sheldon Press, London 1995,
ISBN 0-85969-727-4
✦ *Living with Asthma and Hay
Fever*; John Donaldson, Penguin,
London 1994 (revised edition),
ISBN 0-14-023126-9
✦ *The Which? Guide to Managing
Asthma*; Mark Greener,
Which? Books, London 1997,
ISBN 0-85202-661-7
✦ *Your Child: Asthma*, Erika
Harvey, Element Books, London
1998, ISBN 1-86204-207-1

Chemical allergies
✦ *Allergy to Chemicals and
Organic Substances in the
Workplace*; GW Cambridge &
BFJ Goodwin, Science Review,
Northwood 1984,
ISBN 0-905927-51-6
✦ *The Chemical Connection*,
Louise Samways, Greenhouse
Publications, Ellwood Victoria
1989, ISBN 0-86436-224-2
✦ *The Consumer's Good Chemical
Guide*, John Emsley, WH
Freeman, Oxford 1994,
ISBN 0-7167-4505-4

Coeliac disease
✦ *Coping with Coeliac Disease*;
Karen Brody, Sheldon Press,
London 1997,
ISBN 0-85969-738-1

Complementary medicine
✦ *The Complete Medicinal
Herbal*; Penelope Ody, Dorling
Kindersley, London 1993,
ISBN 0-7513-0025-X
✦ *The Complete New Herbal*;
Richard Mabey, Penguin, London
1991, ISBN 0-14-012682-1
✦ *Encyclopedia of Aromatherapy*;
Chrissie Wildwood, Healing Arts
Press, Rochester, Vermont, 1996,
ISBN 0-89281-638-4
✦ *The Family Guide to
Homeopathy* (revised edition);
Dr Andrew Lockie,
Hamish Hamilton,
London 1998,
ISBN 0-241-13572-9
✦ *The Family Medicine Chest*;
Michael van Straten, Weidenfeld
& Nicholson, London 1998,
ISBN 0-297-82450-3
✦ *Handbook of Over-the-Counter
Herbal Medicines*; Penelope Ody,
Kyle Cathie, London 1996,
ISBN 1-85626-235-9
✦ *Neal's Yard natural remedies*,
Susan Curtin, Romy Fraser, Irene
Kohler, Arkana (Penguin)
London 1997 revised edition,
ISBN 0-14-019543-2

Eczema
✦ *Coping with Eczema*;
Dr Robert Youngson, Sheldon
Press, London 1995,
ISBN 0-85969-736-3
✦ *Eczema and other Skin
Disorders*; Dr Jovanka Bach,
Grafton, London 1987,
ISBN 0-246-12947-6
✦ *Eczema and Psoriasis, How your
Diet can Help*; Stephen Terrass,

Thorsons, London 1995,
ISBN 0-7225-3148-6
✦ *The Eczema Handbook*; Jenny
Lewis, Vermilion, London 1994;
ISBN 0-09-178377-1
✦ *Eczema in Childhood: the Facts*;
David J Atherton, Oxford
University Press, Oxford 1994,
ISBN 0-19-262398-2
✦ *Family Health Guide, Eczema*;
Patsy Westcott; Ward Lock,
London 1997;
ISBN 1-7063-7527-0
✦ *The Natural Way with Eczema*;
Sheena Meredith, Element,
Shaftesbury 1994,
ISBN 1-85230-493-6
✦ *Your Child: Eczema*;
Maggie Jones, Element,
Shaftesbury 1998,
ISBN 1-86204-209-8

Food Allergy
✦ *The Additives Guide*; Dr
Christopher Hughes, John Wiley
& Sons, Chichester, 1987,
ISN 0-471-91507-6
✦ *Complete Guide to Food Allergy
and Intolerance (3rd Edition)*;
Dr Jonathan Brostoff and
Linda Gamlin, Bloomsbury,
London 1998,
ISBN 0-7475-3430-6
✦ *Beating Food Intolerance: How
to Recognise It, How to Cure It*;
Charles Lee, Allergy Shop,
Hayward's Heath 1992,
✦ *E for Additives (2nd edition)*;
Maurice Hanssen with Jill
Marsden, Thorsons, London
1988, ISBN 0-7225-1562-6
✦ *Food Allergy: Adverse Reactions
to Foods and Food Additives (2nd
edition)*; ed Dean D Metcalfe,

Hugh A Samptosn & Ronald A
Simon, Blackwell, Cambridge
Massachusetts 1997,
ISBN 0-86542-432-2
✦ *Food and Food Additive
Intolerance in Childhood*;
TJ David, Blackwell, Oxford
1993, ISBN 0-632-03487-4
✦ *Food Chemical Sensitivity*;
Robert Buist, Prism Press, Dorset
1987, ISBN 0-907061-99-0
✦ *Managing Food Allergy and
Intolerance, a Practical Guide*;
Janice Vickerstaff Joneja, Canada
1995, ISBN 1-55203-000-8
✦ *Secret Ingredients*; Peter Cox
and Peggy Brusseau,
Bantam, London 1997,
ISBN 0-553-50554-8
✦ *Was it Something You Ate?
Food Intolerance, What Causes It
and How to Avoid It*; John
Emsley and Peter Fell, Oxford
University Press, Oxford 1999,
ISBN 0-19-850443-8

Hay fever
✦ *The BMA Family Doctor Guide
to Allergies and Hay Fever*;
Professor Robert Davies, Dorling
Kindersley, London 1999,
ISBN 07513-0675 4
✦ *Complete Guide to Hay Fever*;
Dr Jonathan Brostoff and
Linda Gamlin, Bloomsbury,
London 1993,
ISBN 0-7475-1291-4
✦ *Coping successfully with Hay
Fever*; Dr Robert Youngson,
Sheldon Press, London 1995,
ISBN 0-85969-720-7
✦ *How to Beat Hay Fever*; Dr
Mark Payne, Thorsons, London
1998, ISBN 0-7225-3630-5

+ *Living with Asthma and Hay Fever*; John Donaldson, Penguin, London 1994 (revised ed), ISBN 0-14-023126-9

Headaches and migraine

+ *Coping Successfully with Migraine*; Sue Dyson, Sheldon Press, London 1991, ISBN 0-85969-626-X
+ *Headaches, the Complete Guide to Relieving Headaches and Migraine*; John Lockley, Bloomsbury, London 1994, ISBN 0-7475-1462-3
+ *Migraine and Headaches*; Dr Marcia Wilksinson, Macdonald Optima, London 1991, ISBN 0-356-19732-8
+ *The Migraine Handbook*; Jenny Lewis, Vermilion, London 1998, ISBN 0-09-181666-1
+ *Mind over Migraine*; Belinda Hollyer, Headline, London 1994, ISBN 0-7472-4477-4

IBS

+ *IBS, a Complete Guide to Relief from Irritable Bowel Syndrome*; Christine P Dancey and Susan Backhouse; Robinson, London 1997, ISBN 1-85487-910-3
+ *Irritable Bowel Syndrome*; Dr Sarah Brewer; Thorsons, London 1997, ISBN 0-7225-3392-6
+ *Overcoming IBS*; Christine P Dancey and Susan Backhouse; Robinson, London 1993, ISBN 1-85487-175-7

Miscellaneous

+ *The British Medical Association Complete Family Health Encyclopedia (2nd edition reprint)*; ed. Dr Tony Smith, Dorling Kindersley, London 1998, ISBN 0-86318-438-3
+ *The Good Housekeeping Family Guide to Over-the-Counter Medicines*; Ebury Press, London 1999, ISBN 0-09-186851-3
+ *The Good Housekeeping Family Guide to Prescription Medicines*; Ebury Press, London 1999, ISBN 0-09-186973-0
+ *The Hamlyn Encyclopedia of Family Health*; ed. Dr Michael Apple, Hamlyn, London 1999, ISBN 0-600-59254-5
+ *Handbook of Over-the-Counter Medicines*; Dr Mike Smith, Kyle Cathie, London 1994, ISBN 1-85626-151-4
+ *Handbook of Prescription Medicines*; Dr Mike Smith, Kyle Cathie, London 1993, ISBN 1-85626-105-0

Psoriasis

+ *Beat Psoriasis*; Sandra Gibbons; Thorsons, London 1996, ISBN 0-7225-3357-8
+ *Coping with Psoriasis*; Professor Ronald Marks, Sheldon Press, London 1981, ISBN 0-85969-690-1
+ *Eczema and Psoriasis, How your Diet can Help*; Stephen Terrass, Thorsons, London 1995, ISBN 0-7225-3148-6
+ *Skin Care for Psoriasis*; Dr V K Dave, Class Publishing, London 1997, ISBN 1-872362-63-X

Appendix 3: Where to find help

Support organisations

Action Against Allergy
PO Box 278,
Twickenham TW1 4QQ
Tel: 020 8892 2711
Can supply information packs and advisory leaflets on a wide range of allergy subjects, including non-allergenic products, and details of your nearest allergy clinic.

Action Asthma
Patient Service
Apartment 900, Freepost,
Bradford, Yorkshire, BD7 1BR
Provides educational material.

Anaphylaxis Campaign
For information, send a stamped addressed envelope to:
2 Clockhouse Road,
Farnborough,
Hampshire, GU14 7QY
Tel: 01252 542029
www.anaphylaxis.org.uk
Offers support and guidance on anaphylaxis. Dedicated to raising awareness in the food industry and the medical profession to ensure that patients get the best possible treatment and advice. Has an information video on anaphylaxis for parents, teachers and child carers.

Arthritis Care
18 Stephenson Way
London, NW1 2HD
Tel: 0800 289170
(12pm–4pm Monday–Friday)
Arthritis Care offers self-help support, a helpline information service and leaflets on arthritis.

Arthritis Research Campaign
PO Box 177, Chesterfield
Derbyshire, S41 7TQ

The British Allergy Foundation (BAF)
Deepdene House
30 Bellgrove Road
Welling, Kent, DA16 3PY
Tel: 020 8303 8525
Fax: 020 8303 8792
www.allergyfoundation.com
Provides information, advice and support for people with allergies. Publishes details of NHS allergy clinics and the specialists involved. Tests products that may be of practical help to people with allergies and can provide members with information about these. Has local support groups.

British Lung Foundation
78 Hatton Garden
London, EC1N 8LD
Tel: 020 7831 5831
Fax: 020 7831 5832
www.lunguk.org
Provides information on a range of lung diseases, including asthma. Also runs the Breathe Easy Club, a nationwide network which aims to improve the quality of life for people with lung diseases.

British Red Cross
National Headquarters
9 Grosvenor Crescent
London SW1 7ES
Tel: 020 7235 5454
Fax: 020 7245 6315
Website: www.redcross.org.uk
Among many other services, runs
first aid training courses through-
out the UK. Look in your phone
book for details of your local
centre.

British Thoracic Society
1 St Andrews Place
London, NW1 4LB
Tel: 020 7486 7766

The Coeliac Society
PO Box 220, High Wycombe
Bucks, HP11 2HY
Tel: 01494 437278
Fax: 01494 474349
www.coeliac.co.uk
email: admin@coeliac.co.uk
(please include name & address)
Has a range of information and
support services for people with
coeliac disease, including a list of
gluten-free manufactured products.

Department of the Environment
Pollution Hotline
Tel: 0800 556677
For information on air quality.
Information also available on
BBC Ceefax, pages 410-417.

Digestive Disorders Foundation
3 St Andrews Place
London, NW1 4LB
Tel: 020 7486 0341
Fax: 020 7224 2012

Registered Charity No 262762
www.digestivedisorders.org.uk/
index.htm

Food and Chemical
Allergy Association
27 Ferringham Lane
Ferring, West Sussex
Helpline: 01903 241178

Health Information Service
Helpline: 0800 66 55 44
(9.30am-5pm, Monday-Friday)
Provides information on
diseases, treatments, self-help
and support groups, complaints
procedures and availability of
NHS services.

The Hyperactive Children's
Support Group
Provides help and support for
hyperactive (ADD AD/HD)
children and their families.
HACSG
71 Whyke Lane, Chichester
West Sussex, PO19 2LD
Fax 01903 734726
Send SAE, or email
hacsg@hyperactive.force9.net
www.hacsg.org.uk

IBS Network
St John's House
Hither Green Hospital
London, SE13 6RU
Tel: 020 8698 4611

Lactose intolerance
www.dspace.dial.pipex.com/
town/park/gfm11/index.htm

Latex Allergy Support Group
102 Monkseaton Drive
Whitley Bay
Tyne & Wear NE26 3DJ
Tel/Fax: 0191 251 5432
Helpline: 07071 225838
(7pm-10pm, every day)
Information and support for
people with a latex allergy.
Publications include a list
of everyday items that may
contain latex.

**Migraine Action Association
(formerly British Migraine
Association)**
178a High Road, Byfleet,
Surrey, KT14 7ED
Tel: 01932 352468
www.migraine.org.uk
*Information and support for
migraine sufferers. Produces leaflets
and newsletters.*

**National Association for Colitis
and Crohn's Disease**
98a London Road
St Albans, Herts, AL1 1NX
Tel: 01727 844296
(10am-1pm, Mon-Thur)
*Provides information and support
telephone numbers.*

**National Society for
Research into Allergy**
PO Box 45, Hinckley
Leicestershire LE10 1JY
Tel: 01455 851546

National Asthma Campaign
Providence House
Providence Place
London, N1 0NT

Tel: 020 7226 2260
Fax: 020 7704 0740
Asthma helpline: 08457 010203
(local rate calls)
www.asthma.org.uk
*Funds research into asthma
and provides education and support
for people with asthma, their
friends, teachers and employers, and
health professionals. Special club
for children under 12. Local
branches. Publishes booklets,
leaflets and videos (including
videos on self-management of
asthma in several Asian languages).*

**National Asthma Campaign
Scotland**
21 Coates Crescent
Edinburgh, EH3 7AF
Tel: 0131 226 2544
Fax: 0131 226 2401
Asthma Helpline:
0845 7 01 02 03 (local rate)
www.asthma.org.uk

**National Asthma and
Respiratory Training Centre**
Atheneaum, 10 Church Street
Warwick, CV34 4AB
Phone 01926 493313
Fax 01926 493224
*Trains nurses to manage asthma
in general practice and chest clinics.*

The National Eczema Society
163 Eversholt Street
London, NW1 1BU
Tel: 020 7388 4097
Fax: 020 7388 5882
registered UK charity,
No. 1009671
www.eczema.org

Provides support and information, including factsheets and videos, to help improve the quality of life for people with eczema and their carers. Represents the needs of people with carers and raises funds for research to identify causes and potential cures

National Society of Research into Allergy
PO Box 45, Hinckley,
Leics, LE10 1JY
Tel 01445 851546
The society produces a range of booklets and plenty of advice on all forms of allergies and where to get hold of a range of elementary foods and digestive enzymes by mail order. Quarterly magazine. And a list of local allergists.

Pollen Line
Tel: 0870 2402270
For information on pollen counts in the UK.

Psoriasis Association
Milton House, 7 Milton Street
Northampton, NN2 7JG
Tel: 01604 711 129
(9am–5pm, Mon-Fri)
Fax: 01604 792 894
Information on all aspects of psoriasis for sufferers and their families.

The Psoriatic Arthropathy Alliance
PO Box 111, St Albans
Herts, AL2 3JQ
Tel/fax: 01923 672837
www.paalliance.org

St Andrew's Ambulance Association
National Headquarters
48 Milton Street
Glasgow G4 0HR
Tel: 0141 332 4031
Fax: 0141 332 6582
Among other services, offers first aid training for people in Scotland.

St John Ambulance
1 Grosvenor Crescent
London SW1X 7ES
Tel: 020 7235 5231
Fax: 020 7235 0796
Among other services, offers first aid training for people in England and Wales. Look in your phone book for the branch nearest you.

Alternative therapy organizations

Association of Acupuncturists
Tel: 0208 738 0400

Alexander Technique International
142 Thorpedale Road
London, N4 3BS
Tel: 020 7281 7639

British Acupuncture Association
34 Alderney Street
London, SW1V 4EU
Tel: 020 7834 1012

British Acupuncture Council
Park House,
206-208 Latimer Road
London, W10 6RE
Tel: 020 8964 0222

**British Complementary
Medicine Association**
249 Fosse Road South
Leicester, LE3 1AE
Tel: 0116 282 5511

**British Homeopathic
Association**
27a Devonshire Street
London, W1N 1RJ
Tel: 020 7935 2163

**British Institute of
Hypnotherapy**
Tel: 01702 524484

**Chi centre – for traditional
Chinese medicine**
10 Greycoat Place
Victoria, London, SW1P 1SB
Tel: 020 7222 1888

**Council for Complementary
& Alternative Medicine**
Park House
206-208 Latimer Road
London W10 6RE
Tel: 020 8735 0632
Please send an SAE for
information
**International Society of
Professional Aromatherapists**
Tel: 01455 637987

**National Institute of Medical
Herbalists**
56 Longbrook Street
Exeter, Devon, EX4 6AH
Tel: 01392 426022

Society of Homeopaths
2 Artizan Road
Northamptom, NN1 4HU
Tel: 01604 621400

**Society of Teachers of the
Alexander Technique**
2 London House
266 Fulham Road
London, SW10 9EL
Tel: 020 7351 0828

Appendix 4: Food additives

Food additives – colours (E100-E180)

E number and colour	Likely to be found in	Notes	Possible symptoms caused
E100 Curcumin (derived from turmeric)	Curry powder, fats and oils, flour confectionery, ice cream, margarine, fish fingers, processed cheese, savoury rice		
E101 Riboflavin (yellow – vitamin B2, also found in the body)	Dried milk produces, processed cheese, sauces		
E102 Tartrazine (yellow – azo dye)	Cake mixes, confectionery, cordials (e.g. lemon squash), custard powder, ice cream and ice lollies, marzipan, medi-cation, pickles and sauces (e.g. brown sauce, salad cream), ready meals, smoked cod and haddock, soft and fizzy drinks	Banned in Austria, Norway HCSG recommends avoidance	Asthma, breathing problems, hyperactivity, itching, migraine, rhinitis, skin rashes, wakefulness in small children; also affects people sensitive to aspirin
E104 Quinoline Yellow ("coal tar" dye)	Smoked haddock, scotch eggs, ice lollies	Banned in USA, Australia, Japan, Norway HCSG recommends avoidance	Asthma, contact dermatitis, hyperactivity in children; also affects people sensitive to aspirin
107 Yellow 2G (azo dye and "coal tar" dye)	Soft drinks	Banned in USA, Austria, Japan, Norway, Sweden, Switzerland. Proposed ban in EEC – the only EEC country to use it is the UK HCSG recommends avoidance	Asthma; also affects people sensitive to aspirin
E110 Sunset yellow FCF (azo dye and "coal tar" dye)	Biscuits, confectionery, cordials, jams, marzipan, packet soups, tinned prawns, yoghurts	Banned in Finland, Norway HCSG recommends avoidance	Angioedema, asthma, gastric upset, hyperactivity, rashes, rhinitis, swelling, urticaria, vomiting

E number and colour	Likely to be found in	Notes	Possible symptoms caused
E120 Cochineal or carminic acid (red − natural colour from bodies of pregnant scale insects)	Alcoholic drinks, bakery products, biscuits, desserts, icings, red-veined cheddar, sauces, soups	Rarely used − expensive. HCSG recommends avoidance	Hyperactivity, asthma; also affects people sensitive to aspirin
E122 Carmoisine (red − azo dye)	Brown sauce, confectionery, jams, jellies, marzipan, Swiss roll, soup mix, yoghurts	Banned in Japan, Norway, Sweden, USA HCSG recommends avoidance	Angioedema, asthma; also affects people sensitive to aspirin, rhinitis, skin rashes, urticaria,
E123 Amaranth (purplish-red − azo dye and "coal tar" dye)	Cake mixes, gravy granules, ices, jams, jelly	Banned in USA and Norway, only used for caviar in France and Italy. HCSG recommends avoidance	Angioedema, asthma; also affects people sensitive to aspirin, urticaria
E124 Brilliant scarlet 4R (Ponceau − azo dye and "coal tar" dye)	Cake mix, dessert topping, seafood dressing, salami, soup, tinned strawberries, tinned pie filling	Banned in USA, Norway	Asthma; also affects people sensitive to aspirin
E127 Erythrosine (red − "coal tar" dye)	Biscuits, canned cherries and strawberries, chocolate, cocktail cherries, glacé cherries, salami, Scotch eggs,	Banned in USA, Norway	Sensitivity to light
E128 Red 2G (azo dye and "coal tar" dye)	Cooked meats, drinks, jams, sausages	Banned in USA, Australia, Austria, Canada, Finland, Japan, Norway, Sweden, Switzerland The only EEC country that uses it is the UK HCSG recommends avoidance	Hyperactivity
E129 Allura red AC (azo dye)	Biscuits, cake mixes	Banned in Austria, Finland, Japan, Norway, Sweden. The only EEC country that uses it is the UK	Asthma, rhinitis, skin rash

E number and colour	Likely to be found in	Notes	Possible symptoms caused
E131 Patent blue ("coal tar" dye)	Confectionery, biscuits, pickles, potato snacks	HCSG recommends avoidance	Breathing problems, hyperactivity, itching, nausea, rashes, skin sensitivity, urticaria, vomiting, anaphylactic shock
E132 Indigo Carmine ("coal tar" dye)	Biscuits, sweets	Banned in Norway HCSG recommends avoidance	Asthma, breathing problems, hyperactivity, itching, nausea, rashes, urticaria, vomiting,
E133 Brilliant blue FCF ("coal tar" dye)	Tinned processed peas, desserts, confectionery, fish paste, potato snacks	Banned in Austria, Belgium, Denmark, France, Greece, Italy, Norway, Spain, Sweden, Switzerland HCSG recommends avoidance	Asthma, hyperactivity in children
E140 Chlorophyll (Green) – obtained from plants	Confectionery, fats, ice cream, oils, soups, tinned vegetables (naturally green, preserved in liquid)		No known adverse effects
E141 Copper complexes of chlorophyll	Ice cream, parsley sauce, sage Derby cheese, tinned vegetables (naturally green, preserved in liquid)		No known adverse effects
E142 Green S ("coal tar" dye)	Gravy granules, mint jelly and sauce, tinned peas	Banned in Canada, Finland, Japan, Norway, Sweden, USA	
E150 Caramel (dark brown)	Confectionery, crisps, desserts, fish spreads, ice cream, milk puddings, pickles, sauces, soft drinks, spirits, wine		

E number and colour	Likely to be found in	Notes	Possible symptoms caused
E151 Brilliant black BN (azo dye and "coal tar" dye)	Blackcurrant cheesecake mix, brown sauce, chocolate mousse	Banned in Canada, Finland, Japan, Norway, USA HCSG recommends avoidance	Hyperactivity
E153 vegetable carbon (black)	Concentrated fruit juice, jams, jellies, liquorice	Banned in USA.	
E154 Brown FK (mixture of various azo dyes)	Cooked ham, crisps, kippers and smoked fish	Banned in USA, Australia, Austria, Canada, Finland, Japan, Norway, Sweden. The only EEC states to use it are the UK and Ireland HCSG recommends avoidance	Asthma, skin rash; also affects people sensitive to aspirin
E155 Chocolate brown HT (azo dye)	Chocolate cake mixes, confectionery, sauces, seasonings, snacks	Banned in USA, Australia, Austria, Belgium, Denmark, France, Germany, Norway, Sweden, Switzerland	Asthma, skin rash; also affects people sensitive to aspirin
E160(a) Carotene (orange/yellow)	Margarine, soft drinks	Converts to vitamin A in body	
E160 (b) Annatto (bixin, norbixin) (peach colour)	Cakes, crisps, dairy products, fish fingers, ice lollies, smoked fish, soft drinks	HCSG recommends avoidance.	Angioedema, hyperactivity, urticaria
E160 (c) Capsanthin (red/orange) extracted from peppers	Egg yolks, processed cheese slices	Banned in Australia	
E160 (d) Lycopene (red) – extracted from tomatoes		Banned in Australia	
E160 (e) Beta-apo-8'-carotenal (orange)	Cheese slices		No known adverse effects
E160 (f) Ethyl ester of beta-apo-8'-carotenic acid			No known adverse effects

E number and colour	Likely to be found in	Notes	Possible symptoms caused
E161 Xanthophylls (yellow)			No known adverse effects
E161 (g) Canthaxanthin (orange)			No known adverse effects
E162 Beet red, betanin (purplish red)	Desserts, jams, jellies, liquorice, pizzas, sauces	Derived from beetroot	No known adverse effects
E163 Anthocyanins (red, blue, violet)	Confectionery, dairy products, glace cherries, jellies, pickles, soft drinks, yoghurt	Usually derived from grapeskin or red cabbage	No known adverse effects
E170 Calcium carbonate (white)	Biscuits, bread, cakes, confectionery, ice cream, tablets, wine	Naturally occurring mineral	
E171 Titanium dioxide (white)	Confectionery, cottage cheese, horseradish sauce, medication, mozzarella cheese,	Banned in Germany	No known adverse effects
E172 Iron oxides/hydroxides (yellow, red, orange, brown, black)	Cake mix, fish paste, meat paste	Banned in Germany	
E173 Aluminium (metallic surface colour)	Sugar-coated flour confectionery, medication		
E174 silver (metallic surface colour)	Sugar-coated flour confectionery		
E175 Gold (metallic surface colour)	Sugar-coated flour confectionery	Very expensive	
E180 Pigment rubine (azo dye)	Only used for colouring rind of Edam cheese	Banned in Australia	
E181 Tannic acid, tannins (clarifying agent)	Alcoholic drinks		

Food additives – Preservatives (E200-297)

E number	Likely to be found in	Notes	Possible symptoms caused
E200 Sorbic acid	Cheese (processed/surface of hard cheese), confectionery, fermented milk, gelatin capsules, soft drinks, wine, yoghurt		Possible skin irritant
E201 Sodium sorbate	Dried apricots, margarine, pizza, processed cheese	Manufactured by neutralization of E200	No known adverse effects
E202 Potassium sorbate	Cheese spread, dried apricots, fermented milk, glace cherries, margarine, preserves, sauces, soft drinks, wine	Sometimes used instead of E200	No known adverse effects
E203 Calcium sorbate	Concentrated pineapple juice, fermented milk, margarine, yoghurt		No known adverse effects
E210 Benzoic acid	Fruit juices/pulp/purée, jam, margarine, marinated herring, pickles, sauces, syrups, soft drinks, yoghurt	Reacts with sodium bisulphate (E222) E211, 212 and 213 may also be used for these products HCSG recommends avoidance	Asthma, gastric upset, hyperactivity, neurological problems, urticaria
E211 Sodium benzoate (sodium salt of E210)	Caviar, confectionery, orange squash, prawns, sauces, soft drinks	HCSG recommends avoidance	Asthma; also affects people sensitive to aspirin, hyperactivity, urticaria
E212 Potassium benzoate (potassium salt of E210)	Margarine, concentrated pineapple juice	HCSG recommends avoidance	Asthma; also affects people sensitive to aspirin, hyperactivity, urticaria

E number	Likely to be found in	Notes	Possible symptoms caused
E213 Calcium benzoate (calcium salt of E210)	Concentrated pineapple juice	HCSG recommends avoidance	Asthma; also affects people sensitive to aspirin, hyperactivity, urticaria
E214 Ethyl p-Hydroxybenzoate (produced from E210)	Beer, beetroot, coffee essence, dessert sauces, fruit pie fillings, fruit juices, jam, preserved fruit	E215 may also be used HCSG recommends avoidance	Asthma; also affects people sensitive to aspirin, contact dermatitis, hyperactivity, urticaria
E215 Ethyl p-Hydroxy-Benzoate Sodium salt (produced from E210)	See E214	Banned in Australia HCSG recommends avoidance	Contact dermatitis
E216 Propyl p-hydroxybenzoate (produced from E210)	Beer, beetroot, coffee essence, dessert sauces, fruit pie fillings, fruit juices, jam, pickles, soft drinks	E217 may also be used HCSG recommends avoidance	Asthma; also affects people sensitive to aspirin, contact dermatitis
E217 Propyl p-hydroxybenzoate sodium salt (produced from E210)		Banned in Australia HCSG recommends avoidance	Asthma; also affects people sensitive to aspirin, skin sensitivity, urticaria
E218 Methyl parabens	Beer, beetroot, coffee essence, dessert sauces, fruit pie fillings, pickles, sauces, soft drinks	HCSG recommends avoidance	Asthma; also affects people sensitive to aspirin, contact dermatitis, mouth ulcers, urticaria
E219 Methyl p-hydroxybenzoate (produced from E210)		Banned in Australia HCSG recommends avoidance	Asthma; also affects people sensitive to aspirin, contact dermatitis

E number	Likely to be found in	Notes	Possible symptoms caused
E220 Sulphur dioxide	Beer, desiccated coconut, dehydrated vegetables, dried bananas, dried apricots, fruit pie fillings, fruit juices, fruit salad, gelatin, glace cherries, packet soup, sausage meat, soft drinks, wine	Used by Romans and Ancient Greeks to preserve wine HCSG recommends avoidance	Asthma, stomach irritation
E221 Sodium sulphite	Beer, soft drinks, frozen shellfish, frozen chips	HCSG recommends avoidance	Angioedema, asthma, diarrhoea, gastric irritation, nausea, urticaria
E222 Sodium bisulsulphite	Beer, bleaching cod/sugar, frozen shellfish, frozen chips, instant mashed potato, milk, milk products, relishes, soft drinks, wine	HCSG recommends avoidance	Asthma, gastric irritation, urticaria
E223 Sodium metabisulphite	Dried fruit, frozen shellfish, orange squash, pre-packed salad, pickles, puddings, sauces	HCSG recommends avoidance	Asthma, gastric irritation, urticaria
E224 Potassium metabisulphite	Campden tablets, frozen shellfish, frozen chips, wine	HCSG recommends avoidance	Asthma, gastric irritation, urticaria
E226 Calcium sulphite	Cider, fruit juice	Banned in Australia HCSG recommends avoidance	Asthma, gastric irritation, urticaria
E227 Calcium hydrogen sulphite	Beer, jams, jallies	Banned in Australia HCSG recommends avoidance	Asthma, gastric irritation, urticaria
E230 Biphenyl	Citrus fruit skins	E231 and E232 may also be used Banned in Australia	
E231 2-Hydroxybiphenyl	Citrus fruit skins	Banned in Australia	

E number	Likely to be found in	Notes	Possible symptoms caused
E232 Sodium orthophenyl phenol	Citrus fruit skins	Alternatives to E231 Banned in Australia	
E233 Thiabendazole	Citrus fruit skins, bananas	Banned in Australia	
E234 Nisin	Cheese, dairy product, tinned foods		No known adverse effects
E235 Natamycin	Meat, cheese		Nausea, vomiting, diarrhoea and skin irritation
E236 Formic acid (methanoic acid)		Banned in Australia and UK	
E237 Sodium formate (sodium salt of E236)		Banned in Australia and UK	
E238 Calcium formate (calcium salt of E236)		Banned in Australia and UK	
E239 Hexamine	Marinated herrings and mackerel, cheese	Banned in Australia	Gastric irritation, skin rashes
E249 Potassium nitrite	Cooked meat, smoked fish	Curing agent, prevents botulism. Banned in foods for babies under 6 months. HCSG recommends avoidance	Breathing problems, headaches, asthma, nausea
E250 Sodium nitrite	Cured and salted meat products, sauce, ham, bacon, tinned meat, smoked fish, pizza	Curing agent, prevents botulism. Banned in foods for babies under 6 months. HCSG recommends avoidance	Breathing problems, headaches, asthma, nausea

E number	Likely to be found in	Notes	Possible symptoms caused
E251 Sodium nitrate (Chile saltpetre)	Bacon, ham, tinned meats, cheese, frozen pizza	E252 may be used as an alternative. Curing agent, prevents botulism. Banned in foods for babies under 6 months. HCSG recommends avoidance	Breathing problems, headaches, asthma, nausea
E252 Potassium nitrate (saltpetre)	Cured meats, sausages, tinned meats, bacon, smoked frankfurters, some cheeses	E251 may be used as an alternative. One of the oldest known curing agents, prevents botulism. Banned in foods for babies under 6 months. HCSG recommends avoidance	Gastric upset, abdominal pain, nausea,
E260 Acetic acid	Pickles, cheese, sauces, mint jelly, tinned tomatoes, vinegar ("non-brewed condiment"), tinned baby food, tinned sardines, beer, bread		No known adverse effects
E261 Potassium acetate (potassium salt of E260)	Sauces		
E262 Sodium hydrogen diacetate (sodium diacetate)	Bread, crisps		No known adverse effects
E263 calcium acetate (calcium salt of E260)	Packet cheesecake and jelly mix		
E264 Ammonium acetate			Nausea, vomiting

E number	Likely to be found in	Notes	Possible symptoms caused
E270 Lactic acid (found naturally in milk)	Infant formula, confectionery, dressings, jams, pickles, soft drinks, tinned fruit, tinned sardines and mackerel, beer		
E280 Propionic acid	Dairy products, pizza, processed cheeses.	Naturally occurring fatty acid E281, E282 and E283 may also be used	No known adverse effects
E281 Sodium propionate (sodium salt of E280)	Flour products, processed cheeses		Headaches, migraine
E282 Calcium propionate	Flour products, dairy products, processed cheeses		Headaches, migraine; contact dermatitis in bakery workers
E283 Potassium propionate (potassium salt of E280)	Flour products, dairy products, processed cheeses		Headaches, migraine
E290 Carbon dioxide	Fizzy drinks, juices preserved by manual means (apple, blackcurrant, grape)		
E296 Malic acid	Crisps, fruit juice, frozen chips, jams, jellies, tinned tomatoes, tinned peas		
E297 Fumaric acid	Confectionery, instant fruit drinks, instant tea, jams, jellies	Naturally occurring organic acid	No known adverse effects

Food additives – Antioxidants (E300-321)

E number	Likely to be found in	Notes	Possible symptoms caused
E300 Ascorbic acid	Beer, butter, cooked meats, dried potatoes, fizzy drinks, fruit juice, jams, soft drinks, tinned fruit Vitamin C – browning inhibitor		
E301 Sodium ascorbate (sodium salt of vitamin C)	Frankfurters, pork pies, sausages, baby food		
E302 Calcium ascorbate	Bouillon, consommé, scotch eggs		
E303 Potassium ascorbate potassium salt of vitamin C			
E304 Ascorbyl palmitate	Pork pies, sausages, baby food and infant formula, chicken stock cubes	Same function as E300	No adverse effect known
E306 Tocopherol	Vegetable oils, meat pies, Vitamin E		No adverse effect known
E307 synthetic alpha-tocopherol	Sausages, pork pies, Vitamin E		No adverse effect known

E number	Likely to be found in	Notes	Possible symptoms caused
E308 synthetic gamma-tocopherol			
E309 synthetic delta-tocopherol		Destroyed by freezing	
E310 Propyl gallate (extracted from nut galls)	Vegetable oils, margarines, breakfast cereals, instant potato	Banned in foods for babies under 6 months. HCSG recommends avoidance	Gastric or skin irritation, asthma — will also affect those sentitive to aspirin
E311 Octyl gallate	Fats, margarine, oils	Banned in foods for babies under 6 months HCSG recommends avoidance	Gastric or skin irritation, asthma; also affects people sensitive to aspirin
E312 Dodecyl gallate	Fats, margarine, oils	Banned in foods for babies under 6 months HCSG recommends avoidance	Gastric or skin irritation, asthma; also affects people sensitive to aspirin
E315 Erythorbic acid			No known adverse effects
E318 Sodium erythorbate			No known adverse effects
E319 tert-Butylhydroquinone	Fats, oils, margarine		Nausea, vomiting
E320 Butulated hydroxyanisole (BHA)	Biscuits, cheese spread, confectionery, crisps, margarine, savoury rice, soft drinks, vegetable oil	With E321, is the most widely used antioxidant for fats and oils Banned in Japan. Banned in foods for babies under 6 months (except to preserve added vitamin A) HCSG recommends avoidance	Contact dermatitis

E number	Likely to be found in	Notes	Possible symptoms caused
E321 Butylated hydroxytoluene (BHT)	Breakfast cereals, crisps, dehydrated mashed potato, gravy granules, margarine, packet cake mix, salted nuts, vegetable oil	With E320, is the most widely used antioxidant for fats and oils Banned in foods for babies under 6 months (except to preserve added vitamin A) HCSG recommends avoidance	Rashes; also affects people sensitive to aspirin

Food additives – Emulsifiers, stabilizers and thickeners (E322-495)

E number	Likely to be found in	Notes	Possible symptoms caused
E322 Lecithins	Bakery products, chocolate, confectionery, desserts, popcorn, powdered milk, margarine. Usually from soya, but can be from egg, peanuts or maize		
E325 Sodium lactate (sodium salt of E270)	Confectionery, ice cream, jams, jellies, margarine		
E326 Potassium lactate (potassium salt of E270)	Ice cream, jams, jellies		
E327 Calcium lactate (calcium salt of E270)	Jams, jellies, tinned peas, tinned tomatoes, tinned strawberries		Gastric upsets
E328 Ammonium lactate			
E330 Citric acid	Bakery products, beer, biscuits, cheese, cheese spread, cider, frozen fish, ice cream, jam, jelly, tinned fruit and vegetables, soft drink, frozen potato products, tinned sauces, wine	Occurs naturally in citrus fruit	Harmless

E number	Likely to be found in	Notes	Possible symptoms caused
E331 Sodium citrates	Confectionery, ice cream, processed cheese, milk powder, jams, jelly, margarine		No known adverse effects
E332 Potassium citrates	Condensed milk, dried milk, UHT cream, processed cheese, reduced-sugar jam, crisps		No known adverse effects
E333 Calcium citrates	Condensed milk, confectionery, fizzy drinks, processed cheese, saccharine, tinned tomatoes		No known adverse effects
E334 Tartaric acid	Confectionery, fizzy drinks, frozen dairy products, jam, jellies, tinned fruit, tinned tomatoes,		No known adverse effects
E335 Sodium tartrate (salts of E334)	Confectionery, fizzy drinks, jam, jellies		No known adverse effects
E336	Potassium tartrate, lemon meringue pie mix, wine		No known adverse effects
E337 Sodium potassium tartrate (derivated of E334)	Margarine, meat and cheese products		No known adverse effects
E338 Phosphoric acid	Beer, chocolate, cocoa powder, cooked meats, cottage cheese, fizzy drinks, oils and fats		No known adverse effects
E339 Sodium orthophosphates	Cooked meats, processed cheese, instant desserts		No known adverse effects
E340 Potassium orthophosphates	Jelly glazing mixes, packet sauce, instant custard mix, dessert toppings		
E341 Calcium orthophosphates	Cake mixes, ice cream, milk powder, self-raising flour, pastry mix, potato-based snacks, baking powder, tinned tomatoes		No known adverse effects

E number	Likely to be found in	Notes	Possible symptoms caused
E343 Magnesium phosphates			No known adverse effects
350 Sodium malates (sodium salt of 296)	Jams, jellies		No known adverse effects
351 Potassium malate (potassium salt of 296)	Jams, jellies		No known adverse effects
E352 Calcium malates (calcium salt of 296)	Jams, jellies		No known adverse effects
E353 Metatartaric acid (prepared from tartaric acid, E334)	Wine		No known adverse effects
E354 Calcium tartrate			
E355 Adipic acid (Hxanedioic acid)	Drinks, gelatin		No known adverse effects
E357 Potassium adipate			No known adverse effects
363 Succinic acid		Banned in Australia	
E365 Sodium fumarate			No known adverse effects
E366 Potassium fumarate			No known adverse effects
E367 Calcium fumarate			No known adverse effects
E370 1,4-Heptonolactone		Banned in Australia	
E375 Niacin	Bread, breakfast cereals, flour	Occurs naturally in yeast and liver: vitamin B3	
380 Tri-ammonium citrate (salt of E330)	Cheese spread, processed cheese		
381 Ammonium ferric citrates (prepared from E330)	Iron tablets, infant milks		

E number	Likely to be found in	Notes	Possible symptoms caused
E385 Calcium disodium EDTA	Canned fish, canned shellfish, frozen shellfish, tinned mushrooms	Used as a "chelating agent" to bind metal ions Banned in Australia	Vomiting, diarrhoea, abdominal cramps
E400 Alginic acid (extracted from seaweed)	Ice lollies, soft drinks, puddings, jams, yoghurt		No known adverse effects
E401 Sodium alginate (extracted from seaweed)	Ice lollies, soft drinks, soft cheese, puddings, jams, yoghurt, sauces, syrups, beer		No known adverse effects
E402 Potassium alginate (potassium salt of E400)		Rarely used in foodstuffs — E401 tends to be used instead	
E403 Ammonium alginate (ammonium salt of E400)	Icings		
E404 Calcium alginate (calcium salt of E400)	Ice cream, tinned vegetables, processed cheese, tinned ardines, sterilized and UHT cream, ice lollies, yoghurt		
E405 Propylene glycol alginate (derived from seaweed)	Salad dressing, orange squash, tinned vegetables, processed cheese, ice lollies		No known adverse effects
E406 Agar (derived from seaweed)	Ice cream, drinks, baked goods, icings, confectionery, milk, yoghurt, ice lollies		
E407 Carrageenan (Irish Moss — derived from seaweed)	Ice cream, milk drinks, low calorie spreads, dessert mixes, yoghurt, ice lollies, soya milk, biscuits, pastries, toothpaste, glace cherries, pork pies		Colitis, digestive upsets

E number	Likely to be found in	Notes	Possible symptoms caused
E410 Locust bean gum	Jellies, salad dressings, confectionery, cream cheese, tinned vegetables, tinned fish, yoghurt		No known adverse effects
E412 Guar gum	Sauces and dressings, pickles, milk shake, ice cream, frozen fruit, yoghurt, icings		Nausea, wind, abdominal cramp
E413 Tragacanth	Cake decorations, pickles, processed cheese, jam, confectionery, yoghurt		Possible contact allergy
E414 Acacia (Gum Arabic)	Beer, fruit gums, tinned vegetables, wine	Produced by the acacia tree	Irritation of mucous membranes
E415 Xanthan gum (corn sugar gum)	Salad dressings, frozen pizza, pickles, cake mix		No known adverse effects
E416 Karaya gum	Sauces, ice cream, baked goods, drinks,		Asthma, dermatitis, rhinitis, urticaria,
E420 Sorbitol	Dried fruits, confectionery, pastries, ice cream	Banned in foods for babies and young children	Gastric upset
E421 Mannitol (Manna sugar)	Confectionery, ice cream	Banned in foods for babies and young children	Nausea, vomiting, diarrhoea
E422 Glycerin	Liqueurs, confectionery, drinks, baked goods, soft scoop ice cream		Headache, nausea, vomiting, diarrhoea
E430 Polyoxyetheylene (8) Stearate	Bakery foods		Colitis, gastric upset
E431 Polyoxyetheylene (40) Stearate	Bread		

E number	Likely to be found in	Notes	Possible symptoms caused
E432 Polysorbate 20	Bakery products, desserts, dietetic foods	Banned in Australia	
433 Polysorbate 80	Chocolate mousse, artificial cream, bakery products, confectionery, ice cream, drinks		
E434 Polysorbate 40	Cakes, icings, ice cream, frozen desserts	Banned in Australia	
E435 Polysorbate 60	Bread, non-dairy coffee whitener, chocolate coatings, cakes, icings, confectionery, dressings		
E436 Polysorbate 65	Cakes, bread, icings, ice cream, non-dairy coffee whitener, frozen desserts		
E440(a) Pectin	Jams, jellies, puddings, ice cream, frozen products, yoghurts		No known adverse effects
E440(b) Amidated pectin	Jams		No known adverse effects
E442 Ammonium phosphatides	Chocolate products, cocoa		No known adverse effects
E450 Sodium pyrophosphate (sodium salts of pyrophosphoric acid)	Processed cheese, meats, baking powder, self-raising flour, cake mix, frozen chips		Gastric upset
E451 Potassium polyphosphates			Gastric upset
E460 Microcrystalline cellulose	Bread, cake, grated cheese, dehydrated foods		No known adverse effects
E461 Methyl cellulose	Potato waffles, drinks, diet food, soft drinks, sauces, dressings		Abdominal swelling, wind

E number	Likely to be found in	Notes	Possible symptoms caused
E463 Hydroxypropyl cellulose	Glaze on confectionery	Banned in Australia	
E464 Hydroxypropyl methyl cellulose	Frozen potato waffles		No known adverse effects
E465 Ethyl methyl cellulose		Thickening agent. Derivative of cellulose	No known adverse effects
E466 Sodium carboxy methyl cellulose	Packet cake mix, icings, pie fillings, dips, spreads, ice cream, frozen mousses, dressings, frozen chips, processed cheese, puddings, instant mashed potato		No known adverse effects
E469 Sodium caseinate			No known adverse effects
E470 salts of fatty acids	Crisps	Banned in Australia	No known adverse effects
E471 Mono– and diglycerides of fatty acids	Cakes, instant mash potato, crisps, aerosol cream		No known adverse effects
E472 fatty acid esters of glycerol	Packet cheesecake and mousse, bread, nuts		No known adverse effects
E473 Sucrose esters of fatty acids			No known adverse effects
E474 Sucroglycerides		Banned in Australia	
E475 Polyglycerol esters of fatty acids	Confectionery, coffee whitener, dietetic foods		No known adverse effects
E476 Polyglycerol polyricinoleate	Chocolate-coated biscuits, cakes and sweets		No known adverse effects
E477 Propylene glycol esters of fatty acids	Packet cake mix, instant puddings		No known adverse effects
478 Lactylated fatty acid esters of glycerol and propane-1,2-diol			No known adverse effects

E number	Likely to be found in	Notes	Possible symptoms caused
E481 Sodium stearoyl-2-lactylate	Biscuits, bread, cakes		No known adverse effects
E482 Calcium stearoyl-2-lactylate	Gravy granules		No known adverse effects
E483 Stearyl tartrate		Banned in Australia	
E491 Sorbitan monostearate	Dried yeast		No known adverse effects
E492 Sorbitan tristearate	Confectionery		
E493 Sorbitan monolaurate		Banned in Australia	
E494 Sorbitan mono-oleate		Banned in Australia	
E495 Sorbitan monopalmitate		Banned in Australia	

Food additives – Caking agents (E500-579)

E number	Likely to be found in	Notes	Possible symptoms caused
E500 Sodium carbonates	Tinned custard, beer		Gastric upset
E501 Potassium carbonates			No known adverse effects
E503 Ammonium carbonates	Baking powder		Irritation of mucous membranes
E504 Magnesium carbonate	Salt, icing sugar, butter, ice cream	Medical laxative and antacid	
E507 Hydrochloric acid	Beer		
E508 Potassium chloride		Salt substitute	Nausea, vomiting
E509 Calcium chloride	Tinned kidney beans		No known adverse effects
E510 Ammonium chloride	Flour products		

E number	Likely to be found in	Notes	Possible symptoms caused
E511 Magnesium chloride		Essential mineral	
E513 Sulphuric acid	Beer	Banned in Australia	
E514 Sodium sulphate (Glauber's salt)			
E515 Potassium sulphate		Salt substitute	No known adverse effects
E516 Calcium sulphate (gypsum, plaster of Paris)	Beer		No known adverse effects
E518 Magnesium sulphate (Epsom salts)	Beer		
E519 Copper sulphate		Essential mineral	
E524 Sodium hydroxide (caustic soda)	Beer, jams, black olives	Banned in Australia	
E525 Potassium hydroxide	Cocoa products, black olives	Banned in Australia	
E526 Calcium hydroxide	Beer, cheese, cocoa products, crisps		
E527 Ammonium hydroxide	Cocoa products	Banned in Australia	
E528 Magnesium hydroxide	Cocoa products	Banned in Australia	
E529 Calcium oxide (quicklime)	Cocoa products		
E530 Magnesium oxide	Cocoa products	Banned in Australia	
E535 Sodium ferrocyanide			No adverse effects known

E number	Likely to be found in	Notes	Possible symptoms caused
E536 Potassium ferrocyanide	Wine		
540 Dicalcium diphosphate	Cheese, crisps	Banned in Australia. Rarely used in UK	
E541 Sodium aluminium phosphate	Cakes, scones, batters	Banned in Australia	
542 Bone phosphate	Medical tablets		No adverse effects known
544 Calcium polyphosphates		Banned in Australia	
545 Ammonium polyphosphates		Banned in Australia	
E551 Silicon dioxide (silica)	Beer, wine, crisps		No adverse effects known
E552 Calcium silicate	Confectionery, rice, icing sugar, salt		No adverse effects known
E553(a) Magnesium silicates	Confectionery, rice, icing sugar, salt	Banned in Australia	
E553(b)	Talc, polished rice, chocolate, confectionery		
E554 Sodium aluminium silicate	Packet noodles, salt, icing sugar, cocoa powder, milk powder		
E556 Calcium aluminium silicate	Salt, non-dairy creamer	As 554	
E558 Bentonite	Beer, wine		No adverse effects known
E559 Kaolins	Wine		No adverse effects known
E570 Stearic acid			No adverse effects known
572 Magnesium stearate	Confectionery		No adverse effects known

E number	Likely to be found in	Notes	Possible symptoms caused
E575 Glucono-delta-lactone	Bread and bakery products		No adverse effects known
E576 Sodium gluconate		Banned in Australia	
E577 Potassium gluconate			No adverse effects known
E578 Calcium gluconate			No adverse effects known
E579 Ferrous gluconate	Olives, colouring adjunct		

Food additives – Flavour enhancers (E620-635)

E number	Likely to be found in	Notes	Possible symptoms caused
E620 L-Glutamic acid		Similar to MSG	
E621 Monosodium glutamate (MSG)	Packet snacks, sauces, pork pies, packet soup, noodles, processed cheese, cooked cured meats		Headaches, nausea palpitations, asthma; also affects people sensitive to aspirin
E622 Monopotassium glutamate		Low sodium salt substitutes	Nausea, vomiting, diarrhoea, headaches, abdominal cramps, asthma; also affects people sensitive to aspirin
E623 Calcium glutamate	Bouillons, consommé		Asthma; also affects people sensitive to aspirin
E624 Monoammonium L-glutamate			No adverse effects known
E625 Magnesium di-glutamate		Salt substitute	No adverse effects known
E627 Sodium Guanylate	Crisps, gravy granules, cooked cured meats		Asthma; also affects people sensitive to aspirin

E number	Likely to be found in	Notes	Possible symptoms caused
E631 Sodium 5'-inosinate	Crisps, gravy granules, cooked cured meats		Asthma; also affects people sensitive to aspirin
E634 Sodium 5'-ribonucleotides	Frozen potato products	Banned in Australia	Asthma; also affects people sensitive to aspirin

Food additives – (E636-637)

E number	Likely to be found in	Notes	Possible symptoms caused
E636 Maltol	Bread, cakes, ice cream, drinks, jams		No adverse effects known
E637 Ethyl maltol			No adverse effects known

Food additives – Bleaching agents (E900-E1520)

E number	Likely to be found in	Notes	Possible symptoms caused
E900 Dimethyl poly-siloxane (simethicone)	Jams, soft drinks, syrups, soups, frozen vegetables		No adverse effects known
E901 Beeswaxes	Glazes		Allergy
E903 Carnauba wax	Chocolate products		Allergy
E904 Shellac	Cake decorations, confectionery, fizzy orange drink		Skin irritation
E905 Mineral hydrocarbons (Paraffins)	Dried fruit, confectionery		
907 Refined microcrystalline wax	Chewing gum	Banned in Australia	
920 L-cysteine and its hydrochlorides	Flour products, stock cubes		No adverse effects known
924 Potassium bromate	Flour products		Nausea, vomiting, diarrhoea, abdominal pain
925 Chlorine Flour			Gastric problems

E number	Likely to be found in	Notes	Possible symptoms caused
926 Chlorine dioxide See 925			Gastric problems
E927 Azodicarbonamide	Flour	Banned in Australia. Not used in UK	
928 Benzol peroxide			Asthma
E931 Nitrogen			
E932 Nitrous oxide			
E950 Acesulfame potassium			
E951 Aspartame (artificial sweetener)	Low-sugar products		Headaches
E952 Cyclamic acid	Sweetener — drinks, desserts, confectionery, diet foods	Banned in USA, Australia	
E954		saccharines	
E957 Thaumatin (artificial sweetener)			
E965 Hydrogenated glucose syrup (maltitol)	Desserts, ices, jams, jellies, confectionery, cocoa-based products		
E967 Xylitol			E1200 Polydextrose
E1201 Polyvinylpyrrolidone			No adverse effects known
E1202 Polyvinylpoly-pyrrolidone			No adverse effects known
E1400-1450		starches	No adverse effects known
E1505 Triethyl acetate			
E1510 Ethanol			
E1517, E1518 Glycerol acetates			
E1520 Propylene glycol			

Appendix 5: Occupational asthma allergens

Occupational asthma can develop as a result of substances you come across at work. It can take between weeks and years to develop, depending on the type of substance and your own health.

You may notice that your asthma is worse during the working week, it might not occur at work but your symptoms may be worse after work, and get better when you've been away from work for a few days or on holiday. You can prevent occupational asthma by avoiding exposure. For example, your employer may be able to remove sensitizers at work or replace them with a safe alternative. If it isn't possible, your employer may be able to reduce the risk with improved ventilation (such as extractor fans); if that isn't possible, you should wear equipment such as masks to stop you inhaling the sensitizer.

Your employer has a legal duty to deal with respiratory sensitizers in the workplace, this is set out in the Control of Substances Hazardous to Health regulations 1994.

If you suspect that you have occupational asthma, you should see your GP, who may send you to a specialist to confirm the diagnosis. If you do have occupational asthma, your GP will advise your employer to move you away from the respiratory sensitizer. You may also be eligible for compensation in the form of Industrial Injuries Disablement Benefit; talk to your local Benefits Agency about how to make a claim.

Occupation/industry	Potential asthma allergen
Adhesive handlers	Acrylate, epoxy resin
Animal handlers/breeders	Animal hair and dander, animal proteins, animal urine, animal saliva, feathers
Carpenters	Airborne particles (wood dust)
Cleaners and janitors	Chloramine-T, cleaning materials
Detergent workers	Enzymes
Dockers	Airborne particles (chalk dust, coal dust, coffee, cork dust, cotton dust, flour, grains, powdered drugs, silk dust, soya bean dust, talcum powder, tea dust, tobacco dust, vegetable dust, wood dust), grain, grain mite

Occupation/industry	Potential asthma allergen
Drug manufacture/ pharmaceuticals	Antibiotics, drugs, enzymes, gums, medicines
Dye manufacture	Dyes
Electronics workers	Fluxes
Electroplaters/metal refiners	Chromium, cobalt, nickel, platinum salts,
Farming	Grain, grain mite, hay (mould spores),
Food industry (including bakers, manufacturers, millers)	Airborne particles (coffee, flour, grains, soya bean dust, tea dust, tobacco dust, vegetable dust), enzymes, fish and shellfish (particularly those using gutting machines), grain, grain mite, mushroom compost, penicillin
Forestry workers	Wood dust
Healthcare workers	Antibiotics, drugs, formaldehyde, glutaraldehyde, latex, medicines
Hairdressing/beauty industry	Persulphates (henna)
Insulation installers	Isocyanates
Packers	Airborne particles (chalk dust, coal dust, coffee, cork dust, cotton dust, flour, grains, powdered drugs, silk dust, soya bean dust, talcum powder, tea dust, tobacco dust, vegetable dust, wood dust)
Plastics handlers	Anhydrides, epoxy resin, isocyanates, solvents
Polyester resin manufacture	Cobalt
Printing	Gum acacia, solvents, varnish
Shellac/lacquer handlers	Amines
Solderers	Colophony (rosin)
Spray painters	Isocyanates, paint, varnish
Tanners	Chromium
Textile workers	Cotton dust, dyes, silk dust
Tyres/ rubber industry	Cobalt, isocyanates, mercaptobenzothiazole
Vets	Animal hair and dander, animal proteins, animal urine

Appendix 6:
Occupational contact dermatitis

Occupational contact dermatitis can develop as a result of substances you come across at work. You may notice that your dermatitis is worse during the working week and gets better when you've been away from work for a few days or on holiday. Figures from the Health and Safety Executive show that occupational dermatitis (irritant contact dermatitis caused by sensitivity to substances at work) accounts for up to a third of all working days lost by British industry.

You can prevent occupational dermatitis by avoiding exposure – use gloves and protective equipment wherever possible.

Occupation/industry	Potential dermatitis allergen
Agriculture workers	Animal feed, barley, cements, oats, plants, pesticides, plants, rubber, veterinary medications, wood preservatives
Art	Colophony, dyes, epoxy resin, pigments, turpentine,
Builders	Chromates, cement, cobalt, resins, wood
Car and aircraft industry workers	Chromates, cobalt, dimethacrylate resin, epoxy resin, nickel, rubber
Carpenters	Colophony, glues, stains, turpentine, varnishes, woods
Catering industry	Ammonium persulphate, benzoyl peroxide, citrus fruits, colourings, flavours and spices, foods, formaldehyde, garlic, latex (rubber gloves), nickel, onions, sodium metabisulphite, lauryl gallate, octyl gallate, sawdust

Occupation/industry	Potential dermatitis allergen
Cleaners	Latex (rubber gloves), cleaning materials
Electricians	Fluxes, resins, rubber
Electroplaters and metal workers	Chromium, cobalt, nickel
Hairdressers	Dyes, formaldehyde, latex (rubber gloves), nickel, perfumes, persulphates
Horticulture	Latex (rubber gloves), plants, pesticides,
Jewellers fluxes	Epoxy resin, metals, soldering
Medical workers	Anaesthetics, antibiotics, antiseptics, disinfectants, eugenol, formaldehyde, glutaraldehyde, latex (rubber gloves), local anaesthetics, mercury, methacrylates
Painters	Adhesives, chromates, cobalt, colophony, epoxy resin formaldehyde, paints, polyester resins, thinners, turpentine
Photographic industry	Chromates, formaldehyde, latex (rubber gloves), para-aminophenol, sodium metabisulphite
Plastics industry	Acrylics, hardeners, phenolic resins, plasticizers, polyurethanes
Printing industry	Chromates, cobalt, colophony, formaldehyde, glue, leather, nickel, resin, turpentine
Tannery workers	Chromates, dyes, formaldehyde, fungicides, tanning agents
Textile workers	Chromates, dyes, formaldehyde resins, nickel

Index